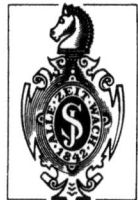

P. Capesius   E. Babin

Radiculosaccography with Water-soluble Contrast Media

With the Collaboration of D. Maitrot

Foreword by M. M. Schechter
Preface by A. Wackenheim

With 228 Figures

Springer-Verlag

Berlin   Heidelberg   New York 1978

Dr. P. Capesius
Département de Radiologie, Centre Hospitalier de Luxembourg, 4, rue Barblé, Luxembourg (Grand-Duché)

Dr. E. Babin
Service de Neuroradiologie, Centre Hospitalo-Universitaire de Strasbourg, 1, place de l'Hôpital, 67005 Strasbourg (France)

ISBN-13: 978-3-540-08559-1   e-ISBN-13: 978-3-642-66832-6
DOI: 10.1007/978-3-642-66832-6

Library of Congress Cataloging in Publication Data. Capesius, P. 1945– . Radiculosaccography with water-soluble contrast media. Bibliography: p.   . Includes index. 1. Nerves, Spinal – Roots – Diseases – Diagnosis. 2. Nerves, Spinal – Roots – Radiography. 3. Lumbosacral region – Radiography. 4. Contrast media. I. Babin, A. Elisabeth, 1938– ., joint author. II. Maitrot, D., joint author. III. Title. RC411.C36   617'.483   77–26014   ISBN 0-387-08526-9

The use of registered names, trademarks, etc. in this publication does not imply, even in the absence of a specific statement, that such names are exempt from the relevant protective laws and regulations and therefore free for general use.
Reproduction of figures: Brend'amour, Simhart & Co., Munchen
Typesetting, printing, and bookbinding by Universitätsdruckerei H. Stürtz AG, Würzburg
2123/3130-543210

Foreword

In the past 30 years roentgen diagnosis has undergone revolutionary changes. Those changes have involved primarily the modality of angiography. The most recent additions to the neuroradiologists' armamentarium has been computed tomography and even more recently total body scanning has been used with promising results. It is obvious that CT scanning has only scraped the tip of the Iceberg in the investigation of the spinal column and its contents.

Doctor Capesius has made a careful study of what he has termed Radiculosaccography. This is the investigation of the lumbar and sacral spine using plain radiography, tomography, and examination of the spinal contents using gas, oily suspensions and water soluble contrast media. A considerable amount of work has gone into this manuscript. Dr. Capesius has compared the advantages of positive and negative contrast medium using oily media and aqueous solutions. A careful analysis has been made of the various contrast media.

This manuscript deals mainly with Radiculosaccography, a technique which displays the roots of the cauda equina and other nerve roots using a water soluble contrast medium.

Radiculosaccography may enhance the techniques already in vague. A comprehensive display of pathology is shown.

New York, January 1978 Prof. M.M. Schechter

V

Preface

Radiological investigation of the lumbar spinal canal has long been neglected because the prominent medullary pathology of the cervical and dorsal segments has monopolized the radiologists' interest. Moreover, the contrast materials, e.g., oily agents and gases, proven quite satisfactory for these two segments, have failed to provide correct information in the lumbar segment. The ability to display the lumbar segment was enhanced considerably by the introduction of water-soluble contrast media.

These new agents have been so widely used in our department that the two main collaborators gained much experience in that field. E. Babin, neuroradiologist, and P. Capesius, general radiologist, report on this extensive study of the roentgenographic systematization of radiculosaccography with water-soluble agents. They also benefitted from constant consultation with neurologists and neurosurgeons.

E. Babin continues the research in this field in our department and organizes post-graduate courses on this subject. P. Capesius, head of the radiological department of the general hospital of his native town, Luxembourg, still participates with E. Babin in the teaching of radiology at the Medical School of Strasbourg.

It is with great pleasure that I write this preface. It is my wish that the authors continue their fruitfull collaboration.

Strasbourg, France   Prof. A. WACKENHEIM

Contents

Part 2   Applications in Different Fields of Pathology

XII

Introduction

General Views Concerning Radiological Investigations of the Lumbosacral Spine

The techniques utilized for the investigation of the lumbosacral spine include plain or tomographic radiography and intracanalicular or intravascular positive contrast examinations. The intracanalicular space may also be visualized with the aid of gas contrast media. Direct nerve root injections are not used currently [27].

Vascular investigations mainly consist of opacification of the spinal extradural plexuses, the indications for arteriography being rare in the lumbosacral area. They are, as a matter of fact, limited to the opacification of the conus medullaris artery in cauda equina syndromes.

Indications for direct opacification of the intervertebral discs are limited to only a few, very definite situations.

I. Plain Radiographs of the Spine

Plain radiography is the basic investigation and should be carried out before any other. It may be supplemented by tomography, preferably with complex motion. The precise contour of the posterior arch is best visualized by axial tomography [15, 23–25, 37], but this hasn't become routine because of the sophisticated equipment needed [5, 38]; moreover, conventional axial tomography is being supplanted by total body computerized tomography [17, 18, 42].

For technical reasons, tomograms in the sagittal plane provide a clear image of the posterior aspect of the vertebrae, whereas axial tomograms give an especially clear image of the posterior arch [40]. Computerized axial tomograms allow correct visualization of all canalicular contours and therefore should permit accurate measurement of the canalicular dimensions for which the conventional technique [12, 19, 41] is inadequate.

II. Subarachnoidal Contrast Techniques

A. Safety

Different schools of thought recommend different contrast agents, either a gas or a positive agent, water- or fat-soluble (see Table 1).

a) *Injection of an opaque agent has the following advantages over use of gases* [14]:
- The examination is simple and does not necessitate special equipment whereas gas myelography necessitates tomography with complex movements.
- The procedure is painless and can be performed quickly.
- The patient can be screened, which allows one to choose the best projection.
- Headache is rarely an immediate post-examination side-effect; it is quite common and severe after gas myelography.

b) *Gas myelography is devoid of early and late complications.* Oily contrast agents

3

Table 1. Comparison of the advantages of the different techniques of myelography

	Type of contrast medium		
	Fat soluble	Water soluble	Gases
Technology	Simple		Complex
Discomfort	Mild		Possibly important
Equipment	Usual		Complex motion tomography
Fluoroscopic control	Helpful		Unhelpful
Immediate complications	None	Irritating for the nerve and the medulla except for metrizamide	None, except for headache
Late complications	Radioclinical signs of arachnoiditis	Radiologic signs of arachnoiditis	None
Three-dimensional representation of the dural sac	Segmental with flow artifacts	Global	Difficult
Opacity of the contrast	Excessive	Good or low	–
Viscosity	High	Low	–
Resorption	Slow and feable	Within a few hours	–
Visualization of the spinal nerve roots			
inside the dural sac	Poor	Good	Bad
outside the dural sac	Inconstant and delayed	Good	Inexistent
Conus visualization	Possible	Impossible, except for metrizamide	Good

have been held responsible for secondary or late arachnoiditis [21, 22, 39] with clinical signs (impotence, cauda equina syndrome, subarachnoid blockage with hydrocephalus), especially when the contrast medium is not or is incompletely withdrawn at the end of the procedure. Water-soluble contrast media also produce late radiologic signs of arachnoiditis [2]. Moreover, they are irritating to the nervous system. This was so much the case with the first agent utilized (Methiodal) that preliminary spinal anesthesia was necessary. Subsequent contrast media (Contrix 28, Dimer-X) have been less and less irritating, and clinical experience with Metrizamide shows that this agent may at a certain dilution be put into contact with the medulla without adverse effect [32].

B. Qualities of the Various Positive Contrast Techniques

When choosing an opacifying medium for the spinal canal, the following points should be kept in mind [14]:
— Myelography with oil media has the advantage of visualizing the conus medullaris region, but this seems now to be also

4

possible with the water-soluble agent Metrizamide.

— The water-soluble media are more fluid and better able to pass through narrow, funnel-shaped parts and to mold the internal contours of the dural sac by reaching the normal and pathologic recesses, i.e., the lateral and posterior recesses. This fluidity brings about a consistent opacification of the radicular sheaths and an early opacification of the cysts and arachnoidal diverticula.

— Iodized oils behave as radiopaque indicators which must be moved to obtain a complete study of the examined region, whereas water-soluble agents opacify the entire thecal sac homogeneously. This allows evaluation of the volume and the three-dimensional deformations of the thecal sac by comparing the pictures obtained in different projections.

— The formation of droplets by the fat-soluble medium and its excessive radiopacity are drawbacks which could be lessened by emulsifying the agent with cerebrospinal fluid. This technique, however, has not proved satisfactory.

— The excessive radiopacity of the iodized oils masks smaller anomalies located within the dural sac. On the other hand, water-soluble media may not be radiopaque enough for obese patients and thus are responsible for suboptimal visualization. This drawback is reduced by varying the dilutation on the injected preparation of Metrizamide [20].

— The resorbability of water-soluble agents allows for a repeat examination if necessary and renders complications such as adhesive arachnoiditis less severe.

In conclusion we believe the water-soluble agents to be the media of choice for the visualization of the cauda equina roots, as well for the intrasaccular roots which are bathed in a moderately opaque fluid, and for the extrasaccular roots which are underlined by the fluid medium penetrating the sheaths. Radicular deformations due to osteoarticular and discal anomalies are thus examined with maximal accuracy.

III. Discography

This direct contrast investigation of the intervertebral disc [11] shows the normal or pathologic condition of the disc [10] and objectifies the intracanalicular leakage of contrast in the case of a degenerated disc. It does not allow conclusions as to the pathogenesis of these anomalies with regard to the roots. To provide correct information this investigation must be carried out at several adjacent intervertebral levels.

Discography is mainly recommended before bone arthrodesis [13] in the case of low back pain or in cases of spondylolisthesis for determining precisely the extent of surgery [29, 31]. It is sometimes used when subarachnoidal investigations are negative or doubtful, e.g., in cases with extreme lateral disc herniations [1, 33, 34].

IV. Lumbar Epidural Venography

This consists of injecting the lumbosacral spinal venous plexuses via the femoral route and catheterizing the ascending lumbar veins [16, 30]. It provides an interesting opacification of the epidural space and may

5

be positive in some cases of negative myelography [26, 35], for example in small and lateral herniations, especially at the L5–S1 interspace where the dural sac is thinner.

We recommend wide use of **Radiculosaccography** (RSG) [7, 9] in cases of sciatica that do not respond to medical treatment and in case of persistent or reoccuring pain postoperatively.

Contrary to some authors [6], we rarely use this procedure in case on nonirradiating lumbalgiae. On the other hand the attitude of those who limit the indications for RSG to peculiar cases [28, 36] seems to us to be out of date when one considers the harmlessness of the contrast media now utilized.

This harmlessness seems primarily due to the rigorous standardization of the technique. As a matter of fact, we perform about 1000 RSG per year, and we have not observed severe complications with the contrast agents since the introduction of new media which do not necessitate spinal anesthesia. We inject a maximal amount of 5 ml water-soluble contrast medium (Contrix 28, Dimer X) diluted in 3–5 ml distilled water. Undiluted contrast medium is never injected. It may sometimes prove insufficiently dense, but we try to mitigate this drawback by an elaborate radiologic technique viz. frontal zonography [3, 4, 8] and several angles of the central beam, adapted to the clinical symptomatology and to the anomalies visualized on the fluoroscopic screen.

In the future, use of Metrizamide will allow more flexibility of total amount and dilution of the injected medium and their adaption to the capacity of the thecal sac or to the obesity of the patient [20].

References of the Introduction see page 139.

Part 1

Chapter 1. Historical Account of Radiculosaccography With Water-soluble Contrast Media

The history of RSG (radiculosaccography) may be divided into four periods due to the utilization of diverse water-soluble contrast media, i.e., sodium monoiodomethane sulfonate (Abrodil, Kontrast U, Methiodal, Skiodan) in 1931, then methylglucamine iothalamate (Conray 60, Contrix 28) in 1967, dimer of methylglucamine iothalamate (Dimer X) in 1970, and, finally, nonionic water-soluble contrast medium metrizamide (Amipaque) in 1973.

I. Sodium Monoiodomethane Sulfonate (Abrodil, Kontrast U, Methiodal, Skiodan)

In 1931, Arnell and Lindström [7] injected a water-soluble and resorbable contrast medium, e.g., sodium monoiodomethane sulfonate, into the lumbosacral dural sac for the first time. This agent was so highly irritating to the nervous structures that it required the preliminary use of a spinal anesthetic. Arnell [4–6] demonstrated the diagnostic value of this method, but it was not as widely used as could be expected because it was felt to be responsible for severe and repeated complications. Those complications were mainly related to the procedure adopted by Arnell. As a matter of fact, he carried out the examination with the patient in the prone position, on a horizontal table, his head and chest raised, so that the contrast medium or the anesthetic could accidentally diffuse up to the medulla and even to the brain.

The technical adjustments developed in 1946 by Lindblöm [64] and in 1951 by Knuttson [60] in Sweden, and in 1948 by Woringer and Langs [88] in France, enabled RSG to become a routine procedure. Both Lindblöm [64] and Knuttson [60] carry out the examination in lateral decubitus on a table, Lindblöm's tilted at 10 degrees and Knutsson's at 35 degrees. Woringer keeps his patient in a sitting position on a rotating chair for the injection of the contrast medium as well as for performing the x-rays [87–89]. The advantage of this method is the prevention of any contact of the anesthetic and the contrast medium with the medulla and the brain. The drawback of the sitting position lies in the fact that it is difficult to maintain in a patient under spinal anesthesia and induces blood pressure changes.

As a result of these new technical adjustments, RSG was also performed outside of Sweden, viz., in France [14–16, 31, 34, 77, 87–89], in Algeria [36], in Germany [72], and in Switzerland [37, 86]. Two monographs have been devoted to RSG with methiodal, one by Ecoiffier [35], the other by Ferrand et al. [36].

But the indications of RSG with sodium monoiodomethane sulfonate remained restricted to very precise cases [75, 76], since this technique was held responsible for two types of severe complications, i.e., marked blood pressure changes [65, 72] and nervous complications such as cauda equina syndrome or paraplegia [3, 65, 69, 71, 81]. Concerning the pathogeny of these complications, it has never been possible to determine exactly to what extent the toxicity proper of the contrast medium or the adverse effects of the spinal anesthesia are the cause. That accounts for the fact that RSG with sodium monoiodomethane sulfonate has not been utilized in the United States where Camp [22] reported a disastrous experiment in dogs — the animals which did not die showed at least paraplegia or hemiplegia.

II. Methylglucamine Iothalamate (Conray 60, Contrix 28)

The experimental studies in 1963 of Kodama et al. [61], those in 1964 of Campbell et al. [23] and in 1966 of Heimburger et al. [52, 53] have demonstrated that methylglucamine iothalamate was the least toxic of the then known water-soluble contrast agents for the central nervous system.

In 1964 Campbell [23] reported the first clinical utilization of ventriculography and RSG. After having carried out about 12 RSG, Campbell concluded that "transient muscle spasms and paresthesiae occurred with sufficient frequency to limit it usefulness." Following these first negative clinical trials by Campbell, Conray 60 was almost never used in the United States thereafter.

In Europe at the VIIIth Symposium on Neuroradiology in 1967 in Paris, Gonsette and André-Balisaux reported [43] the utilization of methylglucamine iothalamate (Contrix 28) in RSG without preliminary spinal anesthesia [42]. Because of the irritating action on the conus medullaris region, Gonsette and André-Balisaux advise following some precautions scrupulously, i.e.,

not using the 28% nondiluted solution, not injecting a total volume of more than 10 ml, and keeping the patient in a sitting position for 6 hours after the examination. A round table was held in Paris in 1968 at the Hôpital de la Pitié where the authors of eight French and Belgian towns pooled their experience of 847 RSG with Contrix 28 [9, 10] carried out with the precautions recommended by Gonsette. No serious complication could be directly related to the method or the contrast medium used. Tonic and clonic muscle spasms of the legs were recorded in 3% of the cases reported, they appeared 2–7 h postinjection and usually responded to an intravenous injection of diazepam. In some rare cases, these tonic or clonic movements may be so violent as to provoke fracture of the femoral neck [39, 40] or collapsed vertebrae [49]. At the worst, they may also lead to status epilepticus requiring treatment with curare and respiratory monitoring [13], and even to coma and death [40]. We ourselves never encountered such severe complications.

III. Dimer of Methylglucamine Iothalamate (Dimer X)

In 1970, Gonsette and André-Balisaux [44] reported on the experimental study and first clinical trial of this new contrast medium elaborated on by the Guerbet research staff. They concluded that this agent was better tolerated in comparison to previous ones, providing a maximal dose of 5 ml was used. Another round table took place at the Hôpital de la Pitié in 1970 pooling 3336 RSG with Dimer X, carried out in French and Belgian departments [47]. A comparison with the results of the previous round table shows that the meningeal signs are more frequent with Dimer X but that the post-

10

RSG hyperalgiae and signs of nervous hyperexcitation (myocloniae, epileptic seizures) are much less frequent with Dimer X than with Contrix 28.

Among all the water-soluble agents utilized for RSG, Dimer X is up to now the most widely used, especially in Europe, i.e., Belgium [40], France [26, 27, 63], Germany [45, 73, 83], Austria [50], Italy [20, 21, 29, 30], Spain [74], Poland [90], Yugoslavia [66], Great Britain [46], and Scandinavia [59], but also in Israel [62].

In the United States, where physicians are still distrustful due to the bad experience made with sodium monoiodomethane sulfonate and methylglucamine iothalamate, Dimer X is presently little used. Lumbosacral spine pathology is mainly investigated by pantopaque myelography.

Until 1976, a large number of publications reported Dimer X to be well-tolerated [11, 18, 33, 40, 59]. In particular, no cauda equina syndrome caused by this method was noted, and the tonic muscle spasms have become so rare that RSG has been employed as a routine exploration technique for patients suffering from sciatalgiae [24, 25], and especially as preoperative exploration for discal herniations [17, 19, 67]. Some authors have even attempted injecting nondiluted Dimer X [50], while others advise that the recumbent position be adopted for the patient immediately after the examination [28, 32].

The year 1976 was marked by two publications, a French one and a Swiss one, which absolutely establish the responsibility of Dimer X for more or less severe and more or less subsiding neurologic complications. Perrigot et al. report four cases of cauda equina syndrome occurring after RSG with Dimer X [48, 70]. On the other hand, Walker et al. record 7.1% of usually subsiding neurologic complications in 355 investigations [85].

In 1970, Autio et al. [8] reported the first case of radiologically diagnosed arachnoiditis following RSG regardless of the contrast media utilized. Statistics from different authors are so varied that it is impossible to establish which of the three contrast media utilized before metrizamide is the most harmless with respect to causing adhesive arachnoiditis.

As for metrizamide, its utilization is too recent to permit forming an opinion on its delayed effects. Since it is admitted that hyperosmolarity is an important factor in the genesis of adhesive arachnoiditis [80], it is to be supposed that metrizamide will avoid them.

Up to now, it has not been established that these post-RSG radiologic signs of adhesive arachnoiditis are correlated with clinical signs.

IV. Metrizamide (Amipaque)

The contrast media formerly utilized were solutions of salts of iodized acids, which were hypertonic. In recent years, attention has been drawn to biological effects ascribed to the hypertonicity of the media [2, 12, 38, 51, 54]. The relation seemed evident between this hypertonicity and the adverse effects of these solutions. Almen proposed chemical modifications in order to synthetize a nonionic material with low osmolarity [1].

Based upon Almen's proposal, a series of nonionic compounds were synthetized in the research laboratories of Nyegaard & Co. (Oslo). One of these compounds was named metrizamide, and this name was later approved by the World Health Organization as the international nonproprietary name.

The experimental and preliminary clinical trials made in four European depart-

11

ments [41, 55, 79, 82] concerning Metriza-mide were published in 1973 in Acta Radio-logica Supplementum 335 [68].

The medium was preconized for use in opaque ventriculography as well as cister-nography and myelography [57]. Up to now, publications concerning its use for lumbar myelography [41, 55, 56, 78, 79, 82] mention that no severe immediate com-plication has occurred, especially no mus-cular spasm or epileptic seizure. Contrari-wise, a few authors report isolated cases of adverse effects like epileptic seizures with the utilization of this material for cervical myelography [58, 84].

References of Chapter 1 see page 140.

Chapter 2. Technique of RSG

I. Generalities

The technique of RSG has varied according to the different contrast media used. We shall not recall the peculiar technical problems due to the use of sodium monoiodomethane sulfonate which were mainly related with the *spinal anesthesia* and which have already been dealt with in Chapter 1.

This Chapter deals with the technical problems of contrast media utilizable without spinal anesthesia, i.e., meglumine iothalamate (Contrix 28, Conray 60), meglumine iocarmate (Dimer X), and metrizamide (Amipaque). The last one, metrizamide, distinguishes itself from the first two in that it may be put into *contact with the medulla* [56]. Therefore, it allows an investigation of the conus medullaris region as well as the cauda equina roots during the same examination.

The *technique for taking the x-rays* does not vary with the contrast media utilized.

The *contrast pattern* obtained is similar for these three media used without spinal anesthesia. The meglumine iothalamate and the meglumine iocarmate are marketed as solutions of salts containing 28% iodine or 280 mg I/ml. They are usually injected after dilution with an equal volume of distilled water or CSF, resulting in a solution of 140 mg I/ml. Metrizamide is often utilized for RSG with that iodine concentration [38, 69], but the mixture with metrizamide may reach 300 mg I/ml without becoming harmful (38, 69), thus providing a contrast pro-

ducing property which for safety reasons could not be achieved with the previous media.

The *osmolarity* of the injected solutions must be known since it is commonly admitted that the biological tolerance of these media depends largely on their osmolarity [6, 35, 60]. With each successive new contrast medium, meglumine iothalamate, meglumine iocarmate, and metrizamide, the osmolarity becomes lower and lower (see Table 2). At a concentration of 170 mg I/mg, metrizamide is isotonic to CSF [39]. The salts meglumine iothalamate and meglumine iocarmate are diluted by some in

Table 2. Comparison of the osmolarities of the different contrast media used in RSG

	Osmo-larity osmol/kg	Refer-ence
Meglumine iothalamate (dilution with distillated water in a ratio of 1/1)	700	[33][a]
Dimer X (dilution with CSF in a ratio of 1/1)	620	[72]
Dimer X (dilution with distillated water in a ratio of 1/1)	480	[72]
Metrizamide 300 mg I/ml	484	[39]
Metrizamide 170 mg I/ml	300 (isotonic to CSF)	[39]

[a] Calculated.

distillated water and by others in CSF. Dilution in distillated water lowers the osmolarity more than dilution with CSF [72].

With these three contrast media, the *resorption times* are much longer than the duration of x-raying. The complete disappearance of the opaque contrast occurs after 5–6 h with meglumine iothalamate and 7–8 h with meglumine iocarmate [33]. Experimentally, the time of resorption of metrizamide is the same as that of meglumine iocarmate [68, 71]. These resorption times may be prolonged in some cases of disturbance of the CSF flow, and especially those related to the megacauda [32].

II. Preparation of the Patient

The relatively aggressive character of the investigation including the lumbar puncture may render the patient apprehensive. He may need to be comforted and instructed of the different steps he will have to undergo. He should also be questioned for a possible intolerance to iodine or any allergic disease, viz., asthma, eczema, etc., so that the physician will proceed knowingly to the injection of a iodized agent.

As a rule, the investigation should not be carried out in the few days following a lumbar puncture so as to leave time for scarring of the dural breach and a return of normal biological conditions in the CSF.

On the morning of the investigation, the patient should have a light meal and no particular premedication is necessary. Some very anxious patients benefit from an anxiolytic premedication, and some who suffer from hyperalgiae may need an antalgic injection just before the investigation. Some authors [45] systematically give a diazepam premedication which combines the advantages of an anxiolytic effect and the prevention of clonic or epileptic complications.

Patients with chronic bronchitis need a particular preparation in order to avoid the occurrence of coughing fits before resorption of the contrast [28, 78].

III. Lumbar Puncture and Injection of the Contrast Agent

A. The Lumbar Puncture

It is preferably carried out with a burred, disposable 0.9 mm gauge needle in order to limit the leak of CSF through the puncture orifice, which is admitted to be a cause of secondary headache [22, 23, 53, 79]. High-level punctures from the L3–4 interspace and higher have the advantage of allowing dilution of the contrast in a longer segment of the dural sac and decreasing the eventuality of an injection at the level or below a blockage.

The outflow of CSF through the needle is not sufficient proof of satisfactory placement of the needle; as a matter of fact, the bevel may be partly in the subdural and epidural spaces. For this reason, it is safer to verify under fluoroscopic control whether the tip of the needle is projected in the center of the canalar area, the patient being in the lateral sitting position.

Before any injection of contrast, we usually withdraw a small amount of CSF to be examined since the cell count and the total protein content may be altered after RSG, whatever the contrast medium utilized (meglumine iothalamate, meglumine iocarmate, or metrizamide) [61].

B. Preparation of the Contrast

It is recommended that *meglumine iothalamate and meglumine iocarmate* not be injected pure [10, 11, 28]; usually 5 ml of the contrast medium are homogeneously mixed with 5 ml of the solvent, i.e., distilled water or aspirated CSF. When the obesity of the patient renders a more important contrast necessary, it is possible to reduce the amount of solvent down to 3 ml; some even utilize Dimer X pure for stout patients [33].

It seems dangerous to increase the amount of meglumine iothalamate or meglumine iocarmate beyond 5 ml, even if the dural sac is large [29, 33, 78].

Some have advised adjunction of a steroid to the contrast medium to prevent the occurrence of headache and other postmyelographic side effects [19, 55], but it is now admitted that this procedure increases the frequency of the post-RSG radiologic features of adhesive arachnoiditis [3, 23].

Metrizamide is available as a freeze-dried crystalline powder which before use is dissolved in a bicarbonate buffer solution in the amount needed to obtain the suitable concentration. The most commonly utilized concentration for RSG is 170 mg I/ml, i.e., the one which is isotonic to CSF. In cases of obesity, the concentration may be increased up to 300 mg I/ml. The necessary amount to opacify the lumbosacral dural sac varies between 10 and 15 ml [39, 69].

C. Injection of the Contrast

Meglumine iothalamate and meglumine iocarmate which are not to reach the medulla are injected with the patient in a sitting or lateral recumbent position on a table tilted head-end up at about 45 degrees.

Metrizamide may be injected with the patient in a lateral recumbent position on a table tilted head-end up at about 10 degrees [39, 69].

The injection is made under fluoroscopic control which ensures, on the one hand, that the contrast medium is in the subarachnoid space and, on the other hand, that it reaches the bottom of the dural sac. When the fluoroscopic control leads to suspicion that the injection is either subdural—opaque stain around the tip of the needle—or epidural—blurred double-track opacity—, one should try to promptly rectify the insertion of the needle, or, if need be, puncture another space.

In cases when there is complete blockage or a very narrow canal, and if one is injecting a medium which is not to reach the medulla, one must stop the injection of the contrast before it reaches the dorsolumbar area.

The occurrence of pain during the injection demands supplementary caution; indeed, this has been reported as a premonitory sign of post-RSG neurologic complications with Dimer X [29, 62].

The injection of the meglumine salts must not be too slow in order to avoid the sedimentation of the contrast at the bottom of the dural sac but also not too quick so that the contrast does not reach the conus medullaris.

Before withdrawal of the needle, it is necessary to verify that the dural sac is opacified at a sufficient height, particularly in case of megacauda, because it may be useful to inject a supplementary amount of diluted contrast. Some prefer to leave the needle in situ while x-rays are taken for diverse reasons, viz., possibility of withdrawing the contrast at the end of the examination, exact marking of the interspace by the sight of the puncture needle on the x-rays and of cutaneous trace of the puncture [49].

IV. X-raying Technique

A. Principles for the RSG Procedure

Up to now, RSG was mainly aimed at the diagnosis of discal herniations. For this reason, frontal and lateral — orthogonal — projections of the dural sac are supplemented by right and left oblique projections in order to visualize the radicular emergences. These oblique projections are performed on either side, generally two of them [24, 50], with the patient rotated at an angle of 15–45 degrees, and they usually prove sufficient to study the anterolateral aspect of the sac (Fig. II,1).

It is not possible to determine the optimal rotation degree of the patient for the realization of these oblique projections. As a matter of fact, the extrasaccular roots have a variable orientation from one patient to the other, and in the same patient from one level to the other [66].

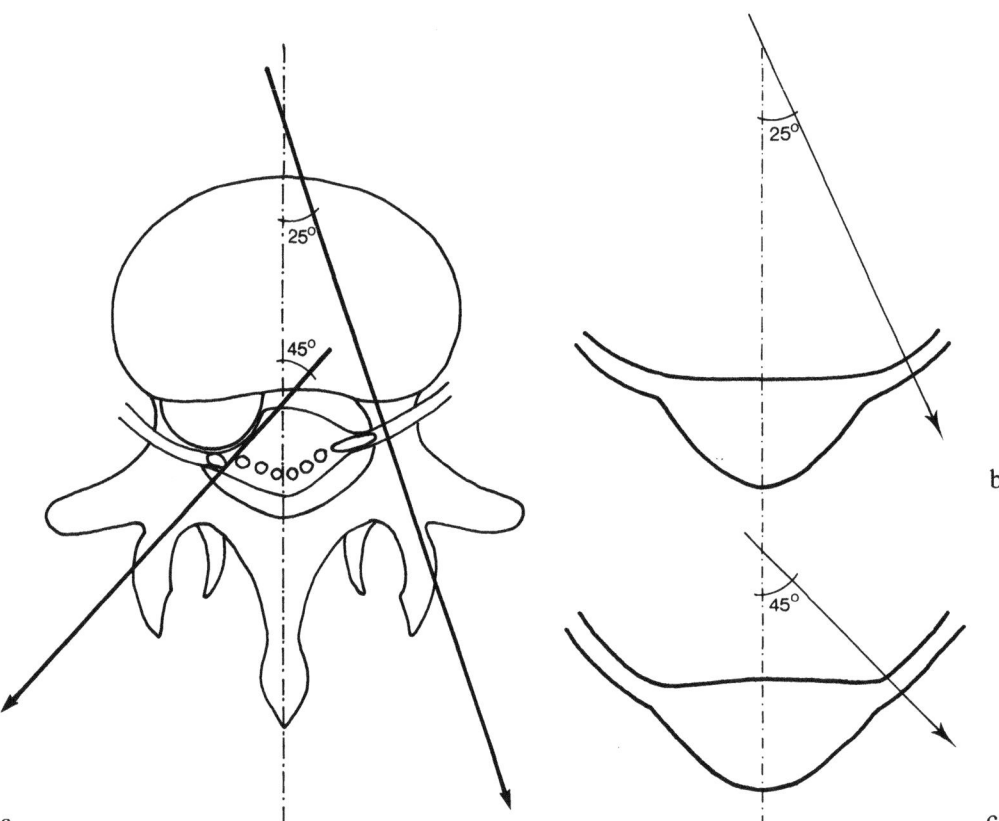

Fig. II,1. **Oblique Projections.** (a) Schematic drawing representing axially the direction of the x-ray beam with regard to the thecal sac in posterior oblique projections. (b) and (c) Schematic drawing representing axially the variable direction of the roots with regard to the frontal plane. Usually, the oblique projections with the patient rotated at an angle of 20–30 degrees are the most informative for the root emergences (b). The central beam is indeed perpendicular to the plane of emergence of the roots. Less oblique projections may be useful for better visualization of the roots when their course is situated in a plane close to the frontal plane. More oblique projections (c) have the advantage of better showing the anterolateral hernial imprints

16

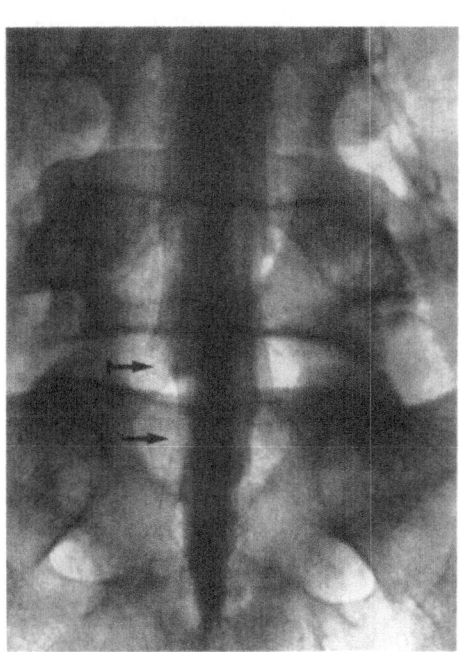
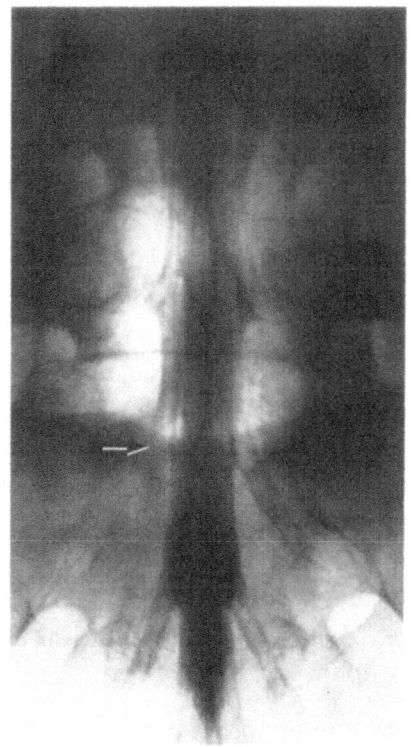

a
b

Fig. II,2. **Usefulness of Ascending Oblique Projections.** (a) Hernial imprint (*arrow*) with nonfilling of the right S1 root at the level of the inferior end-plate of L5 (*crossed arrow*). (b) Nonfilling of the right S1 sheath from the sacral plate on (*arrow*). These projections, in which the intervertebral space is tangentially hit, allow one to precisely locate the level and extent of the hernial compression

The routine projections are adapted to the level pointed out by the clinical signs and to the general conformation of the lumbosacral spine – lordosis, horizontal orientation of the sacrum. For instance, we use an ascending central beam for the lower interspaces in lordotic patients (Fig. II,2).

B. Practical Effectuation of the Projections

1. Basic Projections, i.e., Frontal, Lateral, and Oblique

The x-rays are taken either in the upright or recumbent position on a table tilted head-end up which permits better immobilization and provides a supplementary convenience for lipothymic patients. Nevertheless, the films are preferably taken in the erect position for several reasons [33].

a) The physiologic conditions of the standing position are necessary to demonstrate some discal herniations which might disappear when the lumbar spine does not bear the weight of the body and when the physiologic lordosis straightens out.

b) In case of scoliosis, the injection of the contrast medium or the x-raying in some of the recumbent positions on a tilted table may provoke the contrast to flow up to the medulla [41].

c) The repartition of the contrast due to gravity may mimic a segmental lack of opacification when the patient is recumbent on a tilted table.

d) The erect position allows one to easily perform functional studies, i.e., flexion, extension, and lateroflexion.

Frontal and oblique projections are preferably performed with the patient's back on the table in order to diminish geometric blurring of the image.

Left and right lateral projections are carried out at discretion.

X-rays of the whole lumbar spine and x-rays centered on the lumbosacral interspace, frontal as well as lateral, are useful for adapting the parameters to the strong variations in the thickness which are unavoidable in that area.

2. Complementary Projections, i.e., Zonography, X-rays in the Face-Down Position, Functional Study

The tomographic investigation in RSG may vary according to the available technical equipment and be carried out either in the frontal plane [8, 9, 13, 51] or in both oblique planes [1, 65].

For a better filling of the upper lumbar radicular sheaths, it may be useful to execute a frontal projection in the face-down position on a table tilted head-end up.

As concerns functional study, the flexion-extension is the most informative [50] since it causes variations in the canalar volume and the distance between the dural sac and the posterior aspect of the vertebrae. In fact, one lateral x-ray in the extended position of the patient may be sufficient since it is the one which provides the most valuable data.

V. Postexamination Time

Until recently, the authors who used meglumine salts left their patients in the semirecumbent position for 6–8 h, i.e., for the theoretical resorption delay of the contrast medium.

With Dimer X, Cecile et al. [15, 16] have taken to laying their patients down immediately — even without withdrawing the contrast — in order to reduce the CSF leakage, avoid subsequent headache, and also prevent the occurrence of adhesive arachnoiditis due to a prolonged stagnation of Dimer X at the bottom of the dural sac. They demonstrated that there is no risk in making the patient lie down immediately, provided the amount of Dimer X did not exceed 5 ml.

The most prudent attitude would consist in removal of as much contrast medium as possible at the end of the examination and to lay down the patient afterward.

These different attitudes are bound to become uniform and more simple with the use of a contrast medium devoid of toxicity for the medulla. At the present time, with metrizamide, the patient is made to lie down on a bed immediately after RSG, the head end of which is raised at 10 degrees. In any case, the patient who underwent RSG must remain in the dorsal recumbent position for 24 h.

VI. Adverse Side Effects

The physiopathology of these untoward effects and injuries is not quite clear, and an etiological classification is not yet established [41]. For example, subsequent headache is attributed by some to a meningeal irritation syndrome and by others to the mere hydrodynamic modifications following a lumbar puncture [15]. Severe radicular pain is sometimes considered a sign of neuromuscular hyperexcitability in the same

18

way as muscular spasms, and sometimes a manifestation of toxic radiculitis in the same way as cauda equina syndromes.

The different statistics are not comparable since the practical performance of the investigation is not codified and the criteria for the clinical evaluation vary from one author to the other.

RSG with Methiodal had acquired an unfavorable reputation since the neurotoxicity of the contrast medium necessitated a preliminary spinal anesthesia; severe complications—circulatory collapses, cauda equina syndromes—were frequent [5] and could be attributed either to the spinal anesthesia or to the Methiodal.

The contrast media later utilized (Contrix 28, Dimer X) have been less and less neurotoxic and no longer necessitated a spinal anesthesia but only a simple monitoring of the patient during the few hours postexamination.

The neurotoxicity of metrizamide seems to be attenuated enough so that it may be put into contact with the medulla, even for purpose of diagnosis [56].

Complications are of two types, i.e., those which occur during or just after RSG and constitute the side effects of the examination, and those which are discovered as radiologic signs of adhesive arachnoiditis only after a second RSG has been performed some time after the first one.

Among the early complications, we have isolated those which occur at the time of the puncture or of the injection of the contrast and thus have a specific meaning.

A. Adverse Effects of the Puncture and of the Injection of the Contrast

1. *Lipothymiae* may occur at the mere lumbar puncture and before any injection of contrast medium. It is then a neurovegeta-tive reaction which is usually not severe and could be avoided by atropine premedication and anxiolytic treatment in nervous patients.

2. *Sudden irritating sciatic pains occur during the lumbar puncture* more particularly in cases with narrow lumbar canal or with diffuse compression of the dural sac by an extensive extradural mass [79]. This is an inconsequential incident which is always of short duration and immediately relieved by the displacement of the needle.

3. *Pains occurring during the injection* of the contrast medium should lead to carefulness and eventually to termination of the injection. As a matter of fact, in two of the four cases of cauda equina syndromes reported by Perrigot et al. [62], there was a very strong recrudescence of the lumbar pain or sciatalgiae which may be considered a posteriori a premonitory sign of post-RSG complications.

4. The occurrence of a *collapse* simultaneously with the injection of the contrast medium may be related to an intolerance to iodine which would, in fact, be exceptional during RSG [78].

B. Early Complications

1. The postexamination *headache* is the more frequent complication, occurring immediately or belatedly, short-wearing or tenacious, of variable intensity and frequently unrelieved by symptomatic therapy. These headaches have the drawback of necessitating prolonged bed rest. Two pathogenic mechanisms are considered, with different consequences as to their prevention. The fluid leakage at the puncture point has been demonstrated [53, 79], for instance by isotopic explorations [22, 25]. It is thus advisable to use slender neeedles which provides an argument to those who decided to make their patients lie down in

order to reduce, as much as possible, the deperdition of CSF caused by a prolonged sitting position [15, 18]. Other authors consider the headaches to belong to the more general group of aseptic meningeal reactions, with the argument that they are accompanied by other signs of meningeal irritation – stiffness of the neck, vomiting, fever. They have, moreover, described a high cell count and a lack of balance of the protein content in the CSF, and histologically proved adhesive arachnoiditis. To prevent these aseptic meningeal reactions, the intrathecal injection of steroid (methyl-prednisolone acetate) has been preconized [19, 55], but is is now established that the simultaneous injection of a contrast medium and of a steroid may be responsible for further radiologic signs of arachnoiditis in a subsequent RSG [3, 23].

It is to be noted that Dimer X more frequently produces headache than Contrix 28; this may be related to its slower resorption, the agent being in contact with the meninges for a longer time during a sitting position over several hours (see Table 3).

The frequency of headaches after metrizamide is similar to that after Dimer X [4, 37, 38, 42, 67]. In women, headaches occur more frequently than in men [4, 69].

2. *Meningeal Irritation.* Besides headaches, there may also be other meningeal signs, viz., nausea, stiffness of the neck, febricula.

Experimentally and clinically, all contrast media including metrizamide [27, 70] provoke chemical meningitis with increased cell count and high protein content in the CSF [41, 75]. This symptomatology is usually at its highest 24 hours postinjection and decreases toward the 3rd day [41]. The particular intensity of the symptoms of meningeal irritation with marked fever leads one to suspect a septic meningitis by lumbar puncture inoculation. The hypothesis has been raised that some cases of severe acute meningitis following RSG would be related to a contamination of the CSF with a detergent washing agent [75].

3. *Blood Pressure Changes.* Blood pressure changes were frequent during RSG with sodium monoiodomethane sulfonate.

Table 3. Frequence of post-RSG headache

Authors	Contrast agents		
	Meglumine iothalamate	Meglumine iocarmate	Metrizamide
Clément et al. [17]	8%		
Round table at la Pitié (Paris – 1968) [10, 11]	12%		
Praestholm and Lester [63]	35%		
Lethinen and Seppänen [52]	9%	2%	
Hammer [33]	11%	18%	
Irstam [41]	14%	18%	
Caron-Poitreau et al. [14]		8%	
Round table at la Pitié (Paris – 1970) [28]		20%	
Hindmarsh [38]		21%	21%
Ahlgren [4]		29%	30%
Irstam [42]		34%	34%
Skalpe and Amundsen [69]			31%
Svare and Talle [74]			33%

They were incidently quite important and severe collapses were the major complication in this kind of investigation. With the meglumine salts, the blood pressure changes are, as a rule, moderate—about 20–30 mm Hg—and collapses are almost never seen [41]. Blood pressure changes are usually relieved by raising the patient's legs and giving vasopressors. The recording of blood pressure during RSG with metrizamide did not show any remarkable hydrodynamic change [36].

4. *Painful clonic spasms of muscles* have been reported with the meglumine salts; they were observed more often with meglumine iothalamate than with meglumine iocarmate. The clinical findings are consistent with the experimental studies. The publications concerning RSG with metrizamide do not mention the occurrence of muscular spasms [69, 70, 74].

Those observed with the meglumine salts occur about 3 h after the injection and are usually relieved by an intravenous injection of diazepam. There exist a few case reports about spasms so severe that they provoked fractures of the femoral neck [16, 26, 41, 78] or vertebral collapses [30].

The statistics of the literature vary greatly because of the different techniques used by the different authors. The best statistics are reported by Hammer [33, 34], who takes the following precautions with Dimer X: under fluoroscopic control, an optimal, i.e., individually varying, minimal amount of contrast medium is injected, the level of which must never rise as high as the medullary conus. Usually 5 ml are sufficient, an amount which is rarely exceeded. Fluoroscopic controls indicate the time needed for disappearance of the contrast.

The most unfavorable statistics are those of Lethinen and Seppänen [52] who utilize a different technique than all the other authors, in so far as they x-ray their patients in the recumbent as well as in the erect position, moreover with functional studies—bending and Lasègue's tests. Several factors may account for the unfavorable statistics of Ahlgren [2], viz., injection of a too large amount of a too highly concentrated contrast medium—7.5 ml of meglumine iothalamate mixed with 2.5 ml of CSF—the patient being on a table tilted head-end up at only 15 degrees (see Table 4).

5. *Epileptic Seizures.* With the meglumine salts, epileptic seizures are very rare [19–21, 26, 28, 78] and are not reported in some important statistics [2, 33, 42, 52].

In two cases reported in the literature, the epileptic seizures have evolved toward a status epilepticus [26, 38, 78], with fatality in one case [26].

Recent statistics concerning metrizamide do not mention epilepsy, but the utilization of this contrast agent in cervical myelography has already brought about three cases of postmyelographic epilepsy [40, 58,

Table 4. Frequency of clonic muscular spasms

Statistics concerning meglumine iothalamate

Round table in La Pitié, Paris (1968) [10, 11]	3%
Clément et al. [17]	4%
Praestholm and Lester [63]	4.4%
Ahlgren [2]	6.4%

Statistics concerning meglumine iocarmate

Round table in La Pitié, Paris (1970) [28]	1%
Caron-Poitreau et al. [14]	2%

Comparative statistics

	Meglumine iothalamate	Meglumine iocarmate
Hammer [33]	1.7%	0%
Irstam [42]	4%	2%
Lethinen and Seppänen [52]	14%	5.5%

76]. Transient EEG abnormalities may be recorded in some RSG with meglumine iocarmate [45] and with metrizamide [27, 48, 70].

Exceptionally, clouding of the consciousness has been reported as a sign of intolerance of the central nervous system [41, 78].

6. *Cauda Equina Syndromes.* Up to 1976, no case of cauda equina syndrome has been reported after the use of meglumine salts or metrizamide. At the most, transitory micturition disturbances lasting for 1 or 2 days have been described and may be considered minimal symptoms of the cauda equina [78]. They have been reported with the three contrast media, i.e., meglumine iothalamate [63], meglumine iocarmate [28, 78], and metrizamide [38, 69].

Suddenly, in 1976, two publications considered meglumine iocarmate to be responsible for severe complications of the cauda equina, i.e., four cases of Perrigot [62] and 13 of Walker [78]; all these cauda equina syndromes were not entirely reversible and some of them involved the lower segment of the thoracic medulla [62, 78]. In these two publications, the injected amount of dimer X was occasionally more than 5 ml and even up to 10 ml.

Neurologic complications may also occur when RSG is performed after a lumbar traumatism with ruptured dura mater [77].

C. Delayed Complications: "Post-RSG Arachnoiditis"

Since the publication by Autio et al. (1972) [7], it is known that RSG with water-soluble media may cause delayed radiologic signs of adhesive arachnoiditis which are disclosed during a second RSG. Those signs are:

1. Poor visualization of the lumbosacral radicular sheaths, and even nonvisualiza-

tion of the most caudal root sleeves. The amputated appearance of the root sleeves may show clear-cut or blunted round ends.

2. An abnormally opaque and homogeneous contrast pattern of the dural sac which has lost its usual striated appearance and shows sharper margins.

3. A concentric and regular narrowing of the saccular shadow.

Table 5. Radiologic classification of post-RSG adhesive arachnoiditis (Two types according to Jorgensen et al. [47] and three stages according to Slätis et al. [72])

Type 1, nonoperated patients

—Homogeneous contrast pattern without root shadows,
—Nonfilling of the root sleeves,
—Regular and progressive narrowing,

| Stage I |

Obliteration of the sacral root pouches and disappearance of the striated structure normally visible within the saccular area.

| Stage II |

The sacral root sleeves remain unfilled, the fifth lumbar root sleeves are blunted. The dural sac is moderately constricted at the level of the fifth lumbar vertebra.

| Stage III |

All sacral root pouches and the fifth lumbar root sleeves remain unfilled; the fourth lumbar sleeve is blunted. The dural sac is severely constricted at the level of the fifth lumbar vertebra.

Type 2, operated patients

Localized or diffuse arachnoidal proliferation:
'—Filling defects of the root sleeves,
—irregular narrowing, shortening, or occlusion, or even pseudo-diverticular aspect of the dural sac.

22

These signs always predominate at the lower extremity of the dural sac and this intensity decreases progressively cephalad. Three degrees of post-RSG arachnoiditis may be distinguished according to the severity of the above-mentioned signs [72] (see Table 5).

These signs are more frequent and more marked when the patient is x-rayed again after having had a first RSG and operation [3, 43–45, 47, 54]. The signs already described, due solely to the contrast medium (type 1) [47], are associated with the signs due to the operation (type 2) [47], including signs of arachnoidal proliferation, localized or diffuse, i.e., filling defects, irregular narrowing, and shortening or occlusion of the dural sac. Besides, such anomalies may

be seen after an operation without preliminary RSG [47, 54].

As a matter of fact, these post-RSG radiologic signs of adhesive arachnoiditis are not correlated with clinical signs and symptoms [12, 31, 47, 73]. Statistics concerning the frequency of these anomalies vary according to the contrast media utilized, and for a given contrast medium, according to the technique adopted, viz., total amount of contrast, dilution, and delay between the first and second RSG (see Table 6).

Most of the statistics which compare sodium monoiodomethane sulfonate with meglumine iothalamate show that meglumine iothalamate more often causes arachnoiditis than monoiodomethane sulfonate [3, 7, 31, 64]. When comparing the two salts

Table 6. Frequency of adhesive arachnoiditis after RSG

Authors	Contrast agents				
		Monoiodo-methane sulfonate	Meglumine iothalamate	Meglumine iocarmate	Metriza-ide
Autio et al. [7]		0/12 = 0%	6/6 =100%		
Radberg and Wennberg [64]		10/16 =62%	2/3 = 66%		
Halaburt and Lester [31]		1/37 = 2%	12/44 = 24%		
Skalpe and Amundsen [69]					0/19=0%
Nyegaard & Co. (Ahlgren) [59]					0/75=0%
Liliequist and Lundstrom [54]	Total	33/90 =37%			
	Nonoperated	7/45 =16%			
	Operated	26/45 =58%			
Ahlgren [3]	Total	84/240=35%	39/76 = 51%	29/45=64%	
	Nonoperated	11/67 =16%	8/18 = 44%	4/11 =36%	
	Operated	73/173=42%	31/58 = 53%	25/34 =73%	
Irstam et al. [43, 44, 45]	Total	63/111=57%	4/25 = 16%	5/19 =26%	
	Nonoperated	18/51 =35%	1/12 = 8%	0/7= 0%	
	Operated	45/60 =75%	3/13 = 23%	5/12 =42%	

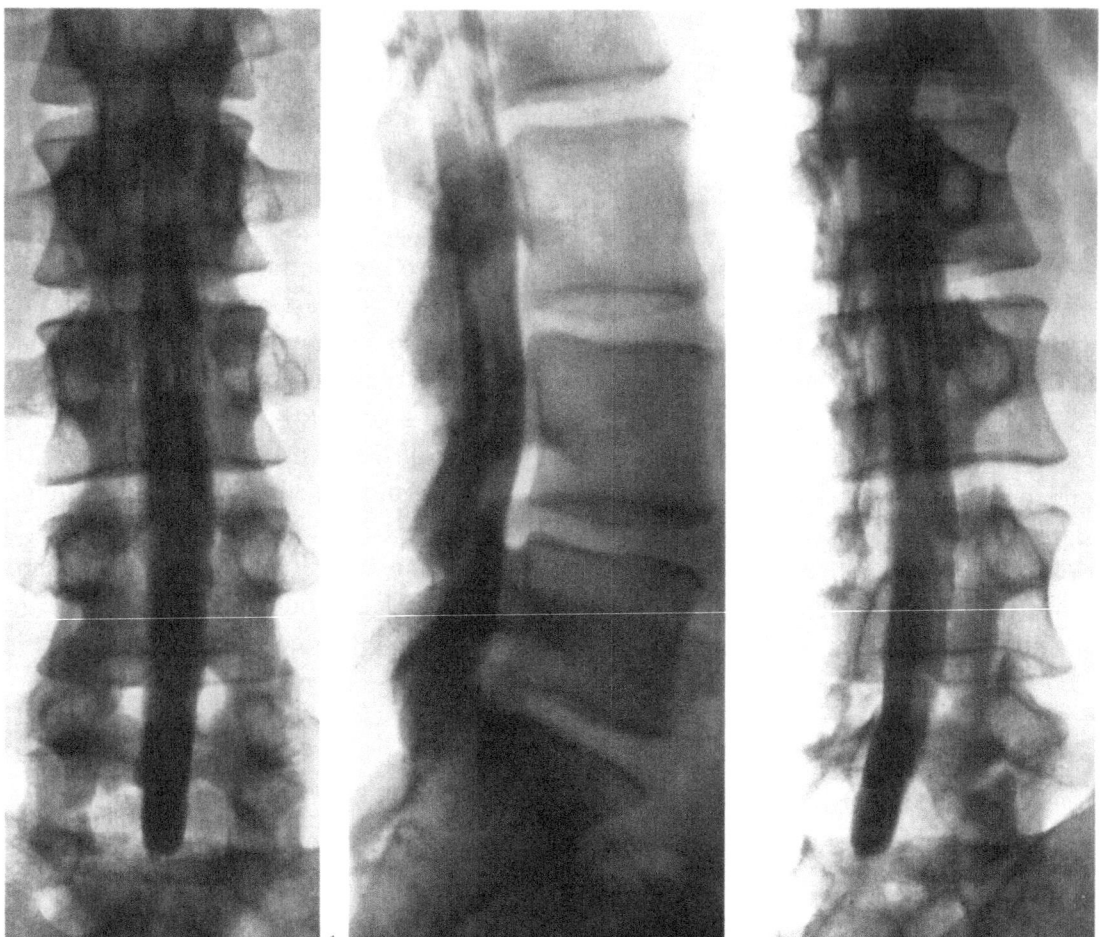

a   b   c

Fig. II,3. **Post-Steroid Arachnoiditis Seen on the First RSG.** 30-year-old male suffering from left sciatalgia for 1 year. During the 6 months before RSG, the patient had seven intrathecal injections of steroids. RSG shows signs of arachnoiditis comparable to those seen after RSG i.e. increased radiopacity of the dural sac which is bare from roots. An amputated appearance of the root sleeve of S1 persists on the right. Linear radiolucencies are visible within the saccular area, nonconsistent with its normal striated appearance. The RSG did not allow the diagnosis of disc herniation and the patient was submitted to operation on the basis of the clinical symptoms. The excision of a left L5-S1 discal herniation was performed. (a) frontal. (b) lateral. (c) left posterior oblique view

of meglumine, one notices that the more recent of the two agents is more often felt to be responsible for arachnoiditis, i.e., meglumine iocarmate [3, 43]. Metrizamide has not been used long enough to allow a precise evaluation of its delayed complications. The first clinical trials [59, 69] would indicate that this medium does not provoke arachnoiditis, a fact that is correlated with its low osmolarity. The theory according to which hyperosmolarity of the CSF is a cause of adhesive arachnoiditis is based on the measurement of the osmolarity at different levels of the dural sac after injection of different contrast media: the highest values for osmolarity were recorded in the lowermost segment L5–S1, in the region where the reactive changes are the most

24

marked [72]. In fact, the clinical statistics on the occurrence of arachnoiditis with the different contrast media refute this theory; successively, the sodium monoiodomethane sulfonate, the meglumine iothalamate, and the meglumine iocarmate have provoked more and more arachnoidal changes though these agents had a progressively lower osmolarity.

It is admitted that the risk of arachnoiditis increases when the amount of contrast medium injected increases [3, 31] and when the CSF already has a high protein content at the moment of injection [3, 31]. Assuming that the stagnation of the contrast medium in the fundus of the dural sac aggravates the risk of arachnoiditis, some physicians have taken the step of making their patients lie down immediately after RSG so as to prevent arachnoiditis [15, 18].

We already saw (see Chap. 2.VI.B.1) that the systematic simultaneous injection of a steroid and a contrast medium, which has been proposed in order to avoid complications [19], has proved to be harmful [3, 23]. Besides, the mere therapeutic intrathecal injection of steroids in cases of sciatalgiae produces features similar to those observed after RSG (Fig. II,3).

Though no correlation has yet been established between those radiologic signs of adhesive arachnoiditis and any clinical symptomatology, these radiologic features nevertheless impede the interpretation of a further RSG [7].

VII. Evaluation of the Technical Characteristics of the X-rays

For the appreciation of the technical quality of the images, one has to take into account the contrast, the geometric deformations, and the false images due to faulty injections.

A. The Radiographic Contrast

The lumbosacral region is known to be a source of difficulties for the radiologist because he has to adjust the parameters to a particularly thick and heterogeneous area and the interpretation may be impeded by the projection of radiolucencies of intestinal origin.

It is all the more difficult to visualize at that level that a water-soluble iodized contrast medium is placed amidst bony structures. The difficulties increase greatly as soon as the patient is either obese or has an increased bone density due to arthrosis. At the worst, in a case of arthrosic narrow canal, the bone condensation may mask the little amount of iodized contrast which has entered the narrowed thecal sac. This drawback consisting in poor images has, however, some value for the diagnosis of narrow subarachnoidal space when the x-rays are correctly performed.

Frontal zonographic sections sometimes allow one to obtain a better image (Fig. II,4).

B. Geometric Deformations

They may be due either to the peculiar configuration of the lumbosacral spine or to a faulty centering of the central beam.

In hyperlordotic patients, who moreover very often tend to have a horizontal sacrum, the frontal image of the dural sac is strongly deformed and shortened on the frontal projection [66].

Spinal desaxations, whether scoliosis or antalgic attitudes, make the radiographic technique very difficult, particularly concerning the positioning of a strict lateral view, or comparative right and left oblique projections.

As a matter of fact, the interpretation of RSG is to perform with x-ray projections

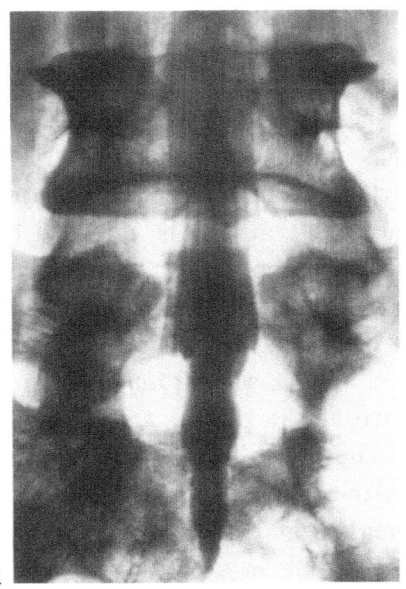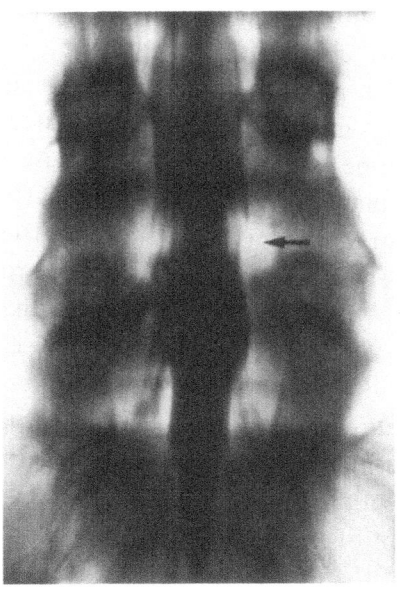

a   b

Fig. II,4. **Usefulness of Frontal Zonography.**
(a) Plain frontal projection. (b) Frontal zonography passing through the pedicles in the same
case. The plain film is doubtful as to the opacification of the L5 and S1 left root sleeves (a).
Zonography demonstrates the correct opacification of the S1 root and the filling defect at
L5 (b) (*arrow*)

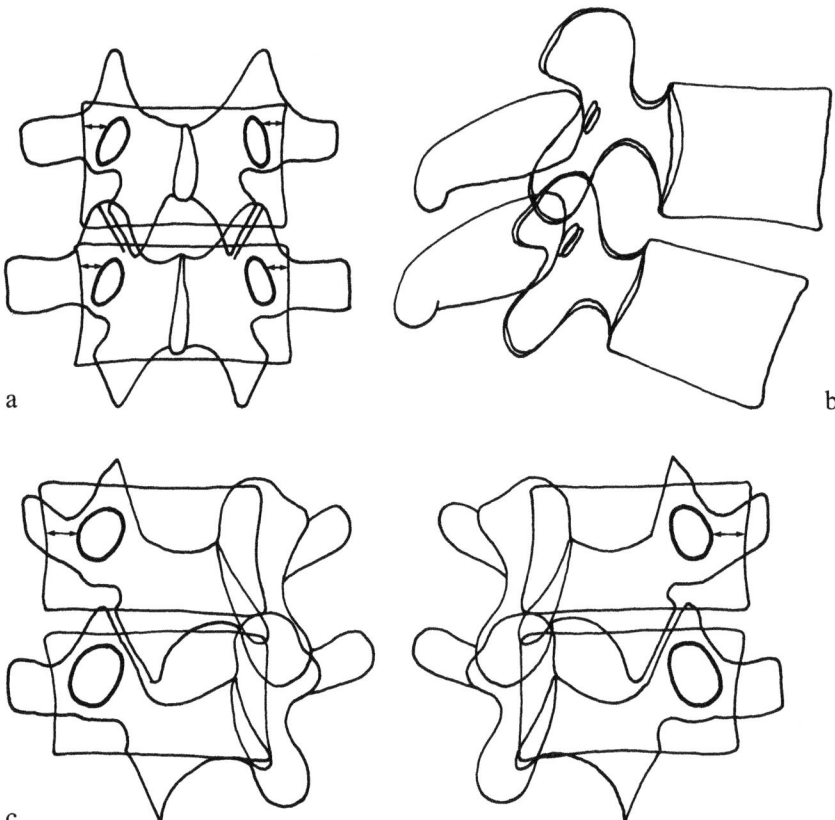

a   b

c

Fig. II,5 **Quality Criteria of the Projections.** (See text). (a) Frontal projection. (b) Lateral projection. (c) Comparability of the oblique projections

26

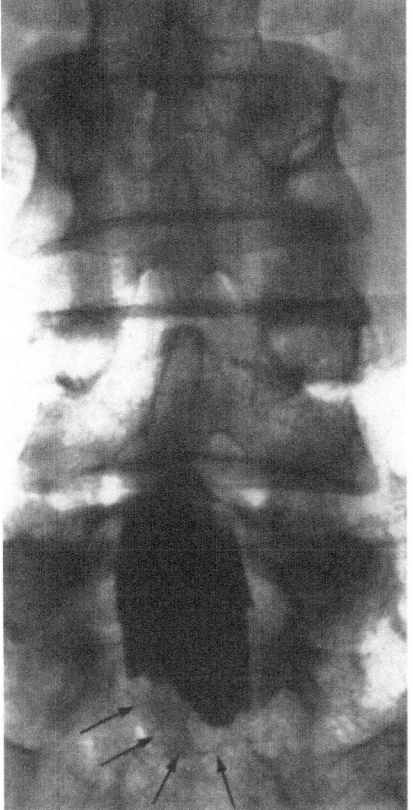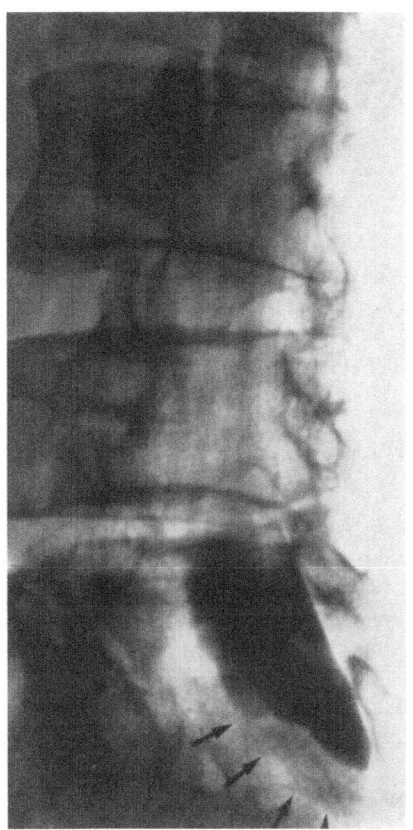

a   b

Fig. II,6. **Subdural Injection**.
(a) Frontal.
(b) Right posterior oblique projections.

The saccular area shows an highgrade contrast. It is a pitfall due to the mainly subdural diffusion of the contrast. The inside of the thecal sac appears slightly opacified (*arrow*)

which are strictly lateral and strictly frontal, and comparable left and right oblique projections. The criterion for a correct frontal projection is the equidistance of the pedicular opacities with regard to the vertebral body contour (Fig. II,5). An x-ray is taken in a strict lateral position when the posterior aspect of the vertebral body and the pedicular shadows are perfectly superimposed. Oblique projections may be considered comparable when the pedicular shadows are equidistant from the anterior margins of the vertebral bodies on the right and left x-rays.

C. Abnormal Images Due to Faulty Injections

A faulty injection may be epidural or subdural.

Subdural injections are visualized as stains of high homogenous density, elongated, and situated either on the anterior or on the posterior aspect of the dural sac (Fig. II,6; Fig. X,4). A localized subdural injection located in the posterior concavity of a vertebral body has to be distinguished from a subarachnoidal accumulation of contrast medium lying above a discal herniation.

An *epidural injection* is displayed as a double-track image, lining anteriorly and

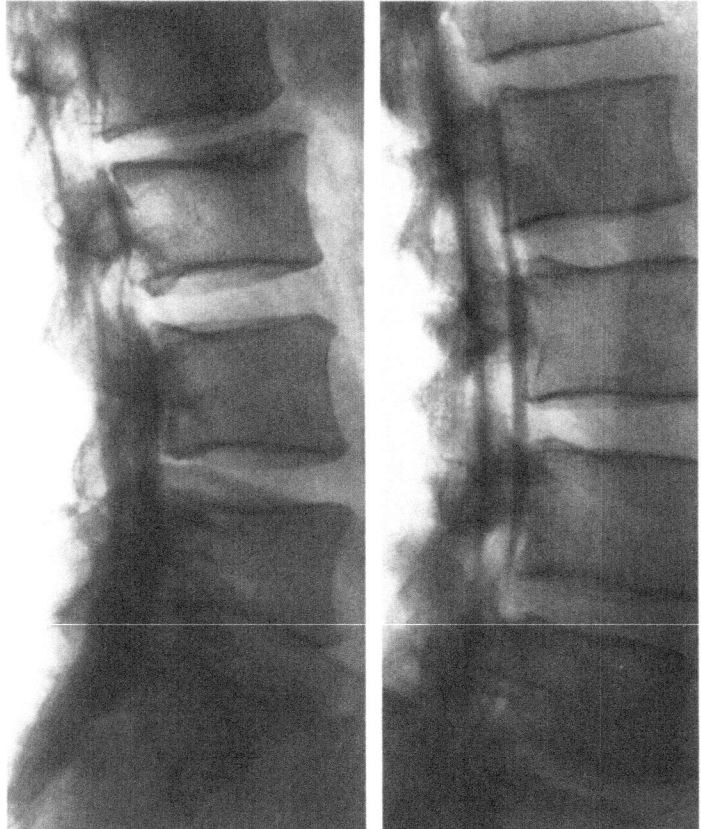

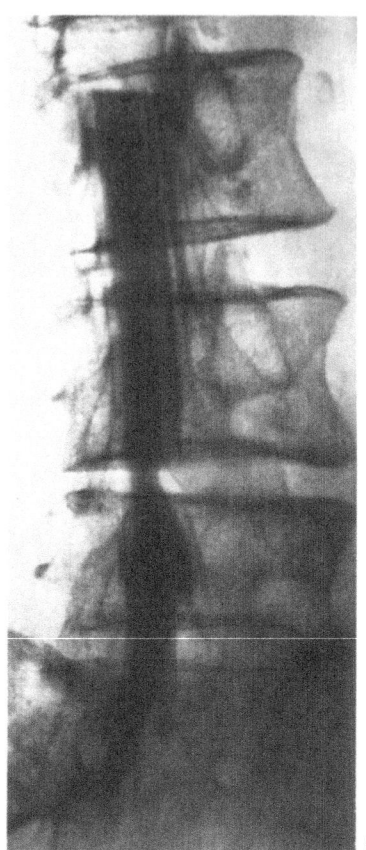

7a
b

8

Fig. II,7. **Extradural Injection**. (a) Partial. (b) Total. In case of total epidural injection, the image on the lateral view is typically constituted by a double-track opacity underlining the anterior and posterior aspects of the canal (b). Partial epidural injection is less readily detected; it results mainly in a blurring of the saccular margins which is prolonged cephalad by similar double-track opacities (a)

Fig. II,8. **Dineric Interface Between the Contrast Medium and the Cerebrospinal Fluid**. The image of the horizontal level corresponds to an artifact due to nondilution of the contrast medium in the CSF

posteriorly the silhouette of the dural sac. It is also visible on frontal projections as a blurred opacity on the canalar area, prolonged in the paravertebral soft-tissues as linear trails (Fig. II,7). The epidural injection has to be distinguished from the image of a very narrow lumbar canal in which the roots are closely bunched and marginated anteriorly and posteriorly by a thin layer of contrast medium.

It may happen that the upper limit of the opaque column is strictly horizontal and linear, witnessing the presence of a dineric interface between the contrast and the CSF, perhaps related to a too slow injection or to an incorrect mixing of contrast medium and water previous to injection (Fig. II,8).

References of Chapter 2 see page 144.

Chapter 3. Some Anatomical Considerations and Clinical Data*

This Chapter deals first with some anatomical considerations concerning the precise structures that are involved in the main pathologic conditions of the cauda equina roots; we shall then consider the clinical pictures of these entities, and finally discuss the indications for RSG.

I. Some Anatomical Considerations

A. The Lumbar Spinal Canal

The lumbar spinal canal is formed by five lumbar vertebrae, each of them constituted by a vertebral body anteriorly, and a posterior arch, joined by the pedicles. These structures delimit the vertebral foramen which is an isosceles triangle in L1 and becomes an equilateral triangle in L5.

The size of the vertebral bodies increases caudad and is the largest at L5.

The lumbar spinal canal [15, 16, 25, 29] is formed by the adjacent vertebral foramina. Its anterior wall corresponds to the vertebral bodies and the interlying discs; its posterior wall is gutter-shaped, formed by the articular processes and the laminae. The deepest part of this gutter corresponds to the junction of the laminae and also to the anterior cortex of the spinous processes.

The lateral walls of the canal are recess-shaped. These walls are alternately constituted by the pedicles and the intervertebral

* This Chapter has been written by D. Maitrot, M.D.

foramina. The superior and inferior articular processes are situated just behind, and thus form the posterior wall of these lateral recesses.

B. The Dural Sac and the Cauda Equina Roots

The dural sac constitutes the duramatral sheath of the cauda equina roots [37]. It extends from the T12-L1 interspace down to S2 or the S2–S3 interspace. Its shape is ovalar at the L1 level and becomes triangular at about the half-height of the lumbar spine, thus adapting to the internal configuration of the bony canal. Below this level, its caliber and its shape vary. It sometimes keeps this triangular shape down to the lumbosacral canal, or becomes cylindrical, tapered, narrow, and detached from the canalar walls.

The cauda equina roots are arranged in an arch of a circle, anteriorly concave, within the dural sac [8, 37]. Thus, at each extremity of the arch are located the right and left roots which are going to emerge at the next underlying level. In the middle of the arch are located the more caudal roots.

At each intervertebral level, on either side, a pair of roots, one dorsal, sensory, and one ventral, motor, pass through the dural sheath toward the intervertebral foramina and constitute the spinal nerve roots surrounded by their radicular sheaths. The external layer—of dura mater—of each sheath is attached on the external margin of the intervertebral foramen, where the fibrous operculum of the external aperture of this opening is also inserted — which is more a canal than a foramen (Fig. III,1).

The emergence level of each root is constant when the dural sac ends at the level of the S1–2 interspace. The emergence levels are the following:

1. The half-height of the vertebral body of the second lumbar vertebra for the second pair of lumbar nerve roots.

2. The upper third of the third vertebra for the third lumbar nerve roots.

3. The upper quarter of the fourth vertebra for the fourth lumbar roots.

4. The upper fifth of the fifth vertebra for the fifth lumbar roots.

5. The L5–S1 disc space for the first sacral roots.

When the dural sac ends at a lower level, each pair of roots emerges lower, and the reverse is true if the dural sac ends more cranially.

C. The Radicular Canal

It is also termed an interdiscoarticular pass and is an anatomosurgical notion [4, 17, 30, 32, 39].

It courses along with the extrasaccular segment of the root. As a matter of fact, it begins where the ensheathed root leaves the dural sac and it terminates by becoming continuous with the intervertebral opening. At this point emerges the spinal lumbar nerve.

Its posterosuperior wall is formed by the ligamentum flavum, the facetal joint, and the lamina of the corresponding vertebra. Anteriorly, it is limited by the disc and the posterior aspect of the vertebral body, both covered by the posterior longitudinal ligament. Its internal wall is represented by the

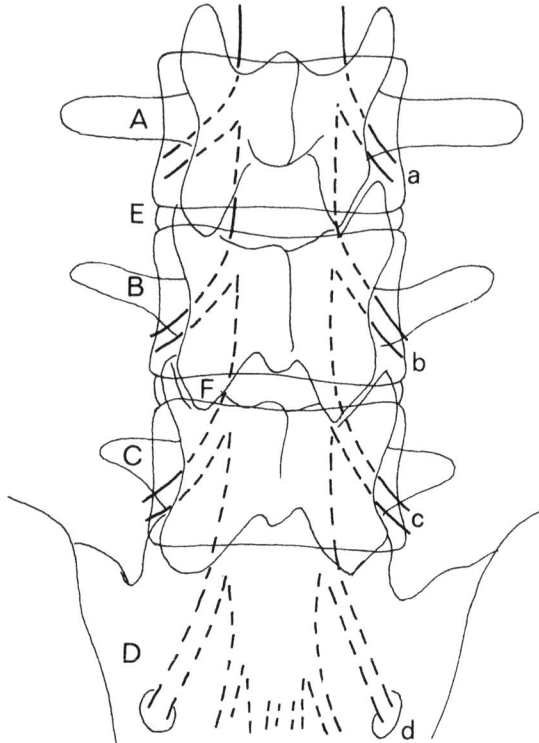

Fig. III,1. **Schematic Representation of the Topographic Relations of the Cauda Equina Roots and the Dural Sac with the Vertebrodiscal Structures Seen From Behind.** (a) L3 root. (b) L4 root. (c) L5 root. (d) S1 root. (A) Vertebral body L3. (B) Vertebral body L4. (C) Vertebral body L5. (D) Vertebral body S1. (E) Intervertebral space. (F) Articular process. This drawing shows the topographic relationship of the disc, not only with the root emerging in its neighborhood, but also with the overlying root, susceptible to being involved by a hernial compression near its entrance into the intervertebral foramen

lateral aspect of the dural sac, and its external wall by the corresponding pedicle — let us recall that each root is numbered like the pedicle with which it has an anatomical relationship (Fig. III,2).

The L4, and chiefly the L5 radicular canals are particularly long and narrow, thus exposing the roots to a discal compression anteriorly, or to a bony compression from backward.

30

D. The Intervertebral Foramen — or Canal

Its anterior limit is constituted by the underlying vertebral body and the disc; its posterior limit by the inferior margin of the lamina of the overlying vertebra, and the facetal joint. Since the articular processes are almost sagittal, the facetal interspace lies in the same plane as the intervertebral foramen.

It has the bilobulated shape of an auricle, the superior part of which belongs to the overlying vertebra, the inferior part to the underlying vertebra.

The transversal axis of each intervertebral foramen is situated at the same horizontal level as the spinous process of the above vertebra.

The diameter of the intervertebral foramina increases in a regular way from one level to the other downward, safe for both L5, which are the smallest of all, though they are traversed by the largest roots [9]. These are also the farthest from the midline.

II. Clinical Data

In this Section we shall summarize the different clinical pictures related to the main pathologic entities which justify the performance of a RSG.

A. Discal Herniations

The conflict between the disc and the root [33, 41] causes a rich and varied symptoma-

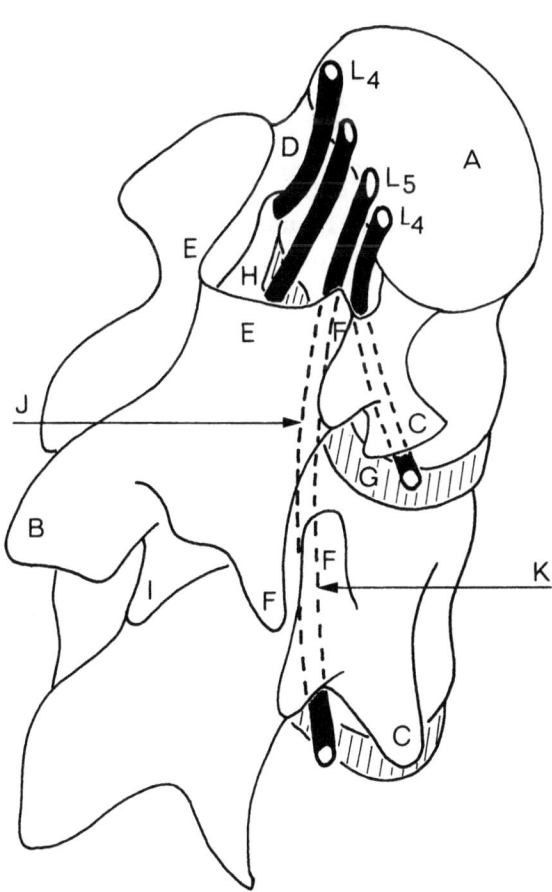

Fig. III,2. **Schematic Representation of the Radicular Canal.** Two vertebrae seen from above and obliquely. The dural sac is not represented. (A) Vertebral body L4. (B) Spinous process L4. (C) Transverse process. (D) Pedicle. (E) Lamina. (F) Articular process. (G) Intervertebral disc. (H) Intervertebral foramina. (I) Interlaminar space. The *right fourth lumbar root* visible in the lateral recess disappears behind the bony structures—pedicle and facetal joint (F)—forming the posterolateral wall of the radicular canal and emerges through the intervertebral foramen. The *left fourth lumbar root* is visible by its medial aspect in the radicular canal. The *left fifth lumbar root* disappears below the L4–5 disc. The *right fifth lumbar root* is represented from the L3–4 interspace on, disappears in front of the L4 lamina (E) to appear again at the level of the L4–5 disc (G) (in front of it). The right L4–5 facetal joint (F) is situated posteriorly and laterally to it, the more so for the superior facet of L5. Thus, it is possible to depict its course through the radicular canal (between two arrows) before it enters into the intervertebral foramen. Note the level of the discoradicular conflict (J) and of the osteoradicular conflict (K)—narrow radicular canal

tology. As a matter of fact, different roots can be concerned with the same pathologic disc, in so far as their anatomical origin and course may vary and the origin of a given herniation may be related to one or the other disc — the disc rupture may occur at various sites and the fragments may migrate in various directions [3, 8, 11, 20].

1. Sciatica [5, 12, 22, 43]

It is characterized by root pain, radiating to the leg, and intensified by motions of the spine and strains rising the CSF pressure within the dural sac. This pain may be accompanied by sensory or motor deficit or loss of a reflex. It is sometimes preceded by acute lumbar pain — "lumbago" — following a strain, and may subside after rest and medical treatment. It may also evolve toward other clinical pictures.

2. Lumbar Paralyzant Radiculitis
[2, 7, 13, 36, 42]

a) Paralyzant Radiculitis in L5
It may at once be paralyzant, the motor deficit is then more significant than the initial pain which sometimes is of short duration.

It may also constitute the evolution of a long-standing sciatica, and in those cases, the radicular pain frequently persists. The functional prognosis of this type of paralyzant radiculitis would be better than in the previous type since the motor deficit regresses more readily after the operation.

It may also be accompanied by loss of the Achilles reflex, and is then rather the symptom of a L5–S1 herniation that has migrated into the intervertebral foramen of the L5 root.

b) Paralyzant Radiculitis in L4
In a great number of cases, RSG does not give evidence of a L3–4 discal herniation; however, it happens that RSG shows another type of conflict between a disc and a root. Then it is often a L4–5 discal herniation which has migrated toward the intervertebral foramen of L4.

c) Paralyzant Radiculitis in S1
This type is less frequent than the L5 involvement. Indeed, it seems that a motor deficit is chiefly observed when a root is compressed from below upward, either in its axillary region or just laterally to it. To produce such a root compression at the level of S1, this root must have its emergence above the L5–S1 interspace, which is only rarely the case.

3. Global or Unilateral Cauda Equina Syndrome

It is then a multiradicular compression which may be accompanied by sphincter disturbances. This multiradicular syndrome is sometimes strictly unilateral, thus adequately termed unilateral cauda equina syndrome [21, 28, 34, 35, 40, 44]. This clinical picture may begin in two ways, i.e.:

a) Acute Cauda Equina Syndrome
This is consecutive to a sudden luxation of the disc. It occurs after a traumatism or a strain due to coughing or sneezing as an acute multiradicular sensory motor deficit with loss of reflexes, accompanied by retention of urine and feces. To ensure improvement, the operation has to be performed at once.

b) Chronic Cauda Equina Syndrome
It differs from the previous syndrome in so far as the multiradicular deficit is often preceded by alternate right and left sciaticae for a certain time, and by incontinence of the urinary bladder, i.e., emptying by overflow.

Whatever the clinical picture, these multiradicular involvements concern mainly the cauda equina roots from L5 on, whether the discal herniation originates in L4–5, in L5–S1, or in L3–4. It may be pointed out that the L3–4 discal herniation more often causes a multiple radicular involvement.

B. The Narrow Lumbar Canal

Its clinical picture is represented by the neurogenic intermittent claudication of the cauda equina [1, 6, 10, 45].

Lumbar or lumboradicular pains appear after a certain distance of walking, which becomes shorter and shorter [18, 27, 38, 46, 47]. They disappear remarkably rapidly when the patient lies or sits down. The sensory disturbances — most often paresthesiae — and the motor deficits — referring frequently to the L5 territory — by and by complete the clinical symptomatology. These pains never reach the intensity of those related with discal herniations.

True radicular deficits may appear but remain for a very long time moderate, though they may sometimes constitute real chronic cauda equina syndromes.

C. The Narrow Radicular Canal

Root compression is not always due to discal herniation. As a matter of fact, the radicular canal may be narrowed either by discarthrosis or by arthrosic hypertrophy of the facetal joints, or of the laminae in their external third, close to the insertion of the facetal joints [4, 17]. The resulting symptomatology may mimic radiculitis related to a discal herniation, save for the fact that the pain is often intensified by walking or prolonged standing, and moreover the objective radicular signs are often mild [32]. This condition most often involves the L4 and L5 roots, owing to the fact that these

course in particularly long and narrow canals (see Chap. 3.I.C).

III. Indications of RSG

Obviously, a precise semiologic analysis very often permits determination of the level of the discoradicular conflict or narrow lumbar canal. However, on the occasion of the study of 700 case reports of sciatica by discal herniation [31], we discovered that the clinical findings were confirmed by surgery in only 65% of the cases; the absence of radiculosaccographic data would thus

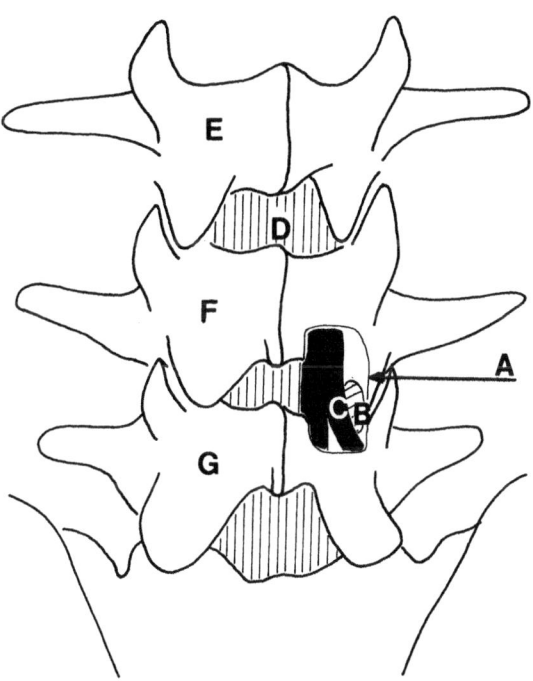

Fig. III,3. **Schematic Drawing of an Operative View of the Spine** — without taking into account the ligamentous and muscular structures: The interlamellar fenestration is often supplemented by an internal facetectomy of the corresponding facetal joint. (A) Removal of the medial part of the corresponding facetal joint. (B) Disc herniation. (C) L5 root. (D) Interlaminar space and ligamentum flavum. (E, F, G) Posterior arches of L3, L4, and L5

have led to a surgical exploration at several levels in 35% of the cases. Besides, the clinical picture does not allow one to foresee the extent of a narrow lumbar canal.

These two failures lead us to consider RSG an indispensable investigation, preliminary to any surgery [3, 23, 24]. This being stated, when should this investigation be recommended, i.e., when is the surgical indication to be discussed?

First, any sciatica without motor deficit, any narrow radicular canal syndrome, or any narrow lumbar canal syndrome must be determined by RSG whenever the painful syndrome does not subside after 2 weeks of medical treatment.

Secondly, a RSG should be promptly performed as soon as signs of motor deficit or sphincter disturbances appear. Thus, the surgical indication could readily be decided so as to ensure good functional recovery.

By giving evidence of the localization [14, 19, 26] and of the precise extent of the conflict between the disc or the bony structures and the root, systematic RSG permits a better adaptation of surgery to each peculiar case. Moreover, it diminishes the risk of negative and even iterative explorations related to forgotten fragments or to a neglected narrow lumbar canal because of its coexistence with a disc herniation.

This attitude has led us to modify the operative tactics, especially as concerns the migrating discal herniations [3] and the herniations causing a cauda equina syndrome, which are often related — as we verified — to the coexistence of a narrow lumbar canal (Fig. III,3).

References of Chapter 3 see page 147.

34

Chapter 4. Normal Radiculosaccography (RSG)

I. Normal Radioanatomy in Routine Projections [3, 9, 11, 16, 21, 22, 24]

A. The Dural Sac

Its full length is only appreciable on *side views*. It occupies the lumbosacral canal down to a variably low level, generally to the S1–2 interspace, but it may already stop at L5–S1 or go lower than S1–2. Its anterior wall runs along the dorsal aspect of the vertebral bodies, bridges the interspaces, and may be slightly indented by the normal bulge of each intervertebral disc. The narrow space situated between the anterior aspect of the dural sac and the posterior aspect of the vertebrae may increase at the lumbosacral level [17]. The dorsal wall of the dural sac lies close to the cortex of the spinous processes and indicates the posterior part of the canal, which is difficult to delineate on plain films.

On *frontal x-rays,* the lower segment of the dural sac appears shortened, owing to the sacral inclination, which is more pronounced in lordotic patients. It lies between the pedicular alignment which indicates the lateral walls of the osseous canal, and its lateral aspects are separated from the cortex of the pedicles by a distance which under normal conditions should be the same on either side.

On the *oblique views,* the dural sac presents a smooth posterolateral aspect in relation to the cortex of the laminae, while its anterolateral aspect is spiky with the off-shoots of the root pockets situated under each pedicular opacity. The nearer the patient is rotated forward by 20–30 degrees, the better these root pockets and the radicular sheaths are visible.

B. The Roots and Their Sleeves

The roots are more or less distinguishable on side views as linear radiolucencies within the opacified dural sac. They become evident only under pathologic conditions.

On the frontal views, the roots are also more or less visible within the sac and become identifiable close to their outpouching as vertical radiolucencies.

Each radiolucency continues towards the intervertebral foramen, passing beneath, and then below each pedicular opacity. The root is visible owing to the surrounding opacity of the subarachnoidal space prolonged within its sheath. On routine x-rays, the L5 and S1 radicular sheaths are the best visible owing to their rather vertical and longer course. A simple method permits identification of these two pairs of roots, viz., the L5 roots pass below the pedicles of the fifth lumbar vertebra, directed caudally and slightly laterally, while the underlying S1 roots descend more vertically toward the first sacral foramina, thus crossing the lumbosacral interspace in its external third (Fig. IV,1).

A better visualization at a definite level may be obtained by means of a complementary view with the central beam parallel

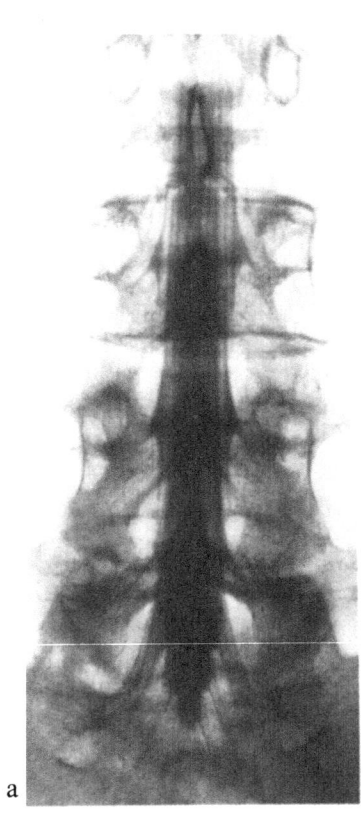
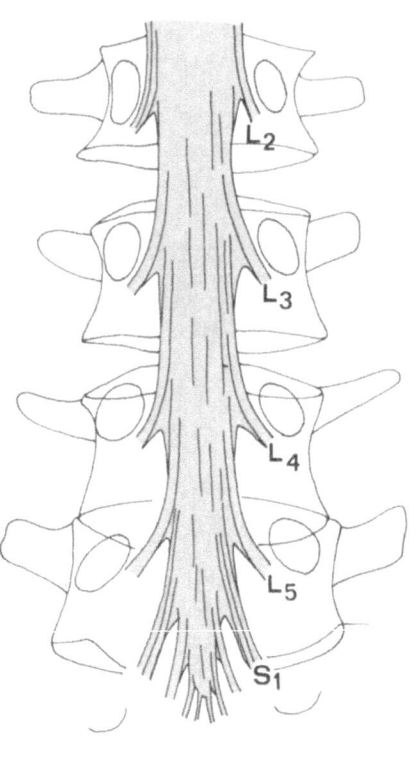

a

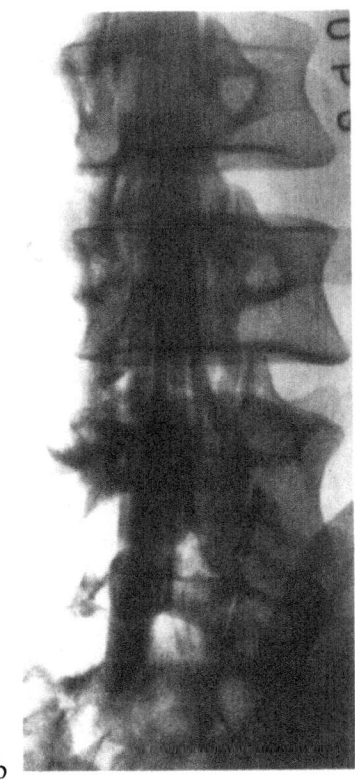
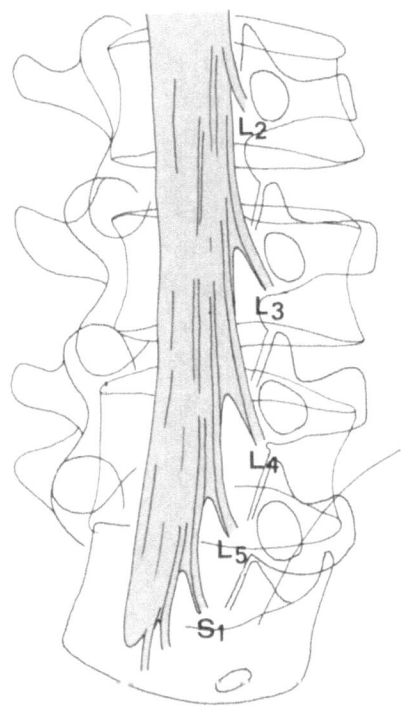

b

36

to the disc concerned. Now, owing to their orientation in a plane oblique with regard to the frontal plane, the radicular sheaths are the best visible on oblique views with the patient rotated slightly forward by 20–30 degrees (Fig. IV,2).

The radiolucency of the root is framed by the overlying and underlying opacity of the root sleeve, the inferior fossa of which is situated in the acute angle formed by the emergence of the radicular sheath and the adjacent dural sac. This fossa decreases gradually in depth and continues laterally with the radicular sheath itself. It also continues caudally toward the supraradicular fossa of the underlying root. This inferior fossa — which we shall term "armpit of the root sleeve" — is prominent for the diagnosis of the compressions on the root. The oblique projections with the central beam at 45 degrees with regard to the frontal plane provide a better image of the anterolateral aspect of the dural sac than of the outpouching sleeves (Fig. IV,2).

II. Complementary Techniques

They are performed for a better visualization, either of the radicular sleeves and their relation to the intervertebral space, or of the walls of the dural sac.

A. Frontal Zonography
[1, 4, 5, 7, 16] (Fig. IV,3)

It provides a better image of the lumbosacral roots — especially at S1 — by eliminating most of the superimposed radiologic shadows. The S1 radicular sheaths are particularly well-defined on such x-rays owing to the fact that they are generally positioned in an almost frontal plane.

Moreover, frontal zonography performed at the appropriate level allows a better delineating of the lateral walls of the dural sac and becomes helpful in defining the shape of an indentation of discal origin.

B. Oblique Ascending Views
(Fig. IV,4)

They are adapted to the slope of the selected intervertebral space and are performed as a complement to a frontal view or even to oblique projections; this latter achieves a double oblique projection and may provide the image of an interruption of a root sleeve. Thus, the relationship of a single root to the corresponding disc can be displayed as well as its possible stop at this level. Note that the geometric deformation of the structures at the adjacent levels impedes their analysis.

Such complementary views are especially indicated in lordotic patients and in cases

___

◁ Fig. IV,1. **Normal Root Emergences.** (a) Frontal projection. The root emergences are symmetric, indicated by triangular opacities corresponding to the fusion of the sub- and supraradicular fossae of two adjacent levels. Each root is termed according to the pedicle below which it passes; thus, the L5 roots are readily identified, passing under the pedicular shadows of the fifth lumbar vertebra. S1 roots have a typical course, running toward the first sacral

foramina (note in this case the double S1 radicular radiolucencies). The underlying sacral roots can rarely be identified. (b) Oblique projections. When the central beam is perpendicular to the plane of the axillary pouches, the oblique projection permits demonstration of the radicular emergences. The roots are termed after the pedicular shadow they run along. The S1 root is directed toward the first sacral foramen

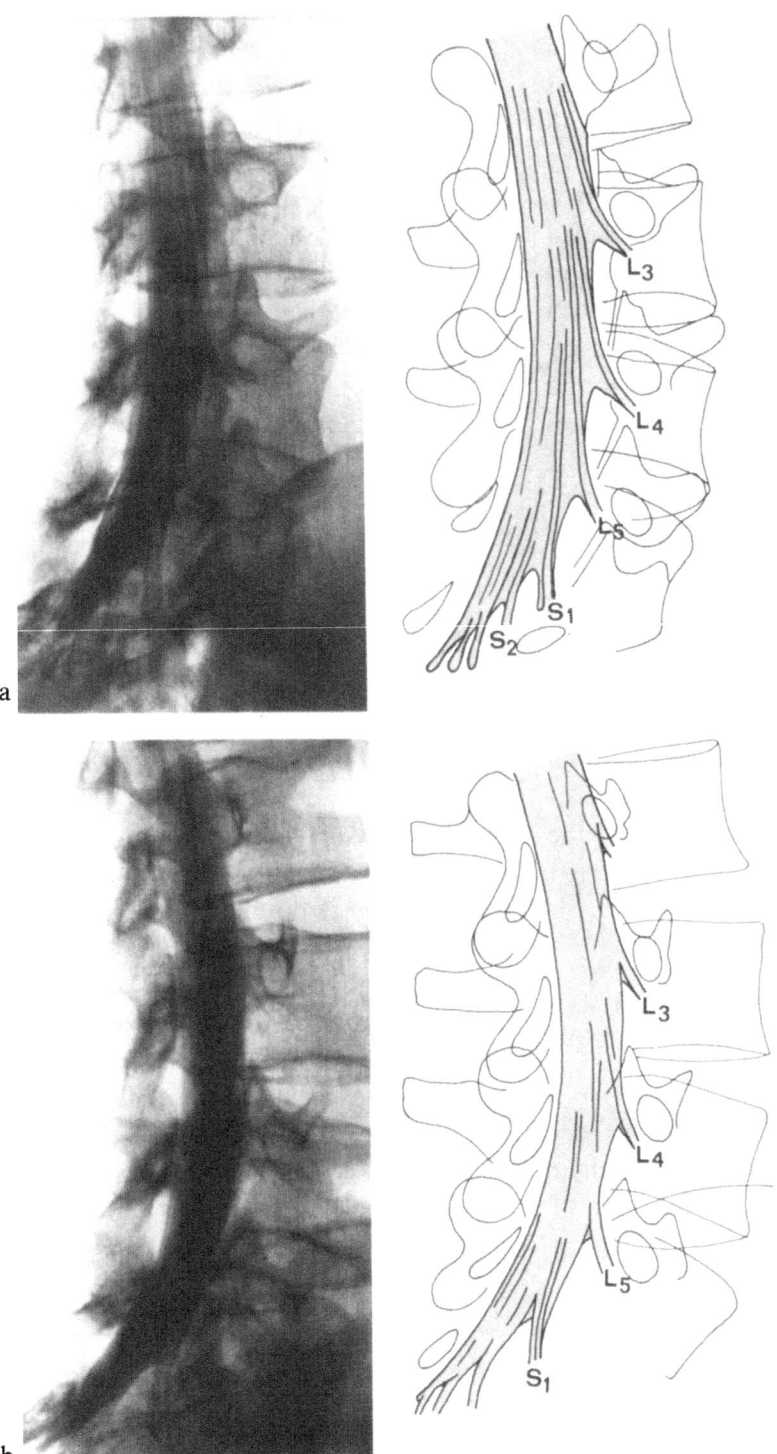

a

b

Fig. IV,2. **Visualization of the Roots With Regard to the Degree of Rotation of the Patient.** (a) Mild rotation (20–30 degrees). (b) More marked rotation (40–50 degrees). It is the same patient in whom the overly pronounced rotation (b) no longer allows visualization of the radicular sheaths and their axillae. Contrariwise, the latter are perfectly visible with the patient rotated at a small angle (a). The importance of the rotation may be evaluated by observing the distance between the pedicular shadow and the anterior margin of the vertebral body

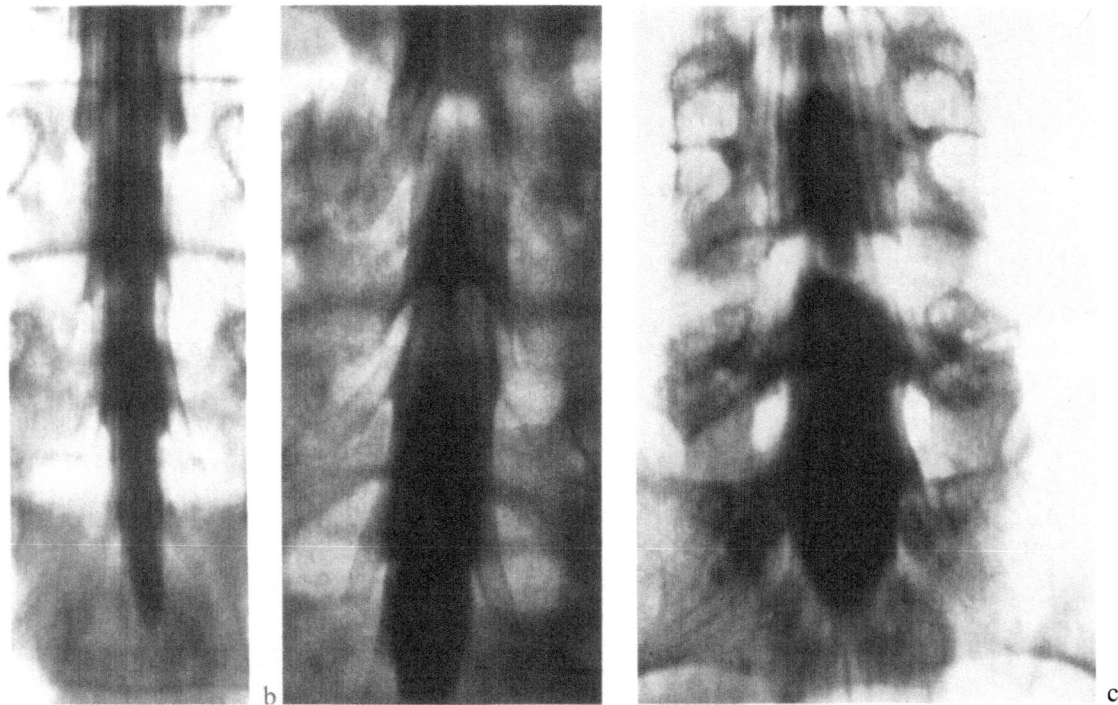

a   b   c

Fig. IV,3. **Frontal Zonograms.** (a) Narrow dural sac. (b) Common type of dural sac. (c) Wide dural sac. The frontal zonography allows a bet- ter analysis of the radicular sheaths and their axillae

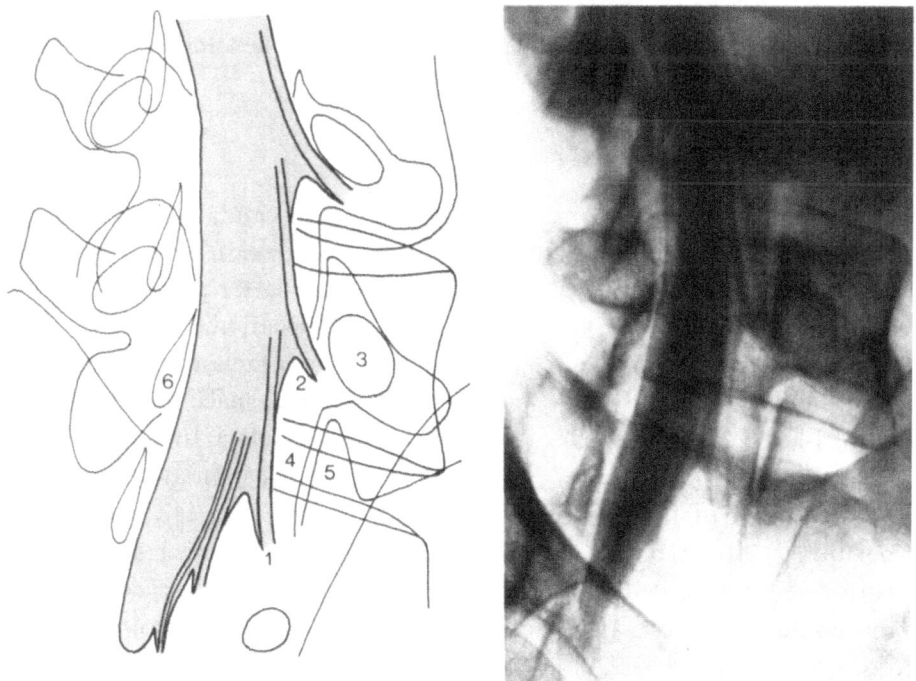

Fig. IV,4. **Ascending Oblique View centered on one Intervertebral Space.** The ascending oblique projection centered on the L5–S1 interspace makes it possible to exactly locate the radicular emergence with regard to the disc. *1* S1 root, *2* L5 root, *3* pedicle of L5, *4* inferior articular process of L5, *5* facet of the articular process of the sacrum, *6* L5 lamina

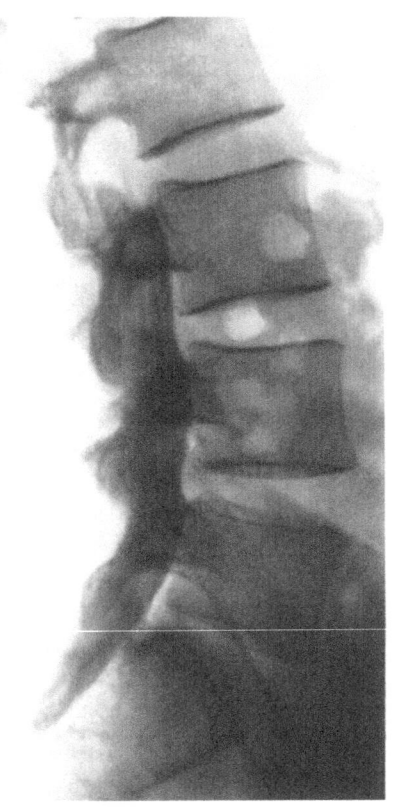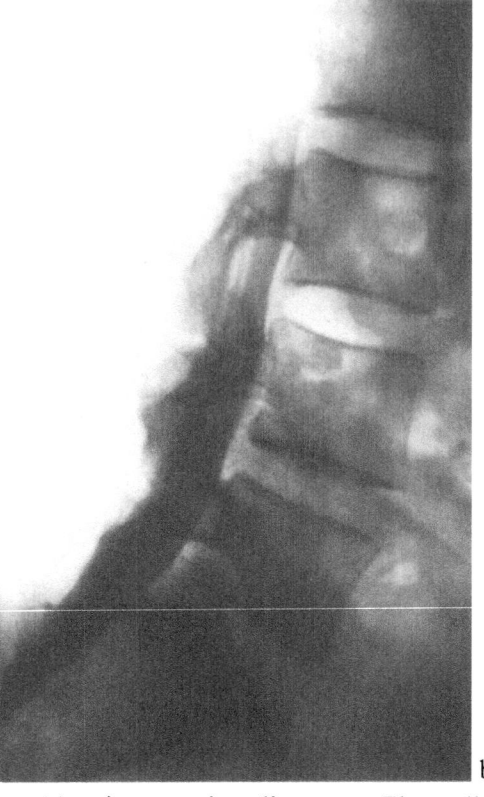

a   b

Fig. IV,5. **Normal Functional Exploration.** (a) Extension. (b) Flexion. During the flexion, the width of the anterior epidural space increases slightly, and the minor discal indentations seen in extension disappear. The radicular radiolucencies visible within the saccular area are stretched during flexion

of mild herniations with minor radiologic signs. They are not useful under normal conditions.

C. Functional Exploration

[6, 8, 14, 19, 23] (Fig. IV,5)

Lateral views of the dural sac in the two positions of flexion and extension performed during RSG may be helpful for the diagnosis of several pathologic conditions (see Chap. 6 and 9). Under normal conditions, the epidural space, seen as a radiolucency situated between the dural sac and the dorsal aspect of the vertebrae, increases slightly from the upper lumbar levels caudad. Moreover, this space increases in flexion and decreases in extension. In the latter position, this space can even disappear, the dural sac coming into contact with the anterior wall of the canal, the epidural space then being very narrow.

Such a functional exploration is useful to substantiate the absence of disc protrusion when the epidural space appears particularly thick behind L5 and S1, and this can be observed more often in patients without physiologic lordosis or even in moderately kyphotic ones. We shall see (Chap. 6) that this functional exploration may reveal a disc protrusion when the epidural space fails to narrow in extension, especially at L5–S1.

III. Normal Variations

A. Variations of the Dural Sac
[21] (Fig. IV,6)

Plain films do not allow us to predict the anatomical type of the dural sac. Indeed, the borderline between normal variations and malformative conditions is not well-defined.

We shall describe separately the variations in length and the variations in width, but these two parameters are roughly correlated, viz., wide dural sacs are also long and conversely narrow ones are also short.

1. Variations in Length

The majority of dural sacs stop at the level of the S1–2 interspace. They are considered short when they end at the level of the lumbosacral interspace and considered long when they extend variably down into the sacral canal.

2. Variations in Width

The ratio between the interpedicular distance at L5 and the width of the dural sac has been proposed as a test of normality [15]. In normal cases, it is almost 1.5, in case of megacauda it is almost 1.

When the dural sac occupies a great deal of space, the epidural space is reduced. Its width is best evaluated on lateral views with

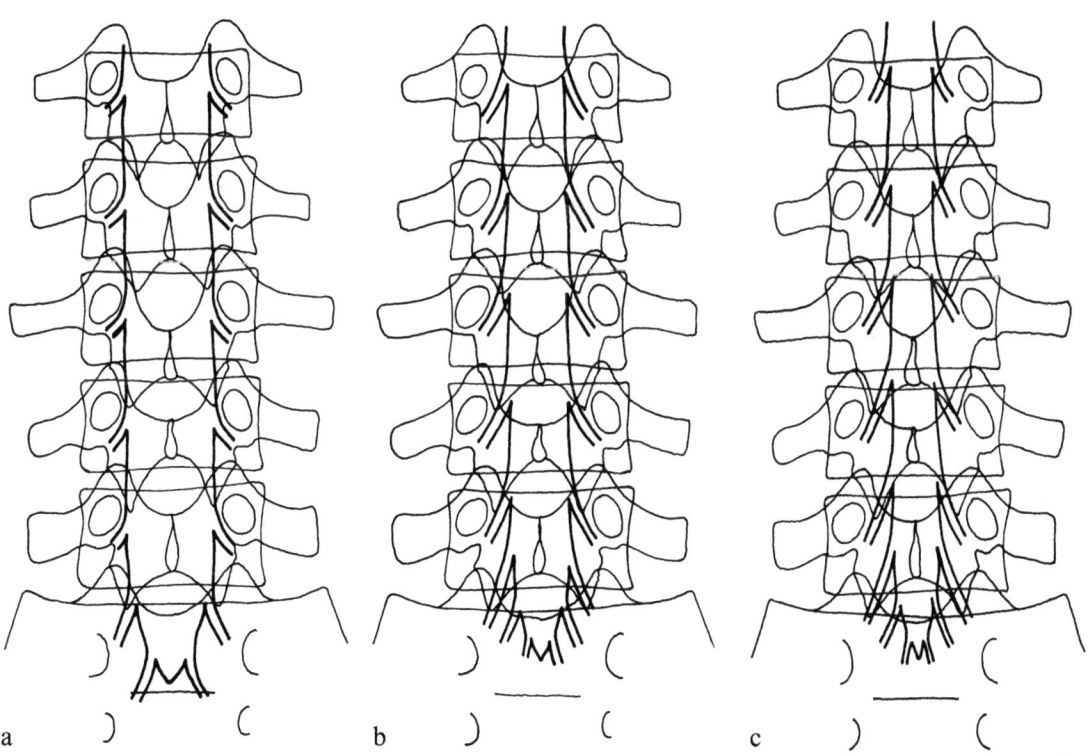

a   b   c

Fig. IV,6. **Variations in the Width of the Dural Sac.** Schematic drawings of: (a) A wide dural sac. (b) A common type of dural sac. (c) A narrow dural sac. The thickness of the epidural space may be evaluated by observing the distance between the lateral margin of the dural sac and the pedicular cortex. Indeed, this thickness depends on the volume occupied by the thecal sac

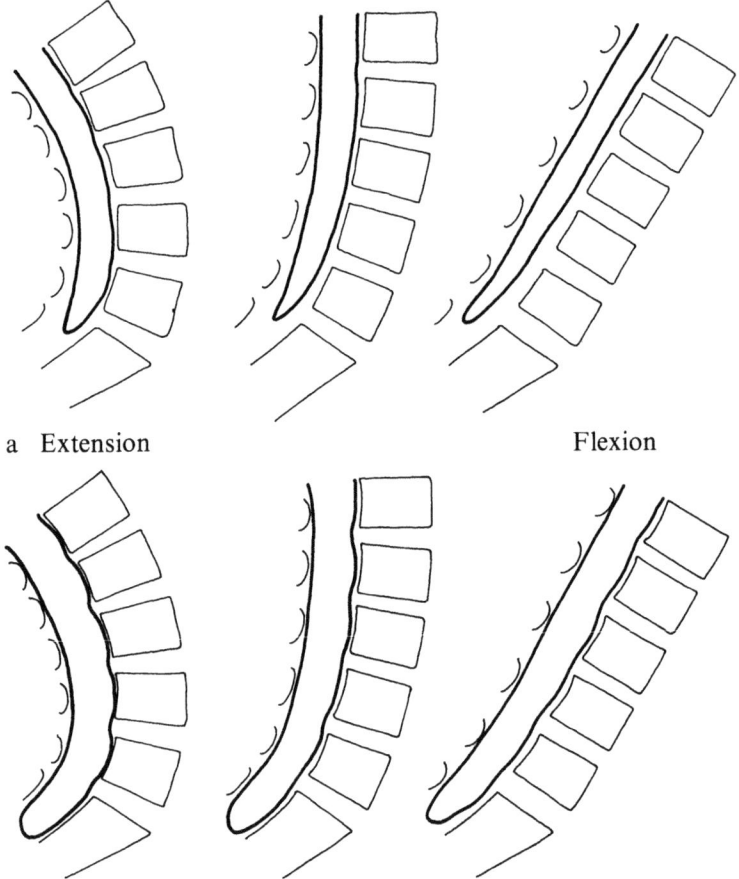

a Extension   Flexion

b Extension   Flexion

Fig. IV,7. **Schematic Diagram of Functional Exploration Under Different Anatomical Conditions.** (a) Narrow and short dural sac. (b) Wide and long dural sac. The anterior epidural space has its maximal width during flexion and is reduced during extension. In the case of a narrow and short sac (a), the maneuver may be useful to detect a herniation. In the case of a large and long dural sac (b), the extradural space is thin all along the lumbar spine. In the extension position, the anterior aspect of the sac is molded against the small disc protrusions which has no pathologic significance

regard to the distance: dural sac — posterior aspect of the vertebrae. Consequently, the narrow cul-de-sac is situated at some distance [17] behind the vertebrae, and is more distant the more the patient's spine is flexed. Conversely, the so-called megacauda lies close to the anterior wall of the canal, so that extension will bring it into close contact with the vertebrae, even molding their posterior concavities (Fig. IV,7).

B. Variations of the Roots and Their Sheaths [21]

Variations of the dural sac go along with variations in the level of emergence and general orientation of the roots. Though these variations have been known for 10 years, their importance has only been recently recognized as helpful for diagnosis. Thus, the status anatomicus is responsible for the kind of discoradicular conflict and possible varieties of migrating herniae (see Chap. 6).

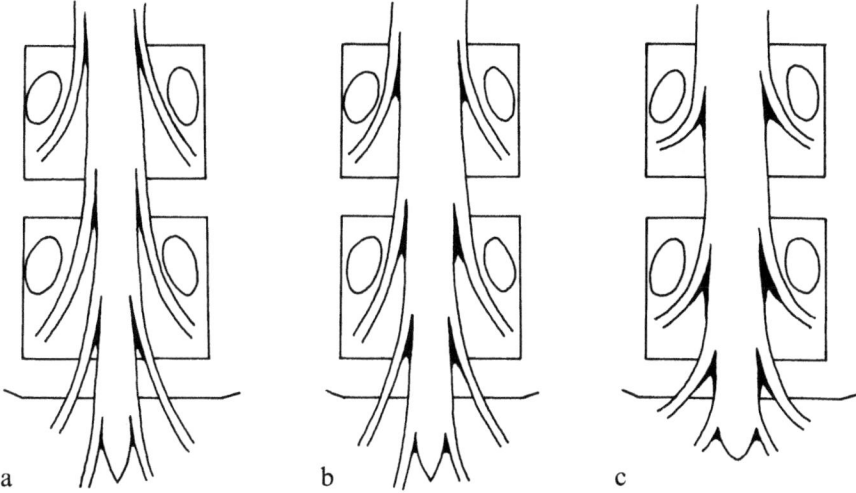

Fig. IV,8. **Variations in the Mode of Emergence of the Root Sheaths.** (a) High originating sheaths, with a rather vertical course. (b) Common type. (c) Low originating and horizontal sheaths

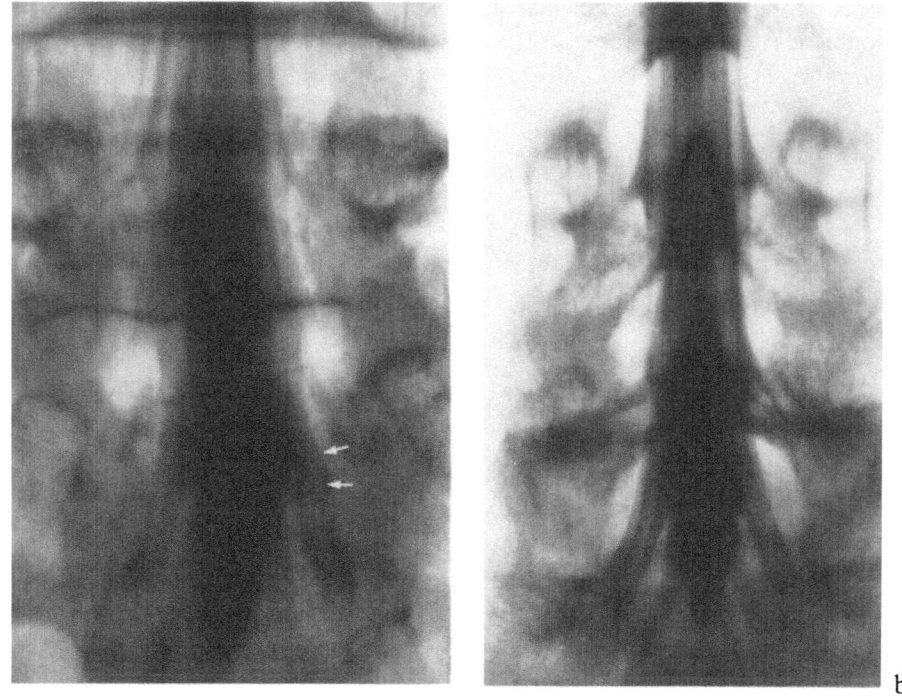

Fig. IV,9. **Nonpathologic Anomalies of the Extrasaccular Segments of the Roots.** (a) The left S2 root is sinuous just distal to its emergence (*arrows*). (b) Doubling of the S1 radicular translucency, best visualized on the right side

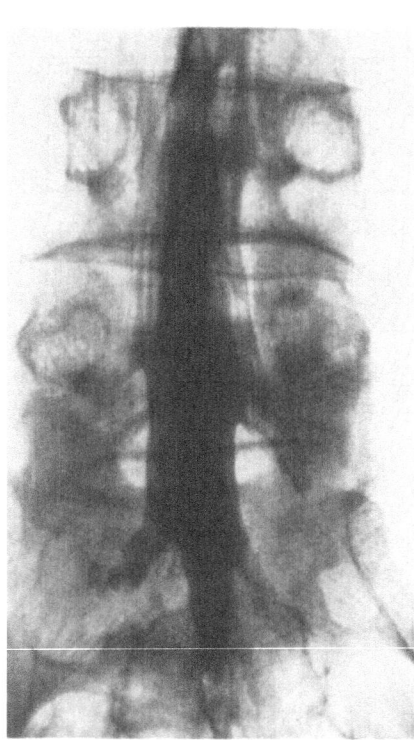

Fig. IV,10. **Abnormal Emergence of the Radicular Sheaths.** On the left side, the L5 and S1 roots have a common origin situated at the half-height of the contralateral emergence points of the same roots. Moreover, several radicular sheaths show doubling

Generally, the L5 roots originate at the half-height of the fifth lumbar vertebra and the S1 roots just above the L5–S1 disc. When the dural sac is narrow and short, the roots can be expected to have a higher origin and a rather vertical direction, and conversely a wide and long dural sac has low originating roots, more horizontally directed toward the intervertebral foramina (Fig. IV,8).

Other anomalies [10] may predominantly affect the lower lumbar and sacral root sleeves. Some of them are common, such as diffuse or cyst-like dilatations of the root sleeves, duplication or sinuosity (Fig. IV,9) of the radiolucency of the sleeves. Other anomalies are very rare, such as common dural origin of two nerve roots also called gun-barrel-like coupling of the spinal nerve roots [20] or common exit of two nerve roots through the same intervertebral foramen [2], or connection between two roots with otherwise normal course [12, 13].

References of Chapter 4 see page 149.

Chapter 5. Analytic Radiosemiology in RSG

The systematic analysis of RSG includes the study of the thecal sac as well as of the area between the sac and the bony canal.

I. The Thecal Sac

A. Terminology and Radiologic Geometry

The radiologic projection of an opaque volume varies according to the geometry of its walls and the direction of the central beam which is utilized.

If one of the walls of the *x-rayed volume* presents a flat surface and if this surface is hit tangentially by the central beam, the *margin* which represents the radiographic projection of this *wall* is clear-cut, and the adjoining area is uniformly opaque. If one of these two previous conditions is lacking, i.e., unflat surface or nontangential central beam, the outline of the x-rayed volume presents a shading-off toward the periphery and even to the extent of margins getting blurred.

In RSG, the x-rayed volume is either a cylinder, an ellipsoid, or a trihedral with rounded angles.

The *trihedral* has three flat aspects, each of which projects as a clear margin on one film: the one which is attained with a tangential beam. On each of these three preferential films, the opposite margin of the sac shows a shading-off, similar to the two margins of the radiographic projection of the same volume on any other film (Fig. V,1 a).

Contrariwise, there is no preferential direction of the beam for the *cylinder* since its silhouette shows a marginal shading-off and less clear margins on all its projections (Fig. V,1 b).

The *ellipsoid* has a lateral view with relatively clear margins and a frontal view with relatively blurred margins (Fig. V,1 c).

According to the topography of the deformation of the sac with regard to its axis, the morphologic type of dural sac, and the orientation of the beam, the margins of its outline may have a more or less shaded-off opacity. But usually each of these deformations will be best shown on one of the routine projections of the RSG.

In practice, these theoretical considerations are altered by the presence within the dural sac of roots causing the opacity to become heterogenous.

The analysis of the deformations of the margins of the silhouette of the thecal sac on the routine projections is followed by the synthesis which permits localization of the direction of the compression, and eventually the shape of the dural sac on which this compression is exerted. This localization of the deformation of the sac provides indications about the origin of the compression, since anterolateral compressions are frequently of discal origin, whereas posterior compressions are mainly of bony origin (Fig. V,2).

A radiologic study of the dural sac includes the appreciation of its overall sil-

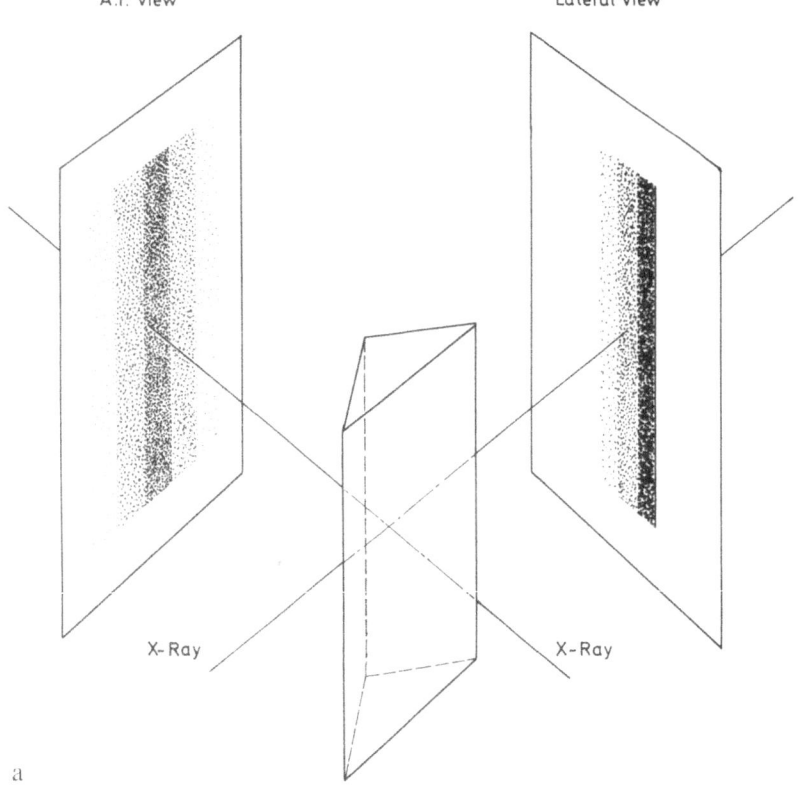

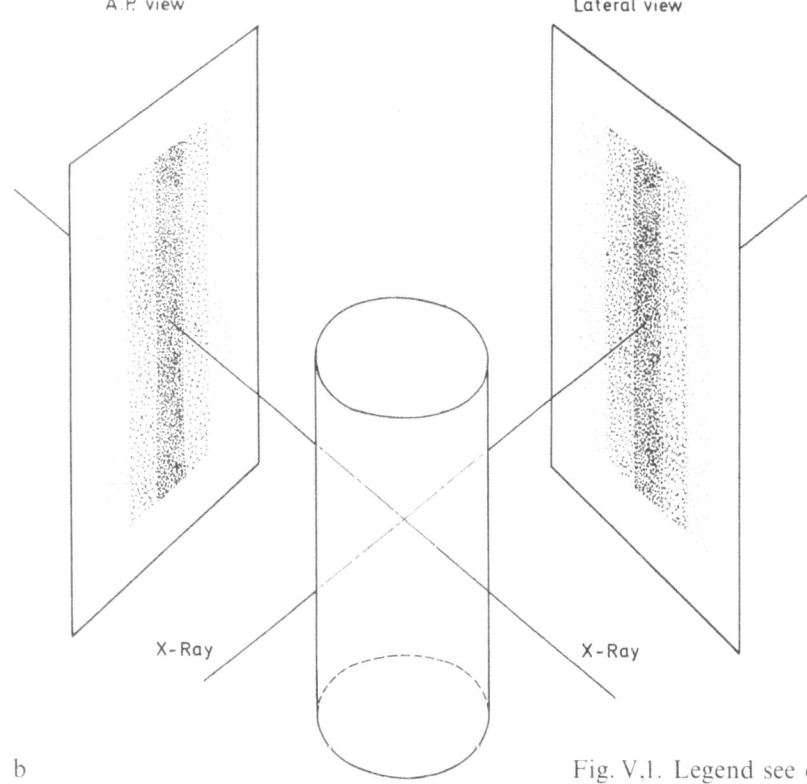

Fig. V.1. Legend see opposite page

A.P. view   Lateral view

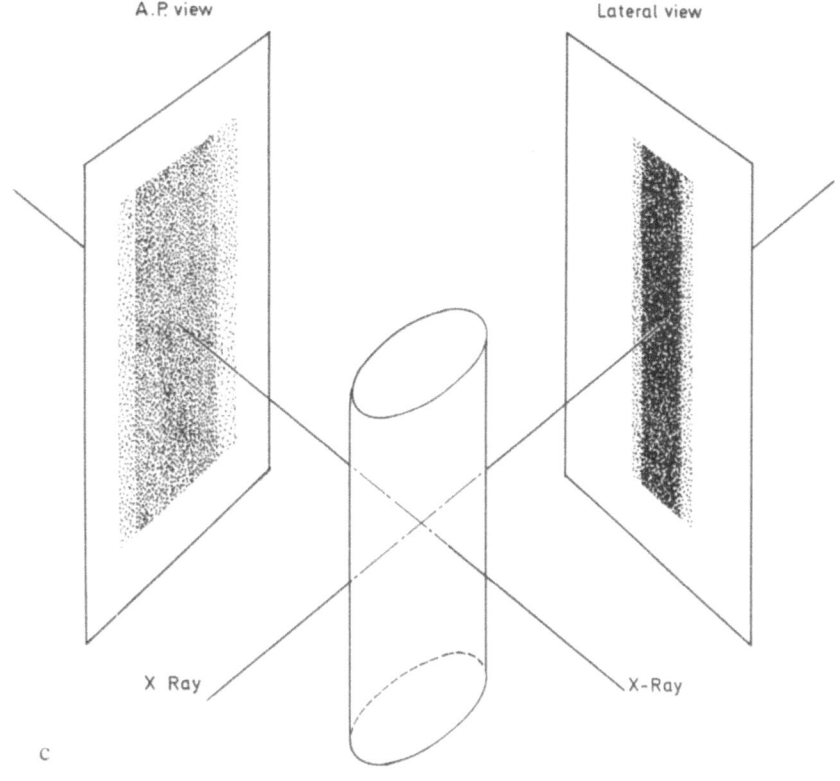

X Ray   X-Ray

c

Fig. V,1. The Margins of the Projection of an Opaque Volume. (a) *Trihedral:* Let us take for example an isosceles trihedral, the basis of which is parallel to the central x-ray. On this —lateral—projection, its base is projected as a clear-cut margin whereas the opposite margin of its silhouette shows a shaded-off margin. The orthogonal—frontal—projection falls perpendicular to the basis of the trihedral and the margins of the radiologic projection of the volume are shaded-off. (b) *Cylinder:* The existence of a symmetry axis causes the two orthogonal projections to be identical, the absence of plane aspect involves a shading-off of the margins of the silhouette in all the projections. (c) *Ellipsoid:* It is supposed to be x-rayed along its two symmetry axes. Along the greater axis—lateral view—the shading-off of the margins of the silhouette is feeble whereas on the orthogonal projection—frontal view—the silhouette is less dense on the whole and has more shaded-off margins.

This schematic geometry of the thecal sac allows one to explain the variable degree of distinctness of the margins of its silhouette.

The usually trihedral shape with blunted angles accounts for the anterior margin of the thecal sac being the most distinct in most of the cases.

The excessive tapering of the lateral recesses may explain the shaded-off blurring of the lateral margins (frontal projection)

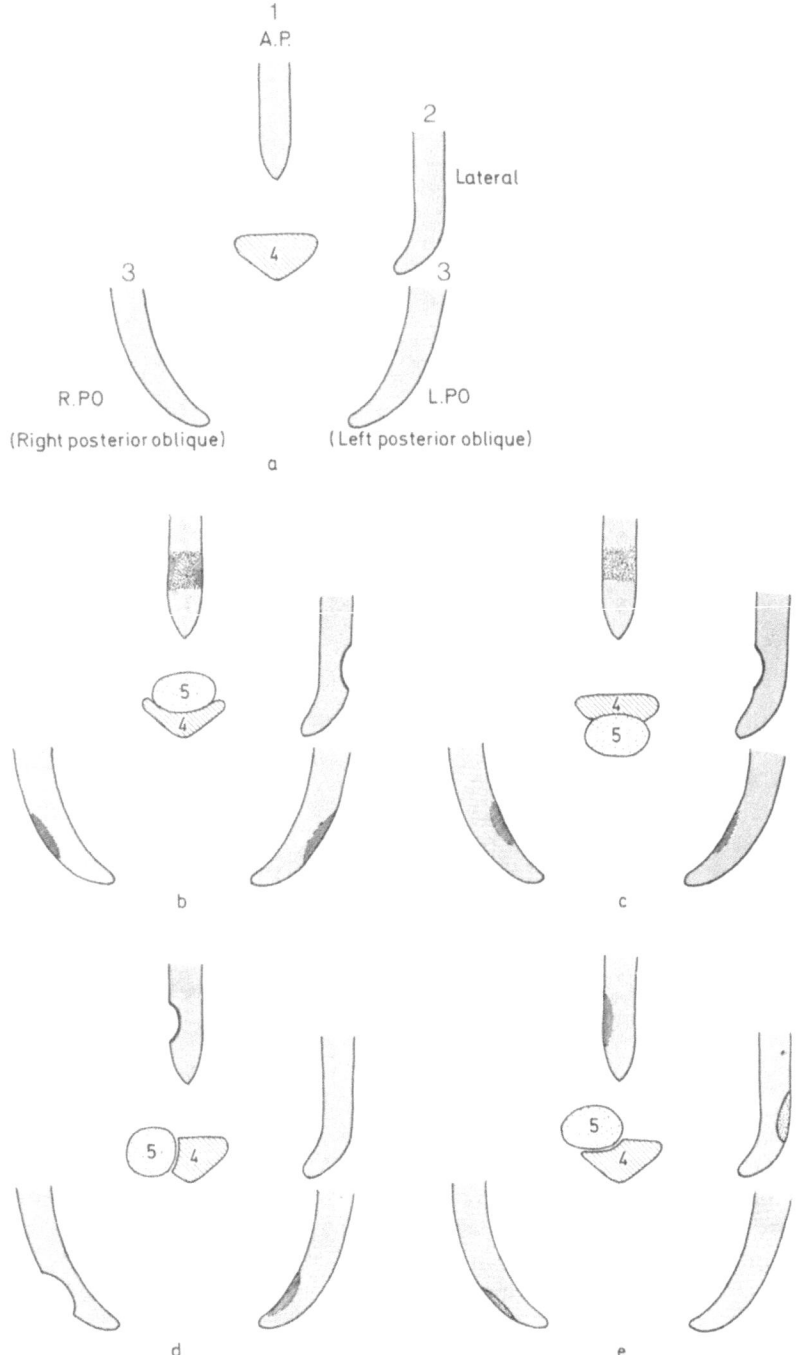

Fig. V, 2. **The Different Types of Compression of the Dural Sac as Seen Schematically on Routine Projections.** (a) Absence of compression. (b) Anterior compression. (c) Posterior compression. (d) Lateral compression. (e) Unilateral anterior compression. (f) Anterolateral compression. (g) Posterolateral compression. (h) Unilateral bipolar compression. (i) Crossed bipolar compression. *1* frontal projection, *2* lateral, *3*, right and left posterior oblique projections. *4* dural sac, *5* compressive agent.

A voluminous median discal herniation (b) is responsible for a symmetrical blurring of the lateral margins and a clear-cut indentation, without double contour, of the anterior margin also seen on the oblique projections.

A median bony tumor of the posterior arch (c) produces an especially clear indentation of

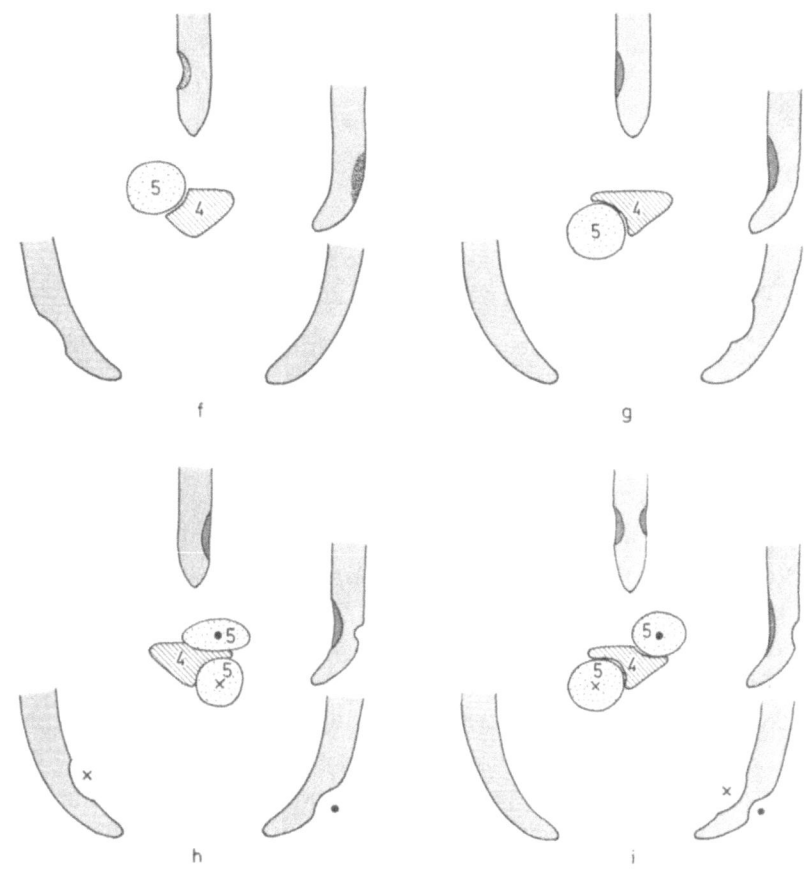

Fig. V,2 (cont.)

the posterior margin, also seen on the oblique projections.

A lateral disc herniation (d) is especially seen as an indentation of the corresponding lateral margin. On oblique projections, it is visualized as an indentation of the anterior margin on the corresponding projection and of the posterior margin on the opposite oblique projection. Such a herniation may not be visible on lateral projections.

A paramedian herniation (e) produces an anterior indentation with double contour. On the other x-ray projections the radiologic signs are minor ones and the diagnosis will be based on the radicular signs.

The usual anterolateral herniation (f) produces an indentation which is similar on the frontal, lateral, and homolateral posterior oblique projections.

An hypertrophic facetal joint (g) produces an indentation on the frontal projection comparable to that of a herniation but it traduces itself moreover by a posterior indentation on the lateral and contralateral oblique projections.

The coexistence on the same side of a backward compression of discal origin and a forward compression of articular origin (h) is mainly seen as a stenosis on the lateral projection and produces dissociated features on the oblique projections.

When this pathologic association is crossed (i), it produces a stenosis of the dural sac on one of the posterior oblique projections

49

houette, the analysis of the margins of this silhouette, and finally of the opaque area within it.

B. The Outline of the Entire Thecal Sac

1. Normal Features

The silhouette of the dural sac varies greatly. The contrast medium becomes diluted in a tubular space situated in the center of the spinal canal. This space is straight on AP views and takes the shape of the lumbar lordosis on lateral views. Its length is measurable only on the lateral views, because of the geometric deformation of the cul-de-sac on frontal projections. It usually ends at the level of S1–2. A large amount of variations are encountered from the L5–S1 space to the lower sacral segments. The bottom of the dural sac progressively tapers out or ends in a glove-finger-like way (Fig. V,3).

Its volume is variable, though not really dependent on the canalar dimensions; there too, a large variations range is seen. Narrow sacs are usually also short sacs, and contrariwise, wide sacs are also the longest. A marked increase of the saccular volume is required to speak about megacauda; this clinical entity means pathologic increase of the volume and may include clinical signs. Conversely, the pathogenic character of too narrow sacs has, to our knowledge, only rarely been reported.

2. Pathologic Features

We will first describe the anomalies in size and shape of the silhouette, next the deformations of the dural sac, and finally the obstructions to the flow of contrast medium.

a) Anomalies of Size; the Megacauda

Up to a certain extent, plain x-rays allow us to predict the existence of a megacauda even before RSG is performed. Attention may be drawn to an abnormal concavity of the posterior aspect of the sacrum. The content of the megacauda is so important that the amount of dye usually injected fails to give a satisfactory opacification whether it is limited to the inferior segment or diffuse but of poor opacity.

The megacauda occupies the largest part of the canalar volume and may show anterior concavities at the level of each disc, its anterior aspect being in contact with the posterior aspect of the discs [13] (Fig. V,4). The emerging radicular sheaths are poorly opacified, their course is short and almost horizontal. The poor intrasaccular opacification, due to an excess of dilution of the contrast medium, and the lack of injection of the sheaths, impedes the diagnosis of discal hernia [17].

b) Anomalies of Shape

Some anomalies in the general morphology of the dural sac may be described separately.

The Molded Dural Sac in a Narrow Canal [5]. In cases with canalar stenosis, the dural sac is cramped into a limited space by the surrounding bony structures in which it is closely embedded. Then, the anterior margin becomes waved by the alternation of concavities at the level of the discs and convexities posterior to the vertebral bodies. The posterior margin of the dural sac shows indentations due to the constrictions of the posterior arches. The indentations of the lateral margins, particularly those due to hypertrophic posterior facetal joints, are visible as stenoses in frontal views. As a matter of fact, the peculiar technical difficulties of the investigation of the narrow canals are responsible for the fact that fron-

50

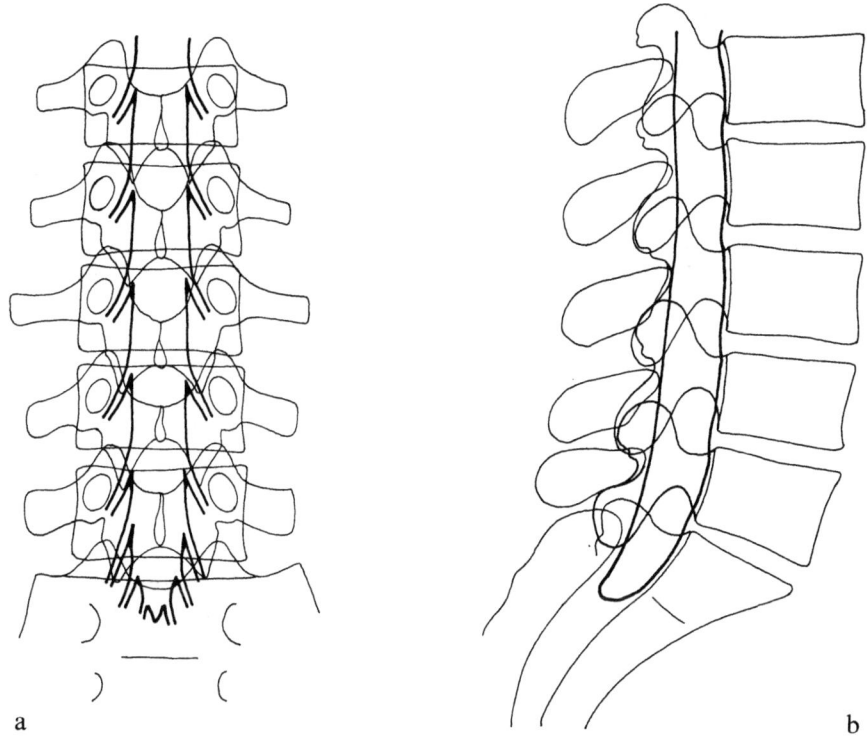

a   b

Fig. V,3. **Schematic Drawing of the Dural Sac Under Normal Conditions as Seen in RSG.** (a) Frontal projection. (b) Lateral projections.

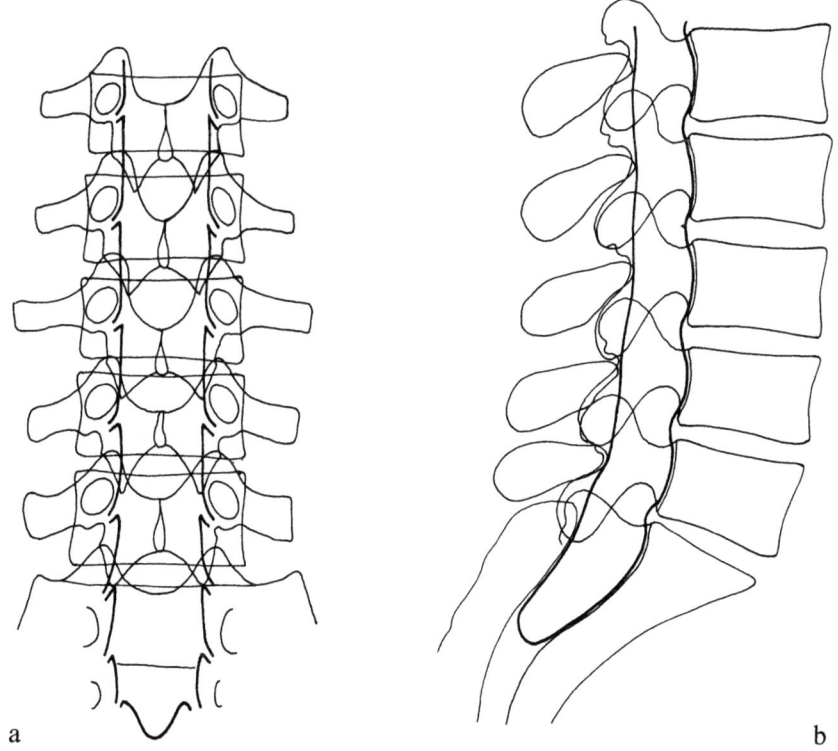

a   b

Fig. V,4. **Schematic Drawing of the Megacauda.** (a) Frontal projections. (b) Lateral projections

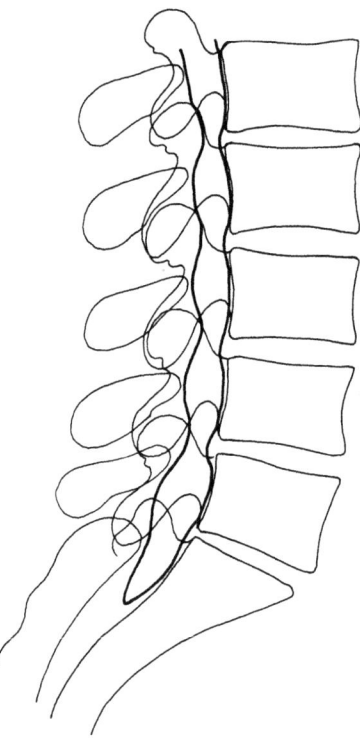

Fig. V,5. **Schematic Drawing of the Dural Sac Molded into a Narrow Canal on a Lateral View**

tal views are less informative than lateral (Fig. V,5).

Localized Stenoses of the Dural Sac. When there is a localized stenosis of the dural sac, this may be of different types depending on the etiology.

The *transverse stenoses,* more or less symmetric, may be consistent with several entities, i.e., discal hernia, bony hypertrophies, and extradural deposit of scar tissue (Fig. V,6). Stenoses due to discal hernia are not compulsorily correlated to a bilateral hernia but may simply be due to a voluminous hernia compressing the sac against the opposite aspect of the canal. The most characteristic stenoses of bony origin are due to the presence of bilateral hypertrophy of the facetal joints which are, moreover, abnormally close to the midline [6]. Stenoses of epidural origin are usually

related to an excess of scar tissue in patients operated upon for discal herniations; this kind of stenosis has irregular margins (Fig. V,8). For the radiologic analysis of transverse dural stenoses, frontal tomograms are useful for visualizing the saccular margins in the stenotic area and their distance to the bony canal.

Anteroposterior stenoses result from the coexistence at a same intervertebral level of a disco-osteophytic protrusion or a true discal hernia with a stenosing hypoplasia or a compressing hypertrophy of the posterior arch.

Concentric stenoses are characterized by the fact that they are visible as hourglass images [21] on orthogonal projections.

c) Desaxations of the Dural Sac
The most common desaxations of the dural sac are only visible on one of the projections of the RSG (Fig. V,7). On the frontal view, such a desaxation intervenes when a voluminous hernia pushes the dural sac against the opposite side of the canal. On the lateral views, the desaxations generally seen are those due to spondylolisthesis. Complex desaxations may result from major bone anomalies of the lumbar spine, viz., scoliosis [12] of degenerative or traumatic origin, neurogenous osteoarthropathies.

d) Peculiar Anomalies of the Cul-de-Sac
Under normal conditions, the culs-de-sac have a variable shape, rather tapered in short sacs and rounded for large ones, but their silhouette is usually regular and symmetric.

Meningeal diverticula may hang at the bottom of the dural sac. When there is only one diverticulum which is median and has irregular margins, it is rather to be related to an arachnoiditis or congenital diverticulum of the dural sac. When the diverticula

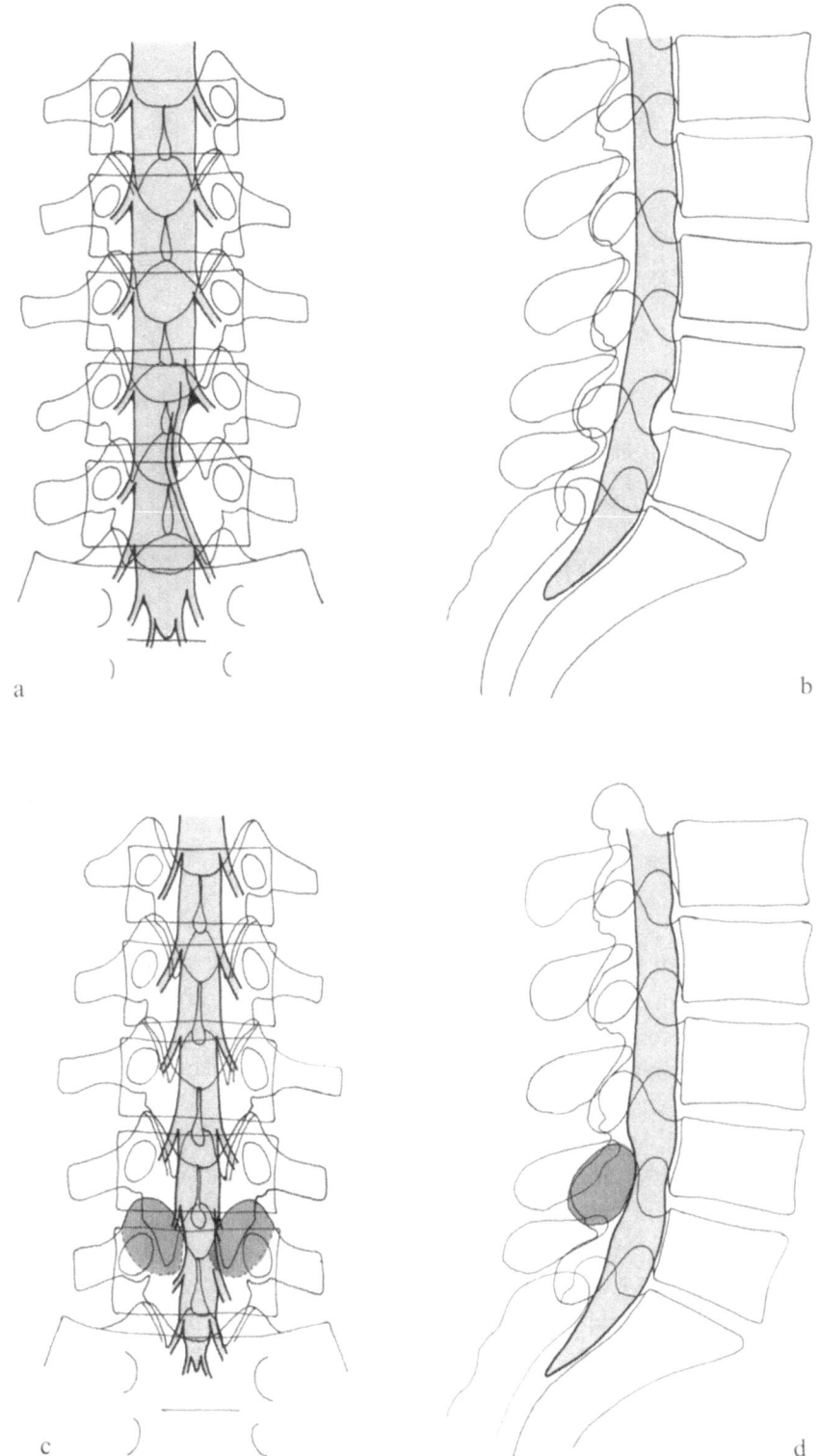

a

b

c

d

Fig. V,6. **Stenoses of the Dural Sac.** (a, b) By herniation of the disc. (c, d) By bilaterally hypertrophied facetal joints. These two pathologic conditions are distinguishable on lateral views by the location of indentation, i.e., anterior in case of herniation, and posterior in case of bony compression

53

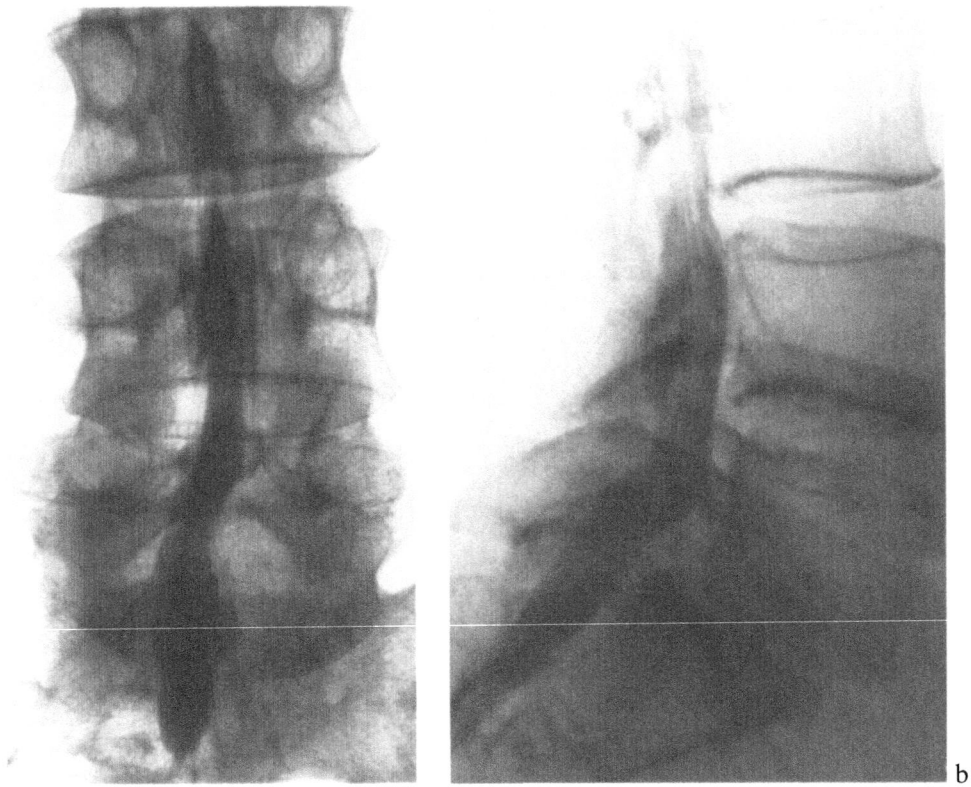

Fig. V,7. **Desaxations of the Dural Sac.** (a) Lateral desaxation due to a voluminous herniation pushing the dural sac towards the opposite internal aspect of the canal. (b) Sagittal desaxation due to mild spondylolisthesis

are paramedian and rather symmetric, it is a matter of variety of dilatation of the sacral nerve root sheaths. These pseudocystic structures are better opacified the later the films are carried out, and they may be embedded in concavities of the posterior aspect of the sacrum.

The distal part of the cul-de-sac may show other major deformities atypical in shape, related with arachnoiditis, and may be associated with pachymeningitis of the dura. These deformations are characterized by the lack of opacification of one or several radicular sheaths which normally are expected to emerge in the concerned region [1, 25], by irregularities in the saccular contour, and by an abnormally dense and homogenous contrast pattern of the sac in the same region. In these cases, the bottom of the dural sac may be either stenosed (Fig. V,8) in an irregular or dilated in an unshapely way.

e) Complete Block of the Contrast Medium

During the intrathecal injection, a complete stop may be disclosed on the fluoroscopic screen. It is usually transient, and on later x-ray films, the passage toward the bottom of the cul-de-sac occurs. When the stop persists, the analysis of its characteristics provides some arguments for its etiological diagnosis [9] (Fig. V,9).

Regular Stops. *Cupula-formed stops* with regular margins at once evoke an intradural rounded tumor, most often a neurinoma, more rarely an ependymoma or another

54

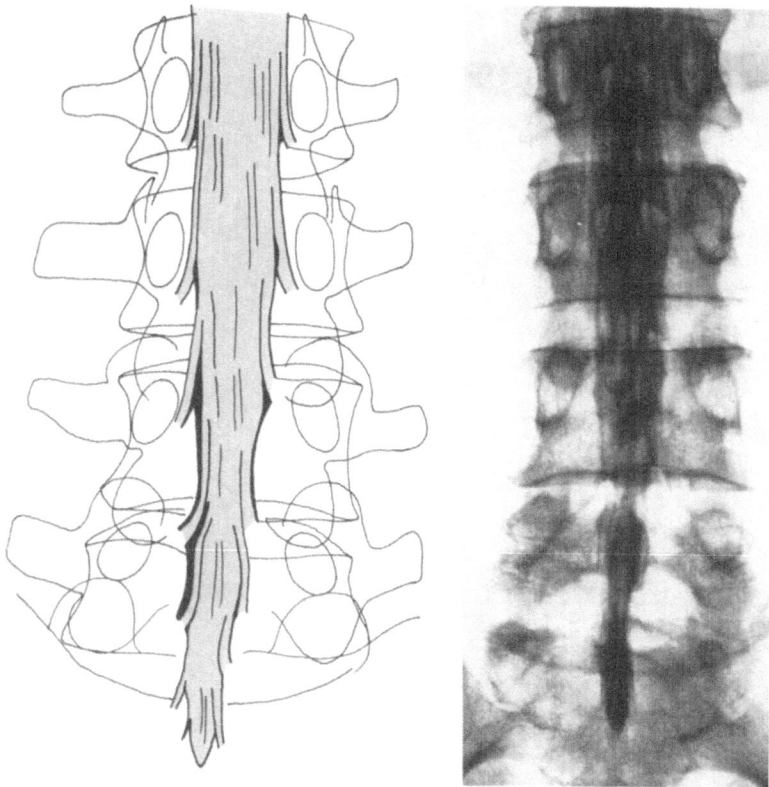

Fig. V,8. **Deformation of the Cul-de-sac by Arachnoiditis.** Below the L3–4 interspace, there is an irregular and symmetric stenosis predominant at the bottom of the cul-de-sac. The radicular sheaths are poorly visualized in the area concerned

type of tumor of the filum terminale. The cupula-like image of these stops is seen on different projections and may be outlined by a fine, linear enhancement of the contrast [9]. The inferior pole of the tumor may be visualized on later x-rays if the bottom of the sac becomes opacified [7].

Bevel-edged stops are due to dural or epidural compression which causes the collapse of the thecal sac just above the stop. These bevel-edged stops occur together with a detachment of the dural sac from one of the internal aspects of the spinal canal. This important radiologic sign permits the localization of the direction of the mass pressure [24].

Exceptionally, one may see a *regular horizontal stop* on a frontal projection, as if cut with a knife, related to a shearing movement of the spine and a consecutive desaxation of the column of contrast at the level of a spondylolisthesis with intact neural arch [19, 22].

Horizontal uneven stops have the same diagnostic value as the cupula-formed stops.

Irregular Stops. Stops of hernial origin are situated at the level of a disc on frontal as well as on lateral projections centrated on the disc. These stops have a dentated margin [15, 20] due to the alteration of radicular translucencies and opacity of the surrounding contrast medium. When there is a detachment of the dural sac or a localized accumulation of the contrast medium just

55

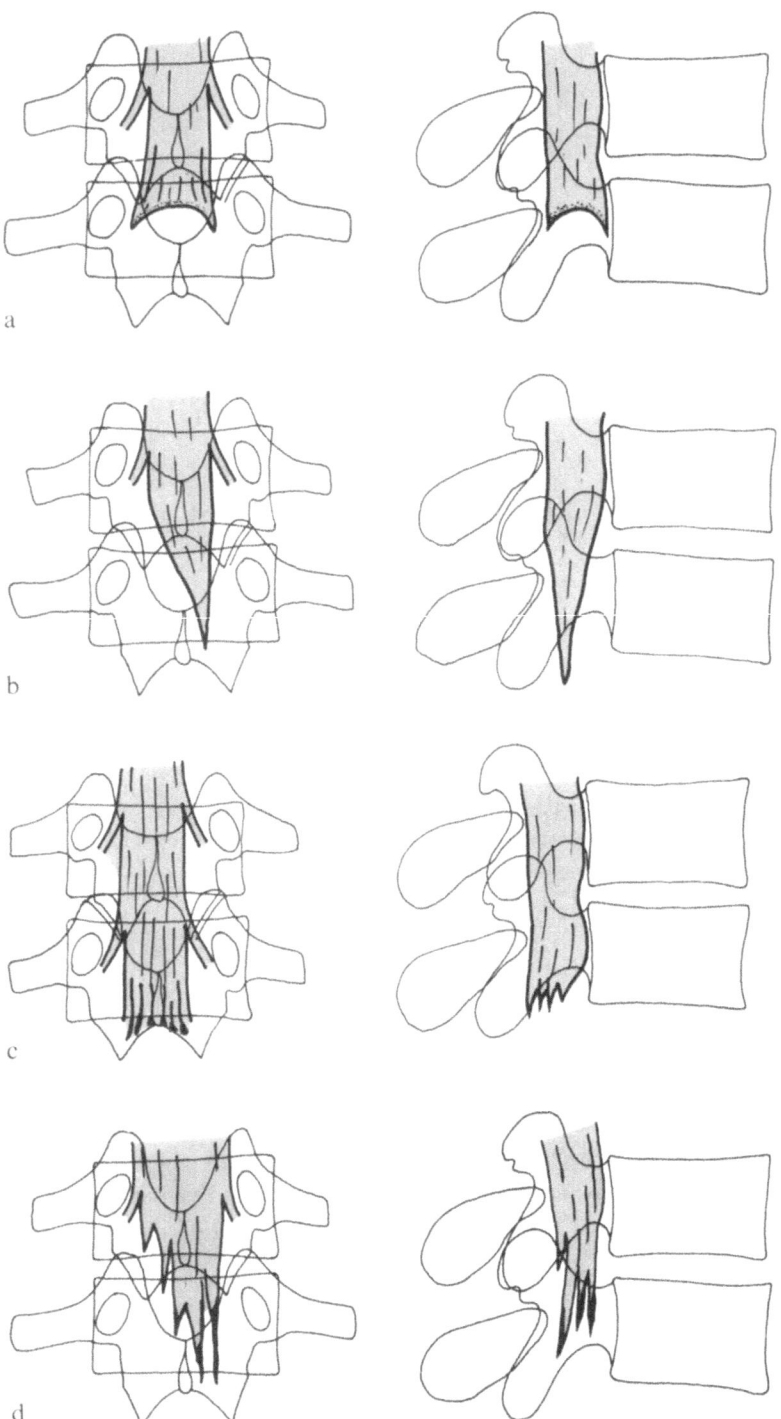

Fig. V,9. **Schematic Drawing of the Different Types of Stop of the Flow of Contrast Medium.** (a) Cupula-like stop. (b) Bevel-edged stop. (c) Fringed stop. (d) Irregular stop. A rounded intradural tumor and particularly a neurinoma is seen as a cupula-like stop on all projections (a). An extradural mass or deposit causes a detachment of the dural sac from the internal wall of the canal situated above the stop (b). Pseudotumoral types of discal herniations are responsible for a fringed horizontal stop situated at the level of the disc (c). The stop due to arachnoiditis is not characteristic but is usually more irregular (d)

above a stop of this kind, this shows the side of the hernia.

More irregular, fringed stops, without relation to intervertebral spaces, are caused by arachnoiditis within the dural sac.

f) Segmental Lack of Opacification

It corresponds to a lower opacity of the contrast column on a more or less short distance [11], either at the level of a very strong compression of the dural sac (narrow canal, voluminous hernia, extradural deposit) or at the level of a poor diffusion of the contrast medium in the meshes of a proliferating arachnoid.

C. The Margins of the Sac

1. Normal Features

We call *margins* of the sac the contours of its image on the different radiculosaccographic projections. In fact, the saccular silhouette has anterior and posterior margins on lateral and oblique projections and lateral margins on frontal projections.

In so far as some sacs have a triangular section surface with an anterior base, the anterior margin corresponds to the tangential projection of its anterior aspect. The posterior margin of the saccular silhouette on oblique projections represents the projection of the posterolateral wall of the thecal sac and is more or less clear-cut, depending on whether the central beam is more or less tangent to this surface.

The margins of the sac are normally smooth, save for the lateral margins which are dentated by the periradicular pouches of the dura mater. The anterior margin of the lateral projection of the dural sac may be slightly indented at the level of normal discs, particularly in lordotic patients or in cases where the sac occupies the largest part of the spinal canal. The posterior margin is always smooth but may be poorly defined because of the superimposition of the bony structures of the posterior arches.

2. Pathologic Features

a) Convexities and Concavities

The margins of the dural sac, as we defined them, may show the following elementary deformations, viz., convexities, concavities, irregularities, and finally blurring. We shall describe them in an analytic way, margin by margin, but it should be understood that an anomaly of the dural sac is preferentially visualized on one incidence but also visible on the others (see above).

Deformations of the Anterior Margin (Fig. V,10). These may be either convex when lying in the posterior concavity of the vertebral bodies or concave when situated behind or in the neighborhood of the intervertebral spaces.

The *convexities* are usually related to the fact that the dural sac occupies the greater part of the spinal canal, whether it is cramped into a small canal or whether it is a megacauda within a normal canal. Then the dural sac occupies the space within the concavities of the vertebrae, which are sometimes important enough to display scalloping of the posterior wall of the vertebral bodies.

The *concavities* are the imprints of discal origin, and may correspond to two pathologic entities:

Multiple and similar concavities may be due to a cramped dural sac which is molded against the normal discs. In these cases, it is only the prominence of one of them which permits determination of disc herniation.

A unique anterior concavity is consistent with herniation of the disc and may be situated strictly at the level of the disc or prolonged upward or downward (according

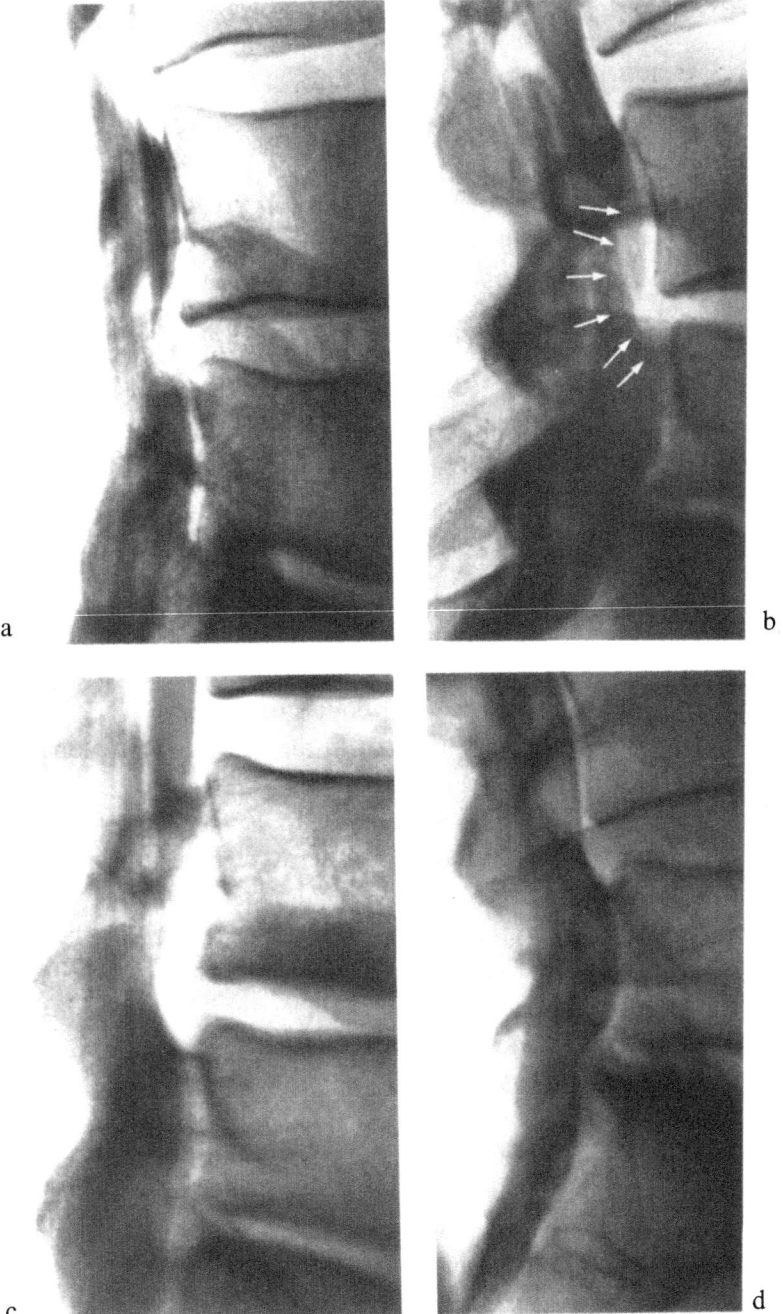

a

b

c

d

Fig. V,10. **Examples of Anterior Indentations of the Dural Sac of Hernial Origin.** (a, b, c) L4–5 herniations. (d, e, f) L5–S1 herniations. (a) Rounded moderate indentation with double contour at L4–5. The mild and regular imprint at the disc lying above may be considered a simple protrusion. (b) This indentation with double contour (*arrows*) accounts for the paramedian location of the hernia. (c) A L4–5 indentation prolonged by a retrovertebral detach-ment in L4 is in favor of the ascending character of a voluminous median herniation. (d) L5–S1 indentation at the level of an hypertrophic ver-tebral bar. (e) Ascending indentation with dou-ble contour due to paramedian L5–S1 hernia-tion which is retrovertebral in L4. (f) Indenta-tion of a descending L5–S1 herniation; the step formation of the anterior margin of the cul-de-sac distinguishes the descending migration from a normal retrosacral detachment of the sac

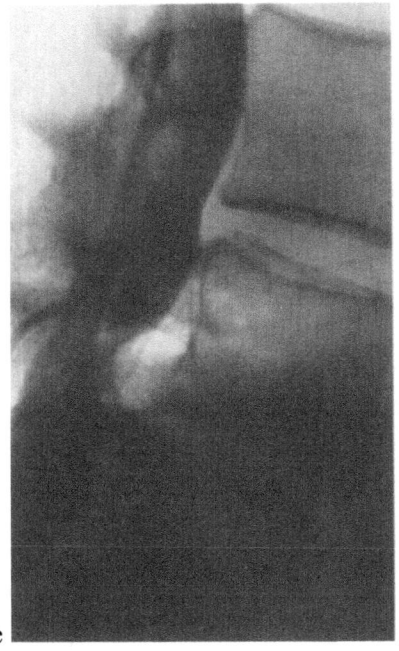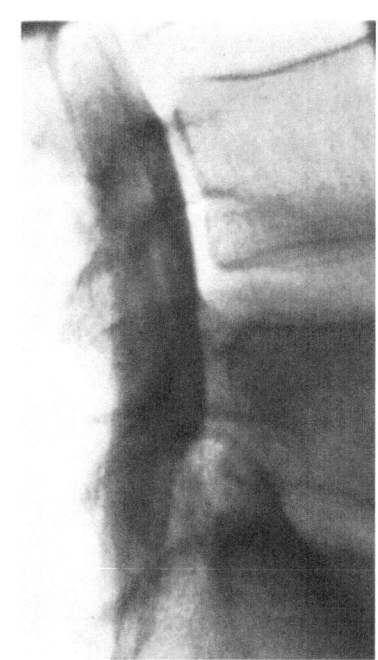

Fig. V,10 (cont.)   e   f

to the direction of the migrating hernia). The existence of a double contour, attributed to the anterolateral situation of the compression, supports the diagnosis of herniation.

Deformations of the Posterior Margin. Posterior *convexities* of the dural sac are only encountered after laminectomies. They correspond to a bulging of the dura at the site of the scar [22, 26]. These scarring features may conversely be seen as irregular defects of the posterior margin and are best visible on oblique projections [8].

The *concavities* have either a bony or a discal origin; an imprint of the posterior margin of the dural sac in oblique projections is to be attributed to one of the osteo-ligamentous structures of the posterior arch [6] (facetal joints, laminae, yellow ligaments) (Fig. V,11). We have to keep in mind the features of the radiologic projections of the bony elements composing the posterior arch in order to establish arguments for the etiological diagnosis. For example, a concavity of the posterior mar-

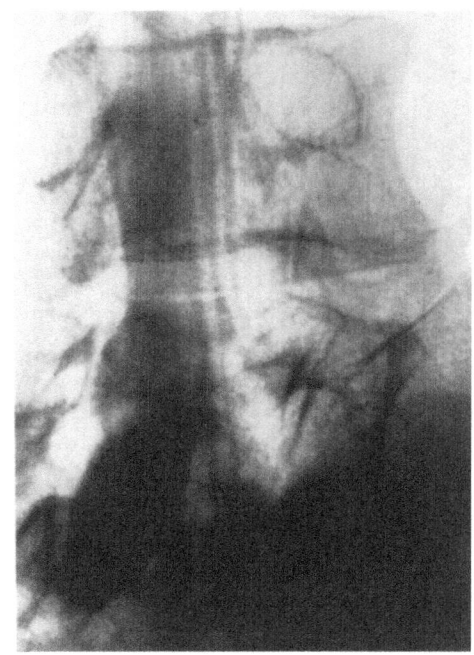

Fig. V,11. **Posterolateral Indentations Due to Yellow Ligaments.** Posterior oblique projection. The location of the posterior indentation between the bony opacities of the lamellae indicates the ligamentous origin of the compression

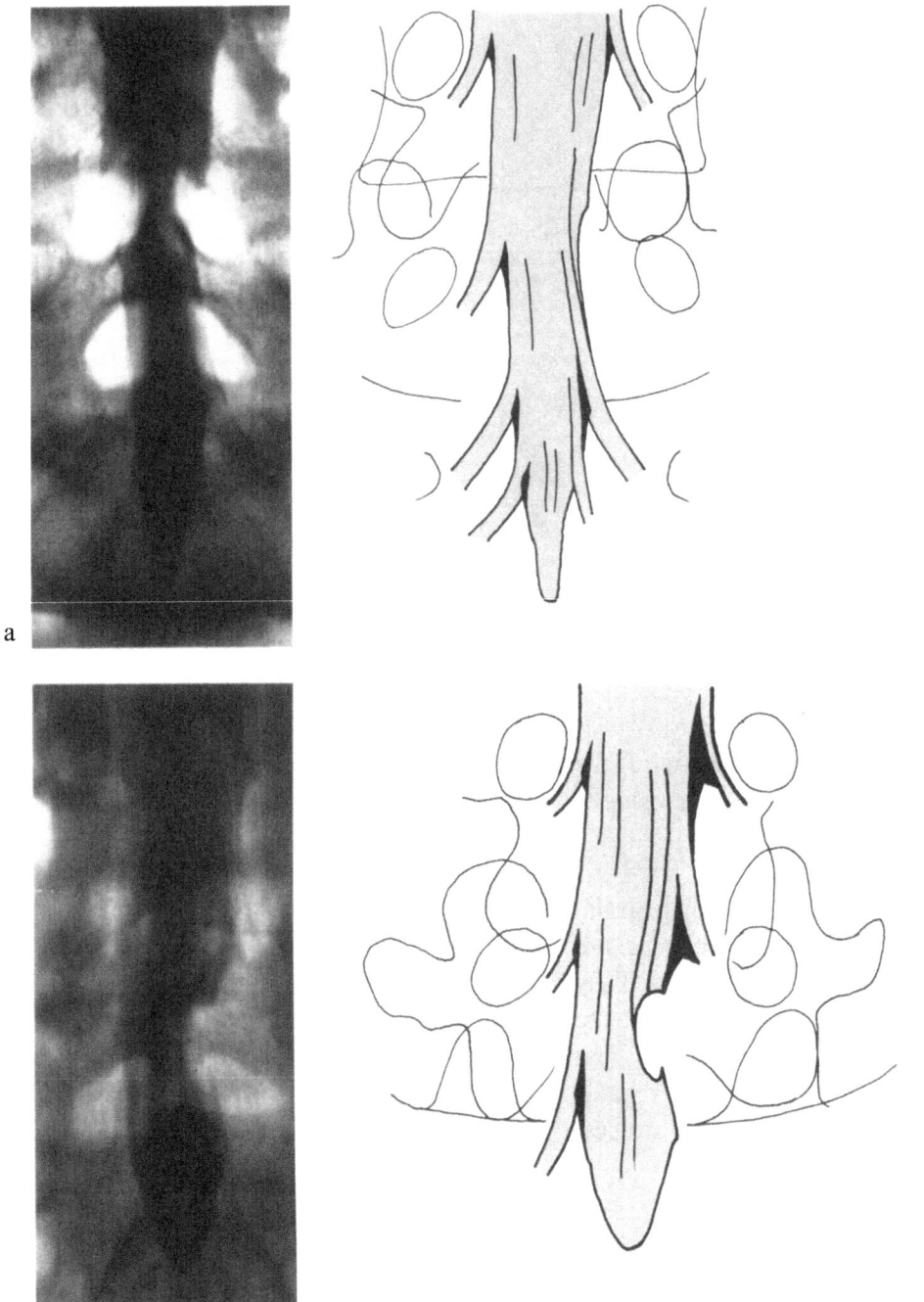

a

b

Fig. V, 12. Legend see opposite page

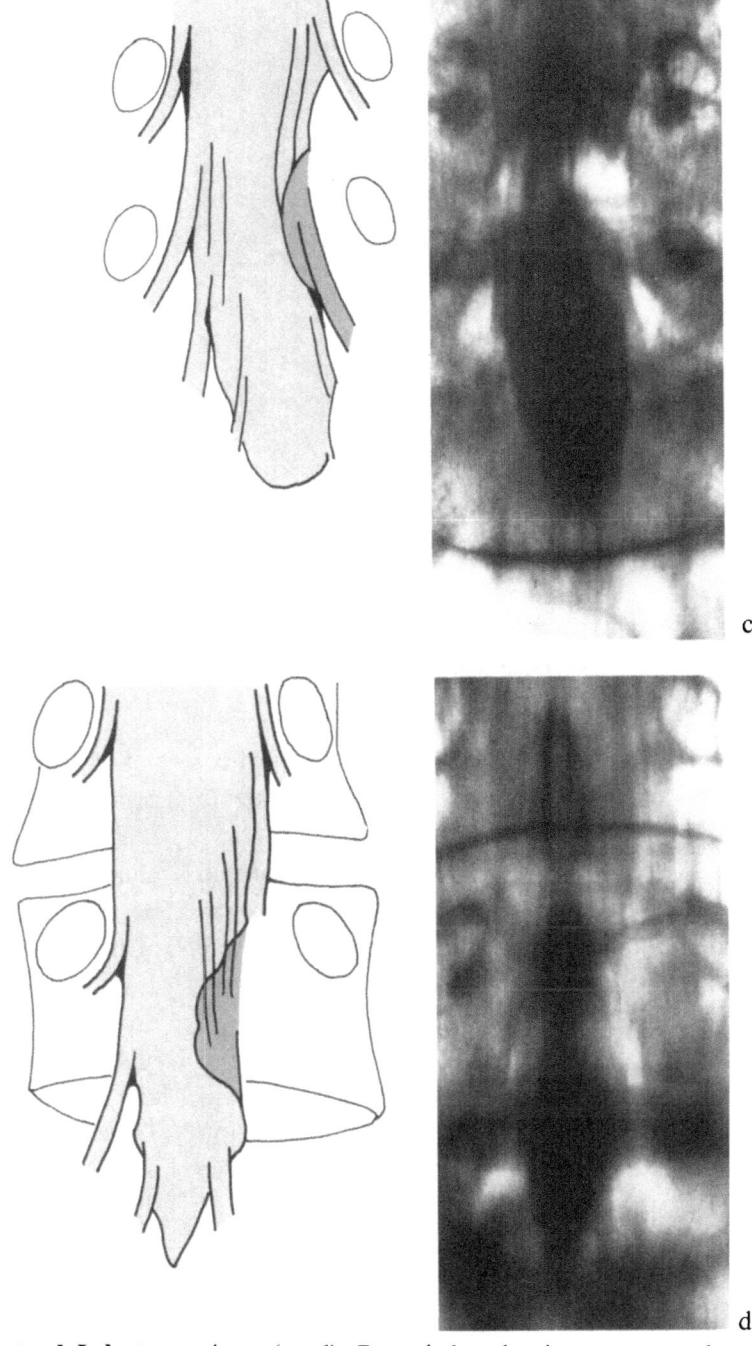

c

d

Fig. V,12. **Different Types of Lateral Indentations in Frontal Zonography.** (a) Flat indentation due to a subligamentous herniation. (b) Characteristic indentation due to a knob-like hernia-tion. (c, d) Rounded voluminous encroachments of regular (c) and irregular type (d). The more irregular is the more evocative of free herniation

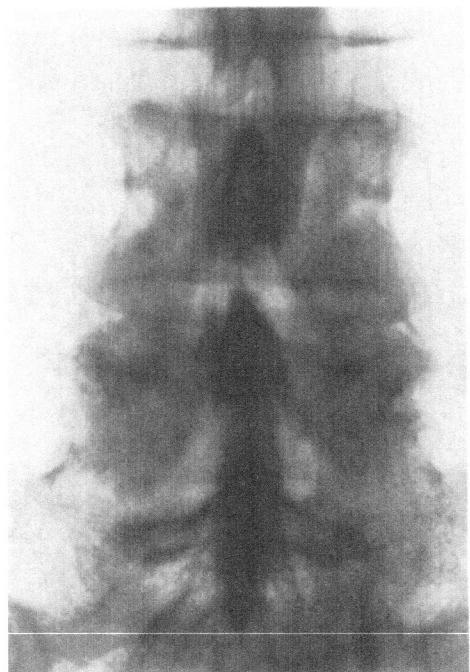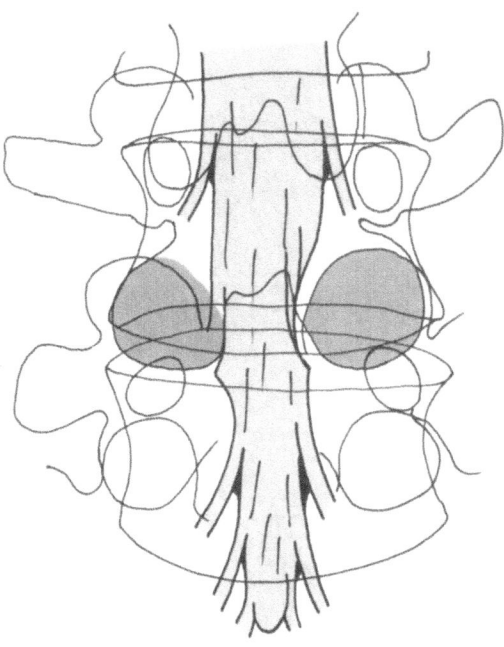

Fig. V,13. **Elongated Indentation at the Level of a Hypertrophic Facetal Joint on a Frontal Projection**

gin of the sac situated between the projection of two laminae is very likely due to the protrusion of the yellow ligament.

A concavity of the posterolateral margin of the sac, thus visible on oblique projections, may be due to a herniation in some cases with horizontal and backward migration of free herniae [18] (see Chap. 6).

Concavities of the Lateral Margins. The anterolateral imprint of a discal herniation is maximal on the corresponding oblique projection, but its features are best analyzed on a conventional frontal projection and especially on tomograms centered on the disc concerned.

Indeed, from the elementary morphology, one may draw indications as to the anatomical type of hernia [2, 3, 4, 18] (Fig. V,12):

Elongated imprint due to *subligamentous herniae,*

Irregular concavity of the margin very likely due to a *free herniation,*

Small indentation in addition to the imprint in case of *knob-like hernia,*

Rounded concavities with smooth margins, consistent with large herniations, do not allow us to predict the anatomical type of hernia.

Lateral imprints of nonhernial origin are rarer. Plain films of the spine, or the study of the bone structures on the RSG, should allow the ready diagnosis of their etiology. These lateral imprints may have a more or less regular shape, only rarely involve the saccular margin, and often be multiple, thus producing an image of stenosis when they are facing each other (Fig. V,13).

b) Irregularities

Irregularities in the margins of the sac preferably involve the bottom, (postmyelographic or postoperative arachnoiditis), and preferably lie on the posterolateral aspect of the dural sac (extradural deposit of scar tissue).

62

c) Blurring of the Saccular Margins

When the saccular opacity is strongly shaded-off toward the periphery, its margins may be blurred on the x-rays for physical reasons, viz., the contrast of the dural sac is then similar to that of the adjoining structures, so that the difference in the absorption of the x-rays is insufficient. Thus, the lateral margins of the dural sac may be blurred in a stenotic area of the canal (see Chap. 9) (Fig. V,14); the use of tomography partially overcomes this difficulty.

D. The Content of the Sac

1. Normal Features

The intrasaccular segments of the roots are barely visible as linear translucencies which are difficult to identify as belonging to a precise root. They are mainly visible on frontal and oblique projections, just above their emergence. They are usually entirely invisible on lateral projections.

The periradicular spaces, in which the contrast diffuses homogeneously, frequently have a stronger shade in the lower part of the cul-de-sac, they are also more opaque at the site of the root emergences, where the root pouches are beginning as infra- und supraradicular fossae. The region of the infraradicular fossa, also called axillary area, is constantly triangular, strongly shaded, and has a symmetric morphology from right to left at a given level.

2. Pathologic Features

a) Abnormal Translucenies

Anomalies of the roots inside the sac are either linear lucencies resembling the roots or rounded or elongated, poorly shaded lacunar areas, rather evoking tumoral masses. Abnormal translucencies of radicular origin may be of three types:

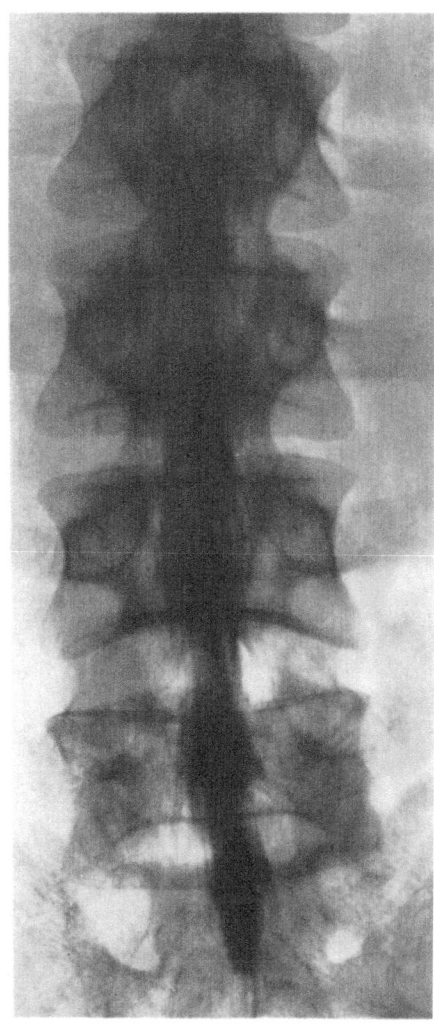

a

Fig. V,14. **Right L5–S1 Herniation in a Narrow Canal.** (a) Frontal projection, (b) Lateral projection. (c) Oblique projection. The dural sac takes in only a small quantity of contrast medium. Its lateral and posterior margins are blurred. This gives evidence of the narrowness of the canal, and is accompanied by a feeble distinctness of the saccular area and a poor injection of most of the radicular sheaths. The right L5–S1 herniation pushes the cul-de-sac toward the left and results in an anterolateral indentation on the dural sac, disrupting the S1 radicular sheath at the upper margin of the intervertebral space

63

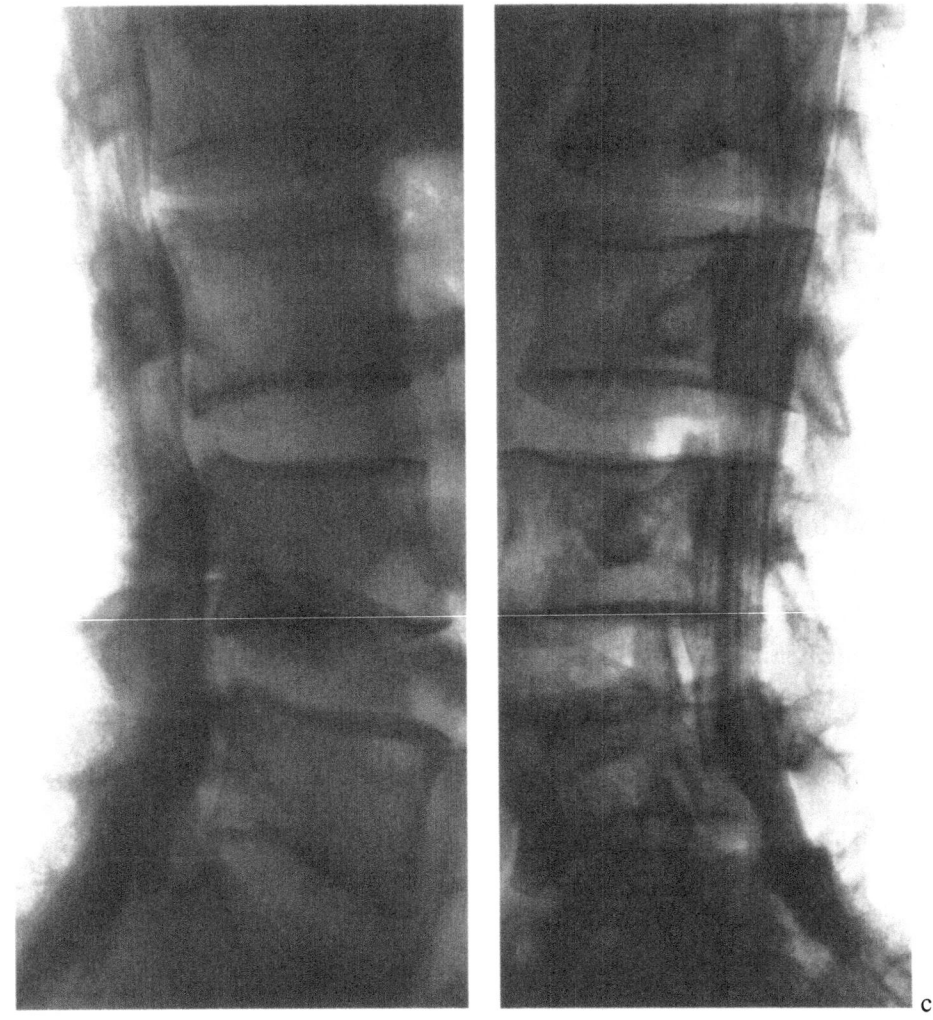

b

c

Fig. V,14 (cont.), Legend see page 63

Unique and rectilinear, adopting the normal course of a root. Thus, in case of disc herniation, the root concerned may be visualized on x-rays as an abnormal linear translucency terminating at the level of the compression of the dural sac [27]. It then becomes visible even in lateral views (Fig. V,15).

Multiple and deviated toward the opposite side of the canal in cases of discal herniation involving part of the cauda equina (curtain-loop sign) [11, 13] (Fig. V,17).

Multiple and sinuous, either in particularly lordotic patients without any pathology [10] or just above a stop in the flow of contrast medium in pathologic cases [14, 23, 26]. These radicular hyperlucencies are even more distinct in cases of lumbar canal stenosis, where they are sometimes gathered to form a unique centrocanalar hyperlucency, only visible on lateral projections and at the level of the stenosis [5] (Fig. V,16). If this phenomenon is very prominent, the clear area becomes homogeneous, the roots are no longer distinguishable within it, and there arises the problem of the differential diagnosis with centrocanalar, ribbon-like translucencies of other origins, such as medullar heterotopia or elongated tumors (neurinomas).

64

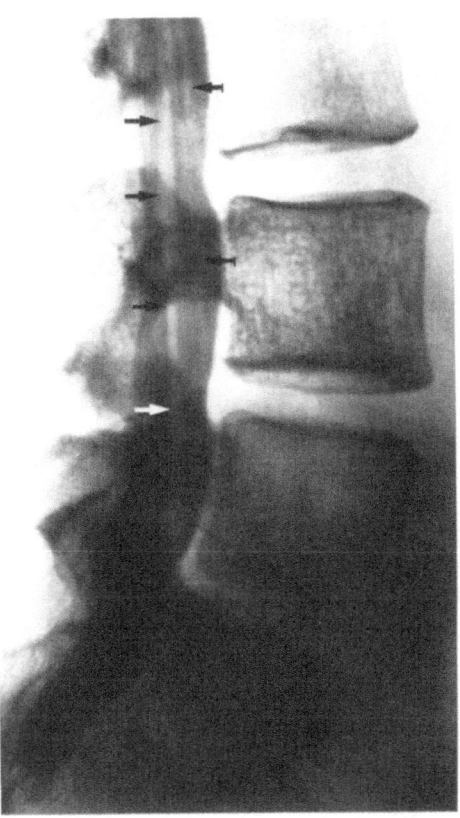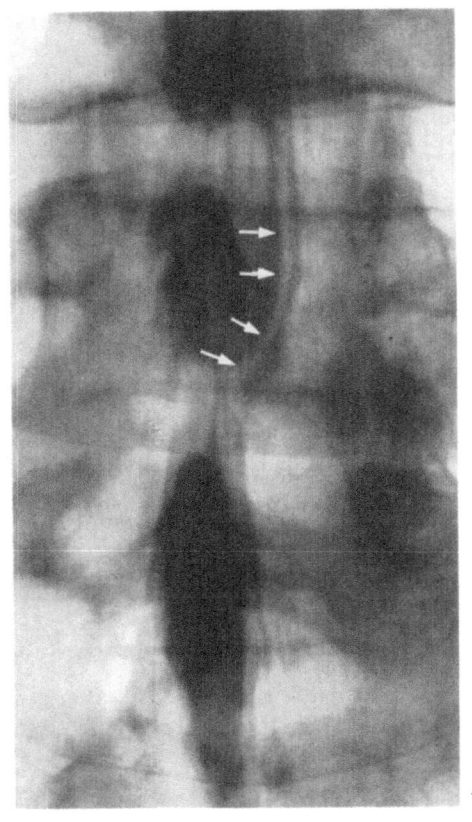

a   b

Fig. V,15. **Large Roots Visible Within the Dural Sac.** (a) Above an L5–S1 herniation (lateral view), the enlarged root (*arrows*) takes on the features of a rectilinear translucency which is directed toward its anterolateral emergence. One of the roots lying above has a normal caliber (*crossed arrows*). Note: the L4 vertebral body is angiomatous. (b) At the level of a left L4–5 herniation (frontal view), the intrasaccular segment of the L5 root (*arrows*) is hypertrophied, inwardly deviated, and sinuous

b) Anomalies of the Periradicular Spaces

The perturbations in the homogeneity of opacification of the periradicular spaces are variable; they may be interpreted as the indirect result of abnormal constraints exerting themselves through the dural sac and bringing about modifications in the topographic relations between the roots (widening of some interradicular spaces at the expense of the others) [5]. Besides, the movements of the spine—lateroflexion, flexion, or extension—may modify these pictures of abnormal distribution of the dye within the dural sac.

The adhesions between the roots due to excessively proliferating arachnoid may account for the occurrence of a unique, ensheating space around the bundle of the roots.

Three main types of abnormal distribution of the contrast medium may be described:

The increased space between two roots at the level of their emergence is seen as an opaque, triangular area which may be considered as the extension of the normal image of the axillary pouch.

The accumulation of contrast in the posterior scalloping of the vertebral bodies is responsible for a *crescentshaped* opacity.

The diffuse pericaudal accumulation of contrast medium is seen on lateral projec-

65

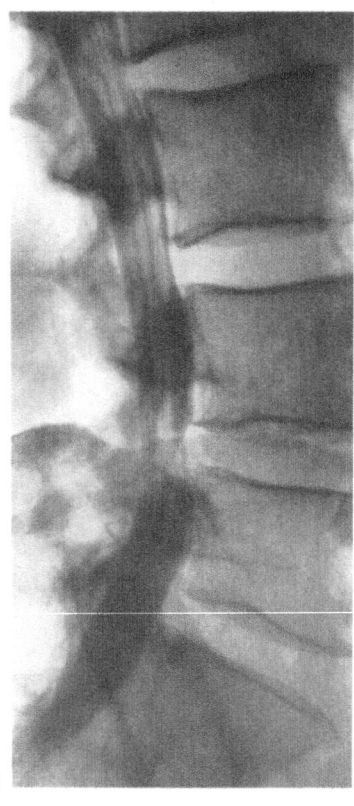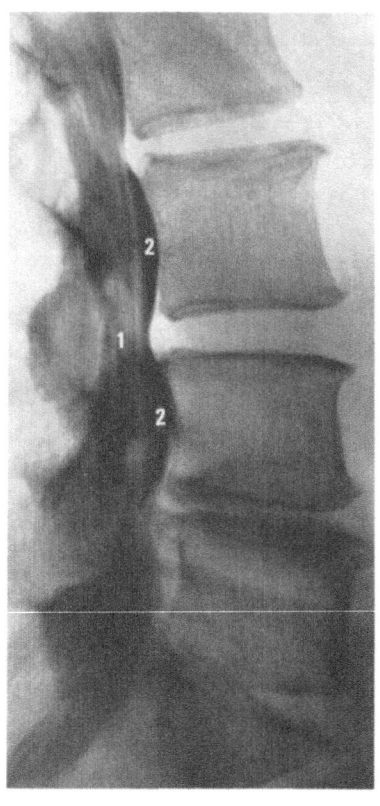

a b

Fig. V,16. **Signs of Intrasaccular Constraint in Cases of Narrow Canals.** (a) Mild signs above a small L4–5 herniation. (b) More marked signs above a larger L4–5 herniation. *1* hypervisibility of the intrasaccular roots, *2* abnormal distribution of the intrasaccular contrast we call retrovertebral stasis

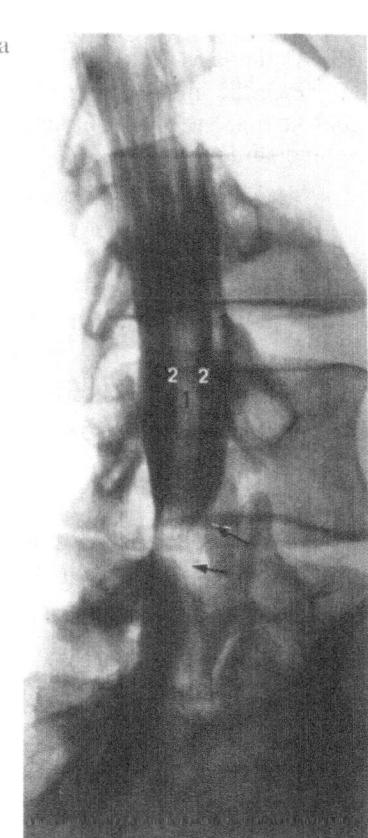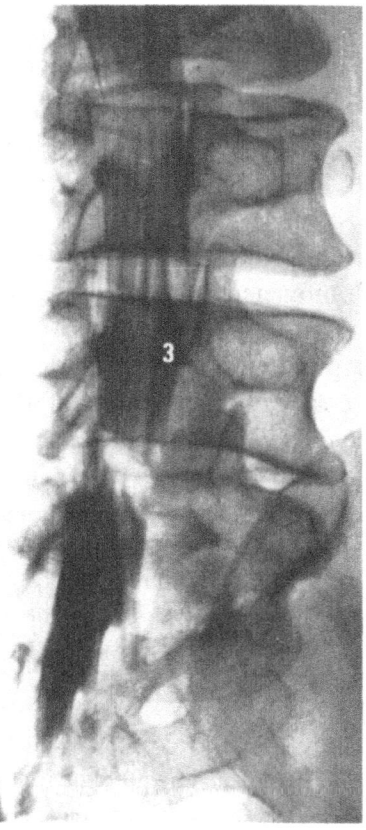

Fig. V,17. **Curtain-loop Sign and Bunching of the Roots.** (a) The bunching of the roots produces a centrosaccular translucency (*1*), surrounded by a dense opacity (*2*) due to accumulation of the contrast. The entire dural sac is stenosed and pushed back by the herniation (*arrow*). (b) In a case of milder compression of hernial origin, the abnormal distribution of the contrast medium is located only in the axillary pouch of the root lying above (*3*)

tions as a *double-track* opacity, best visible in the extension position (Fig. V,16).

II. The Perisaccular Area

It may be interesting to study separately the perisaccular space and the extrasaccular root segments passing through it.

A. The Perisaccular Area Proper

RSG allows us to delineate a space between the opacified silhouette of the dural sac and the structures which form the walls of the bony spinal canal (medial limit of the pedicular cortex on the frontal view, and accessorily on oblique views; posterior aspect of the vertebral bodies and lamellar-spinous junction on the lateral projections) (Fig. V,18).

This space includes the outer layer of the arachnoid, the virtual subdural space, the dura, and the structures constituting the extradural space, i.e., the veins, the roots in their sheaths, and the fatty tissue. It also contains the ligamentous structures inserted in the bony canal and ends with the periosteal lining.

1. Normal Features

Under normal conditions, the dural sac lies at the center of the spinal canal, its anterior aspect may be situated at a variable distance of the vertebral bodies (see Chap. 4). It is very difficult to appreciate the thickness of the perisaccular space posteriorly to the dural sac since the posterior margin of the thecal sac is ill-defined, whereas that of the canal is poorly visible.

2. Pathologic Features

As concerns the pathology, two types of situations may be encountered, i.e., the perisaccular space is either reduced or increased.

a) Reduced Perisaccular Space

Such a reduction is diffuse when the thecal sac is molded within the bony canal, whether this dural sac is of normal size in a narrow canal [5] or whether it is too large in a normal canal.

This reduced perithecal space may be localized in cases of compression of bony origin (dysplasiae and tumors) or when the compressed dural sac is pushed against the opposite canalar margin. The reduction of thickness on one side is then an indirect sign of the presence of a mass on the opposite side (see further in Sect. b). A retractile epidural scar may also be accompanied by a reduction of that space.

b) Increased Perisaccular Space

It is due to the presence of a mass, for instance a discal hernia, a tumoral or inflammatory deposit originating in one of the constituting elements of the extradural space or of its walls.

In case of spondylolisthesis (see Chap. 10), the anterior aspect of the dural sac lies far from the olisthetic vertebra. This detachment may prolong cephalad, whereas the dural sac is abnormally stretched on the posterosuperior angle of the underlying vertebral body or of the body of the sacrum.

B. The Extrasaccular Segments of the Roots, Their Sheaths, and Their Axillary Pouches

1. Normal Features

a) Frontal Projections

General Morphology. Normally the extrasaccular parts of the roots are better visualized the more caudad they are located down to S1 and the longer their course.

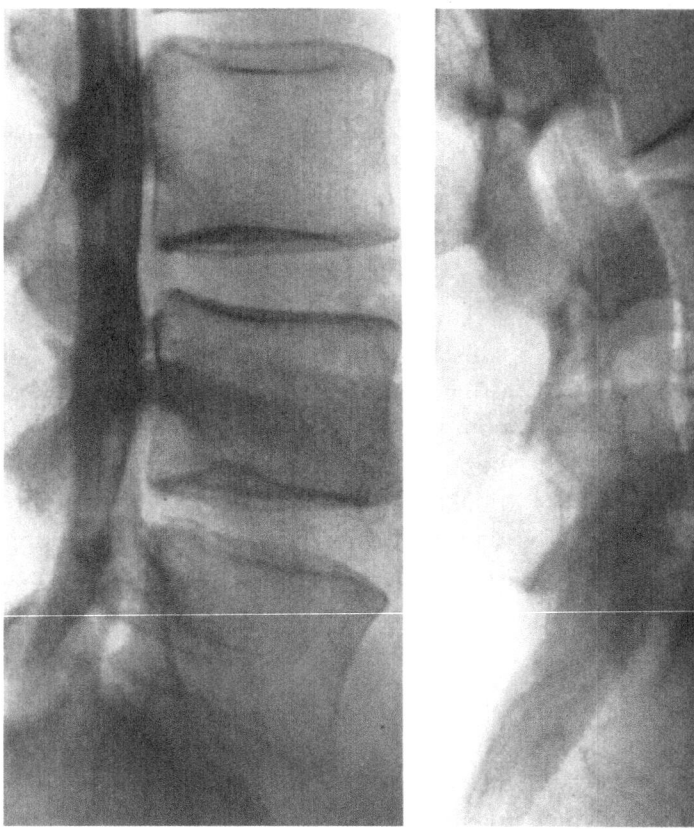

a   b

Fig. V,18. **Thickness of the Anterior Extradural Space.** Under normal conditions, the volume occupied by the dural sac is variable, i.e., a short and narrow sac lies distant from the posterior aspect of the vertebral bodies (a). Conversely, a large and long dural sac is in close contact with this posterior aspect down to the sacral canal (b)

They are seen as a linear radiolucency outlined by the double-track opacity of the cerebrospinal fluid within their sheath.

On frontal projections, the sheaths are directed caudally and somewhat laterally, thus being projected first medial to the corresponding pedicles, and then below them. The L5 and S1 sheaths are the best visible because of their longer course along the roots (see Chap. 4).

Detailed Morphology of the Radicular Emergences. The most common picture of a root is a unique radiolucency underlined by a thin layer of contrast medium on each side. The triangular axillary pouch fuses imperceptibly with the radicular sheath laterally and with the supraradicular fossa of the underlying root caudally. The medial limit of the triangle is given by the intrasaccular radiolucency of the underlying root (see variations in Chap. 4).

b) Oblique Projections

This type of projection has the main advantage of best visualizing the areas of the root emergences and their course. The projections carried out with the patient at an angle between 20 and 30 degrees are the most informative for the root pouches.

c) Lateral Projections

The intrasaccular segments of the roots are completely invisible on lateral projections under normal conditions.

68

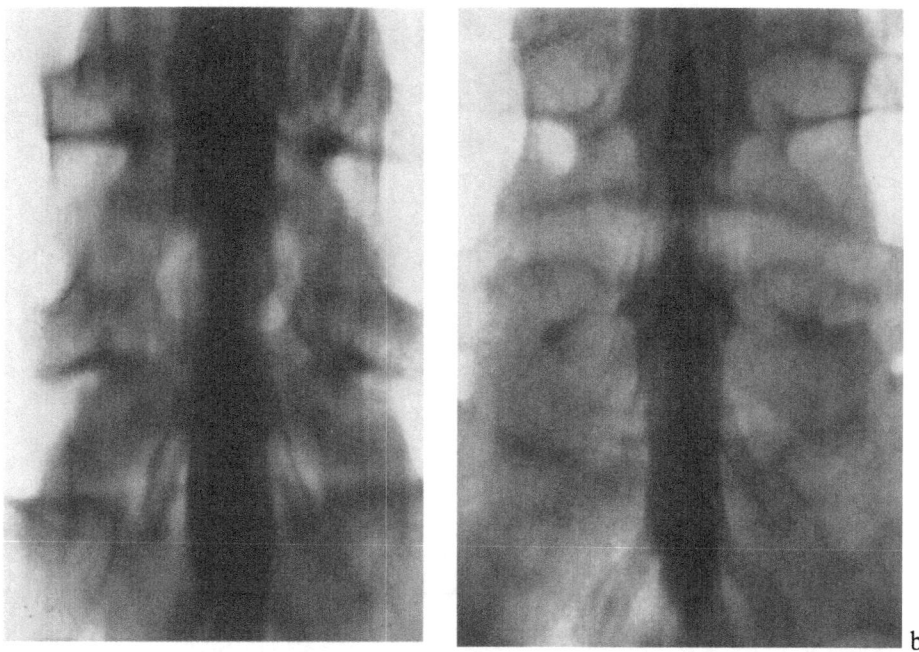

Fig. V,19. **The Radicular Sheath Fails to Opacify.** (a) L5 on the right. (b) S1 on the right. Isolated absence of opacification of a radicular sheath may be the only sign of an utmost lateral herniation

2. Pathologic Features

The roots are located in the neighborhood of the discs; they emerge from the antero-lateral aspect of the dural sac generally just above the intervertebral space and adopt a forward and downward direction that leads them to obliquely cross the posterior aspect of the discs. As a consequence, and besides the intrinsic pathology of the roots (radiculitis, neurinoma), only discal hernia-tions may cause anomalies restricted to one, or at the worst two, radicular sheaths (Fig. V,19). As a matter of fact, these extra-saccular radicular segments are either spared, or diffusely involved by nondiscal pathologic processes.

The first consequence of a hernial com-pression is the collapse of one of the periradicular or axillary subarachnoidal spaces. A further degree of compression causes a deviation of the radicular course, and this deviation cannot be analyzed since the cor-responding sheath fails to opacify. How-ever, indirect signs, and particularly defor-mations of the axillary pouches, are in favor of this deviation.

We shall successively see two types of anomalies of the extrasaccular segments and their sheaths, viz., first, anomalies in the opacification of the sheath and sec-ondly, signs of deviation of the root.

a) Anomalies in the Opacification of the Sheaths

On a given sheath the *filling defects* may be either localized or complete and may predominate on the axillary area or on the sheath itself, according to the site of the compression. Filling defects may also be due, no more to an extrinsic compression (herniation), but to intrinsic pathology (radicular edema) — and that is one of the possible explanations for the "bell-muzzle sign," "signe du tromblon" in French (Fig. V,20) i.e., nonfilling of the radicular

69

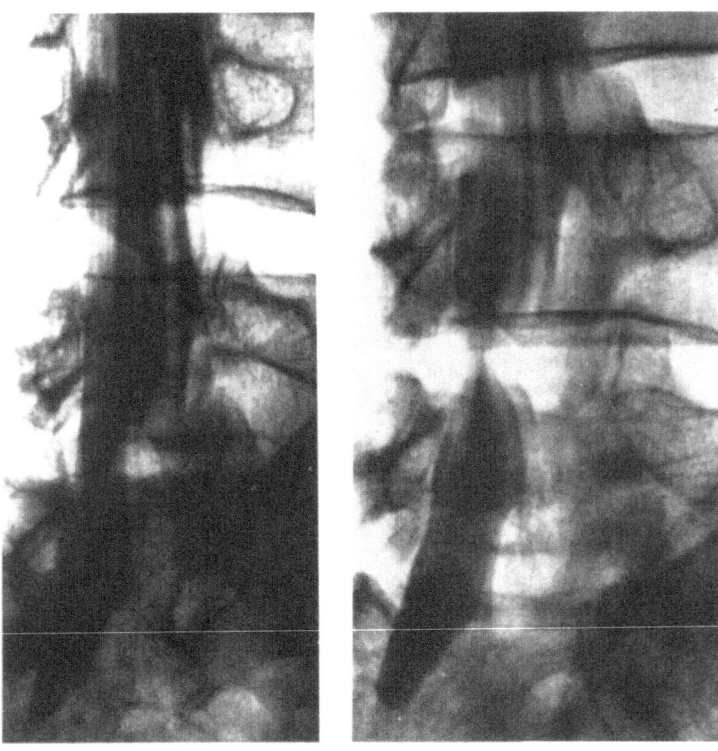

Fig. V,20. **The "Bell-muzzle Sign".** (a) The S1 root radiolucency widens out just before its interruption by a L5–S1 herniation. The S2 root is only moderately deviated by the compression. (b) Bell-muzzle sign located on the L5 root with compression and deviation of the sacral roots at the same level; "curtain-loop sign"

sheath associated with the absence of opacification of one of the infra- or supra-radicular fossae, or of both, so that the radicular radiolucency appears to be enlarged just before its interruption at the exact level of the emergence. This distal flaring is consistent with flattening of the root which is usually confirmed at the operation (Fig. V,21).

Mild discal herniations of the lateral type exclusively cause radicular signs, without imprint on the dural sac [16] (Fig. V,19). Small herniations or sequestrated fragments which have migrated toward the entrance of the intervertebral foramen may produce the same signs. At the utmost, a fragment situated within the intervertebral foramen may have no visible repercussion on the opacification of the sheath because it is too distal, although it is particularly compressive for the root.

A very mild compression may cause localized lack of opacification of the sheaths, either of a margin of one sheath or of one of the angles of an axillary triangle.

Strongly opacified sheaths or axillary pouches are due either to dysplasia, or to a compression.

There are idiopathic dilatations of the radicular sheaths or axillary pouches, smooth and almost regular, bumpy, or even with a distal rounded pouching. These anomalies are predominant on the more caudal roots, which they may involve almost exclusively; as a rule they are bilateral. Their clinical significance is discussed (see Chap. 8). They may help in diagnosis when the nonfilling or the delayed filling of a distal

70

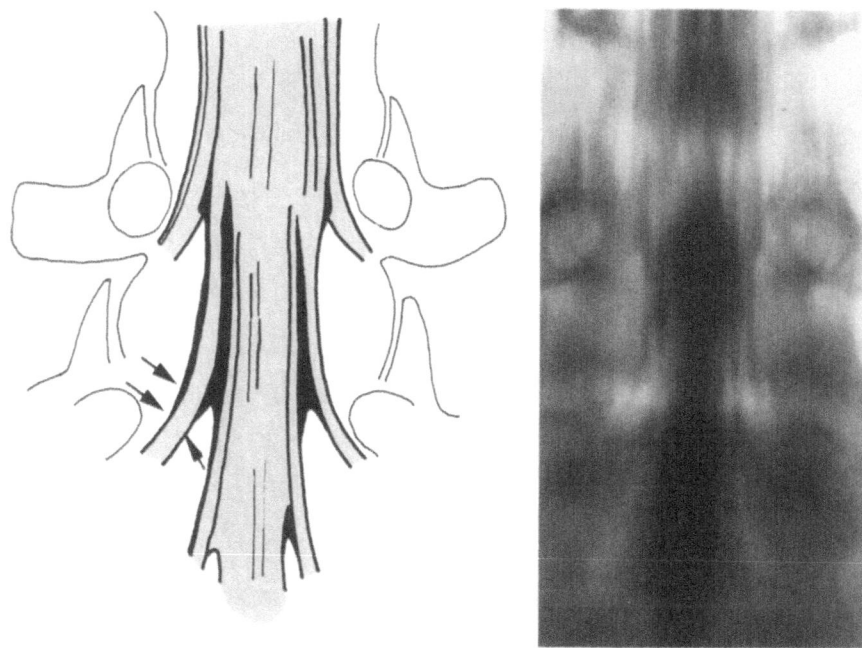

Fig. V,21. **Localized enlargement** of the right L5 radicular sheath. The L5 root is widened at its emergence point due to its flattening on a discal protrusion (*arrows*)

diverticulum is a sign of a proximal compression of the sheath.

The dilatation of a radicular sheath in the neighborhood of a compression is rare and seems to belong broadly to disturbances in the distribution of the contrast medium.

b) Signs Resulting From Deviated Roots

Direct Signs. When the radicular sheath is opacified, the deviation of the root is visualized, i.e., on the frontal view either the medial or the lateral deviation is inferred from the closing or the opening of the angle formed by the root and the lateral margin of the sac.

Left and right oblique projections are rarely comparable and a clear difference between the distances of the anterior edges of the sheaths to the cortex of the pedicles is necessary to conclude a deviation.

Forward or backward root deviation may sometimes be detected on zonograms when two roots belonging to the same pair are visible on different sections.

It is to be kept in mind that the simple radicular deviation may, moreover, mimic an opacification on a longer or shorter course for geometric reasons inherent to the radiographic projection.

Indirect Signs. As a matter of fact, very often the deviated roots also fail to opacify and one has to rely on indirects signs.

The axillary pouch of a nonfilled root sheath may be either widened or narrowed, depending on whether the deviation of the root involved is medial or lateral.

The enlargement of the axillary triangle at the overlying root level bears witness of the ascending character of the discal hernia.

References of Chapter 5 see page 150.

Part 2

Chapter 6. Discal Herniations*

We shall describe successively the anatomical types of herniations and the topographic types, depending on whether the herniation remained near the disc from which it originated or whether it has migrated. These distinctions may seem somewhat far-fetched, but it nevertheless has the advantage of corresponding to frequently encountered radioclinical entities [12]. For instance: L4 radiculitis due to ascending L4-5 herniation [15, 18, 23].

I. Anatomical Types of Discal Herniations

A. Terminology

The main purpose of this Section is to provide definitions of the terms we use, which constitutes a convention facilitating the reciprocal understanding for the members of the surgical and radiologic staffs.

A true herniation is first to be distinguished from a simple protrusion which is only a stage — in principle nonpathogeneous — in the discal degenerative changes and will not be dealt with here.

The anatomical types are distinguished with regard to the relationship between the degenerated part of the disc and the posterior vertebral ligament and the possible existence of a sequestration of a part of the disc (Fig. VI,1).

___
* This chapter has been written with the collaboration of D. Maitrot, M.D.

Subligamentous herniae are usually distinguished from the extraligamentous herniations, an intermedian form consisting in a break of the degenerative discal tissue through the posterior vertebral ligament.

We call *knob-like* herniations those in which the breaking concerns a small portion of the disc through a tiny orifice in the posterior vertebral ligament.

We use the term *extraligamentous* herniations for those in which the major part of the disc passes behind the ligament.

A *free* herniation is characterized by a gap between the discal substance and the disc from which it originates. It is to be noted that this variety of herniations more easily migrates far from its intervertebral space, and the more so when it is extraligamentous. These migrating herniae may also consist in sequestrated fragments (or free fragments). An intradural rupture of a disc herniation is exceptional [5, 21, 33, 34].

B. Radiculosaccographic Signs

To a certain extent, the anatomical type of herniation may be predicted on the view of the radiculosaccographic films [12, 16], from the shape and the importance of its imprint on the dural sac. This imprint is better analyzed on frontal tomographic sections [2, 3, 8, 23].

Subligamentous herniations produce flattened and regular, at the most slightly convex, imprints on the lateral margin of the dural sac. The knob-like herniations are

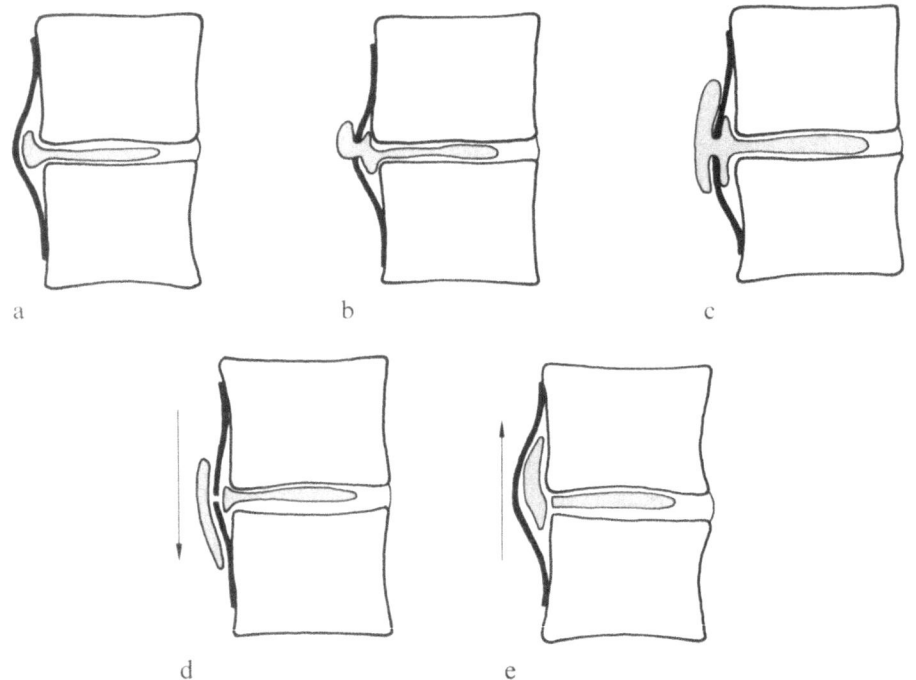

a   b   c

d   e

Fig. VI,1. **Schematic Representation of the Different Anatomical Types of Discal Herniations.** (a) Subligamentous hernia. (b) Knob-like hernia. (c) Extraligamentous hernia. (d) Free extraligamentous hernia. (e) Subligamentous fragment. The two types of subligamentous herniations (a) and (e) have a common feature, i.e., the integrity of the longitudinal vertebral ligament and are distinct from each other by the absence or the presence of a sequestration between the herniated part and the discal material remaining *in situ*.

Ligamentous perforations give way to a variable amount of discal material (b) and (c). After having passed the breach, more or less large fragments may become free (d). These extraligamentous fragments are more able to migrate than the subligamentous (e)

characterized by smooth indentations on which a small rounded imprint is added.

Marked indentations with usually irregular contour and multiple bumps are very likely consistent with extraligamentous or free herniations. This morphology varies slightly according to the level concerned.

II. Topographic Types of Discal Herniations

A. Herniations Facing the Disc From Which They Originate

Though the herniation may have all sorts of locations behind the disc, one may schematically distinguish *anterolateral* herniations from *extreme lateral* herniations on the one hand, and *median and paramedian* herniations on the other hand. As a matter of fact, they are possibly differentiated on behalf of their radiculosaccographic pattern [22].

1. Saccular Signs

Generally (see Chap. 5), the more a herniation is median, the more clearly it is visualized on a lateral projection, viz., a desaxation of the dural sac consisting of an angulated anterior imprint. Conversely, the more lateral it is, the better it is visualized on frontal views. Logically, only anterolateral herniations are responsible for anterior double contour of the saccular silhouette.

Lateral herniations have the peculiarity of producing an indentation along the anterior margin of the dural sac on the corresponding oblique projection as well as along the posterior margin on the contralateral oblique projection. When they are large, they also push the dural sac toward the opposite canalar aspect (desaxation).

2. Radicular Signs

a) Anterolateral herniations are by far the most frequent. Two types of anatomical situations may be encountered depending on the morphology of the dural sac and the mode of emergence of the roots (Fig. VI,2). The herniation is located either laterally to the corresponding root, which it pushes towards the midline (Fig. VI,3), or medially to the corresponding root, which it pushes laterally (herniation into the axilla) (Fig. VI,4). If the origins of the sheaths are situated below the disc level, the root is compressed within the dural sac, just cephalad to its emergence point. In this case, the imprint on the dural sac is more marked than the deviation of the root, and this may even follow a normal course after having emerged (Fig. VI,5).

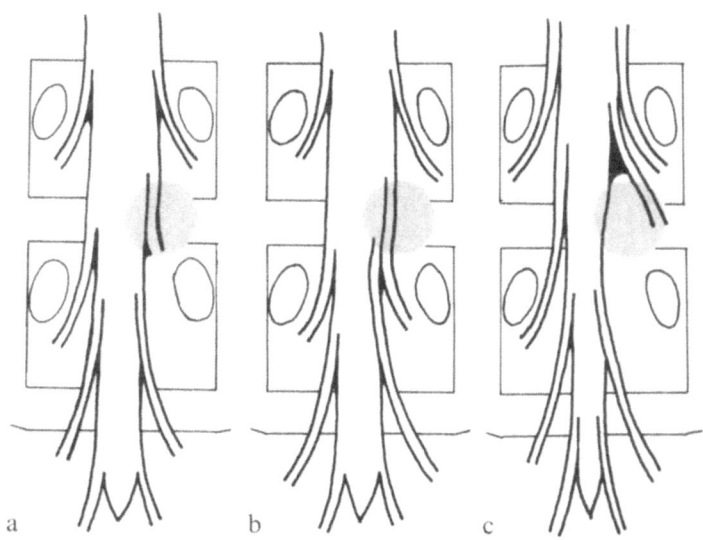

Fig. VI,2. **Schematic Representation of the Location of the Hernia With Regard to the Corresponding Root.** For a same variety of anterolateral herniation, three circumstances may be encountered: (a) The most common is encountered with roots emerging at the level of the disc. Thus, the herniation compresses the roots near its emergence, which brings about the nonfilling of the axillary area and a lack of opacification of the concerned sheath. (b) In case of low origin of the roots, the herniation is located above the emergence region and thus compresses the intrasaccular root segment. The axillary region may be slightly thinner but there is no obstacle to the sheath opacification (supraradicular herniation). (c) In case of high origin of the roots, the herniation is located immediately medially with regard to the course of the root concerned, which is laterally deviated. As a consequence, the axillary region is enlarged (infraradicular herniation)

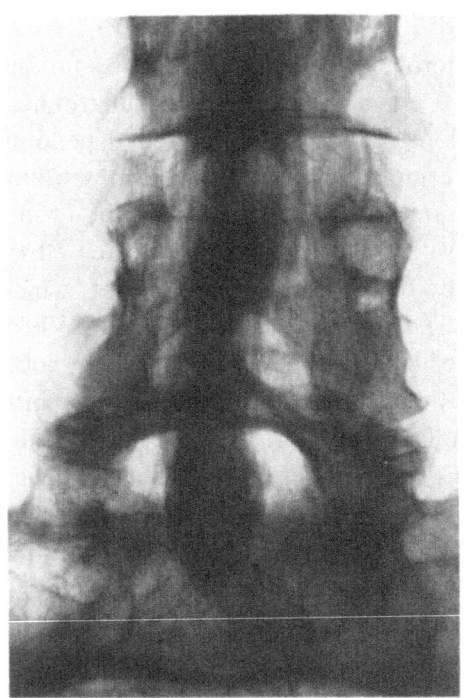

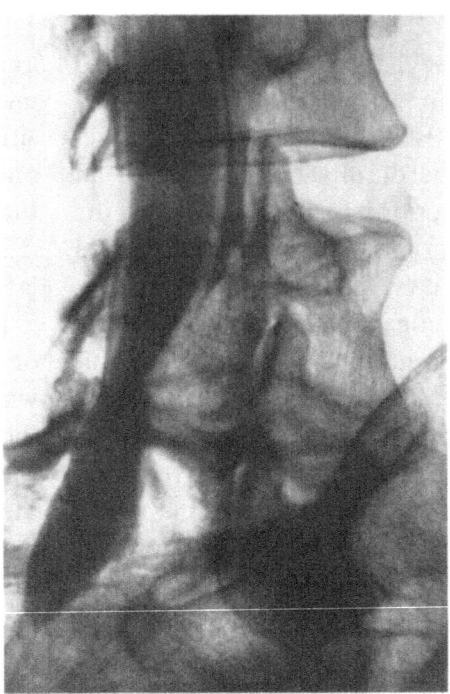

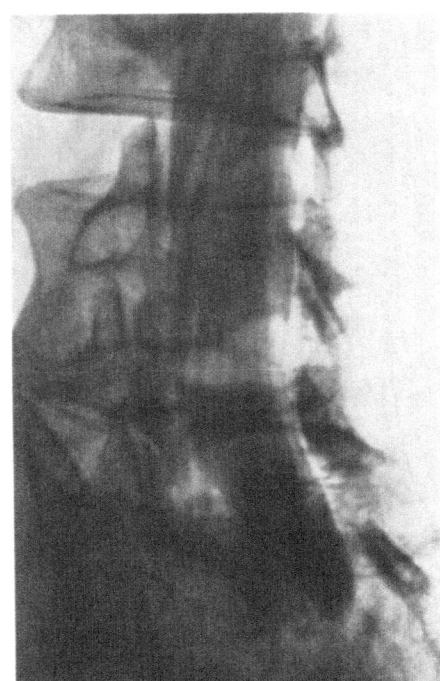

Fig. VI,3. **Voluminous Anterolateral L4–5 Hernia.** (a) Frontal view. (b) Left posterior oblique view. (c) Right posterior oblique view. The marked left lateral imprint on the dural sac, the irregular contour of this imprint, and the deviation of the whole dural sac toward the opposite canalar margin are in favor of the lateral location of the herniation and of its extraligamentous type (a, b). Moreover, there is no imprint on the contralateral oblique projection (c). The extrasaccular segment of the left L5 root fails to opacify and its intrasaccular segment is pushed medially and backward

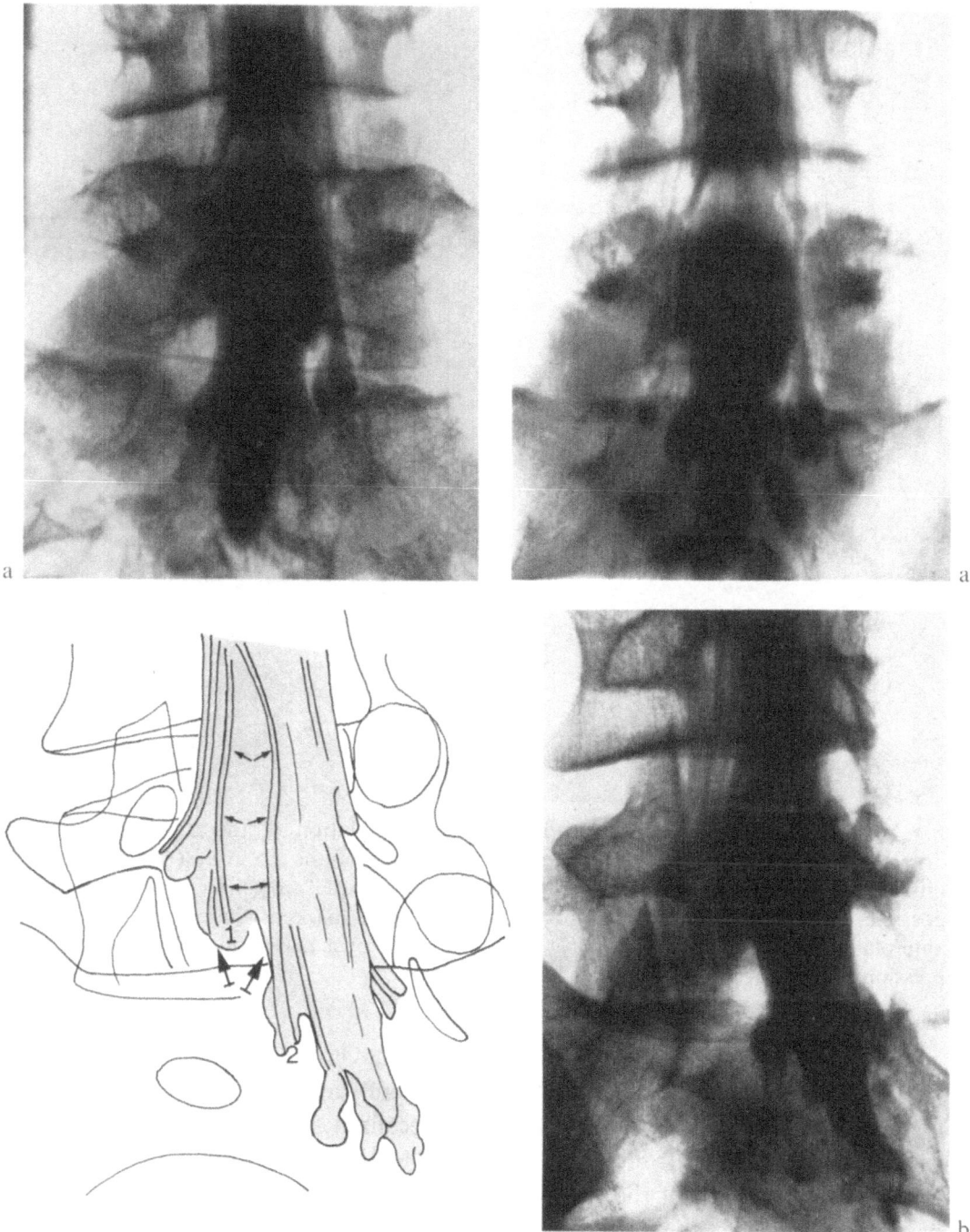

Fig.VI,4. **Herniation in the Axillary Region.**
(a, a′) Frontal view and frontal zonography.
(b) Right oblique posterior view (drawing). In
this case, the cyst-like dilatations of the sheaths
render the radicular signs more obvious. Indeed,
the cyst-like dilatation of the termination of
the left S1 root sleeve has no twin image on
the right side. The hernial imprint on the dural
sac is mild on frontal as well as on oblique
views. The posterior oblique projection on the
same side as the herniation (b) indicates the
exact location of the hernia (crossed arrows)
between S1 (*1*) which is interrupted and laterally
deviated, and S2 (*2*) which is compressed in
the proximal part of its sheath. In addition, the
two intrasaccular S1 and S2 translucencies
clearly diverge (*arrows*)

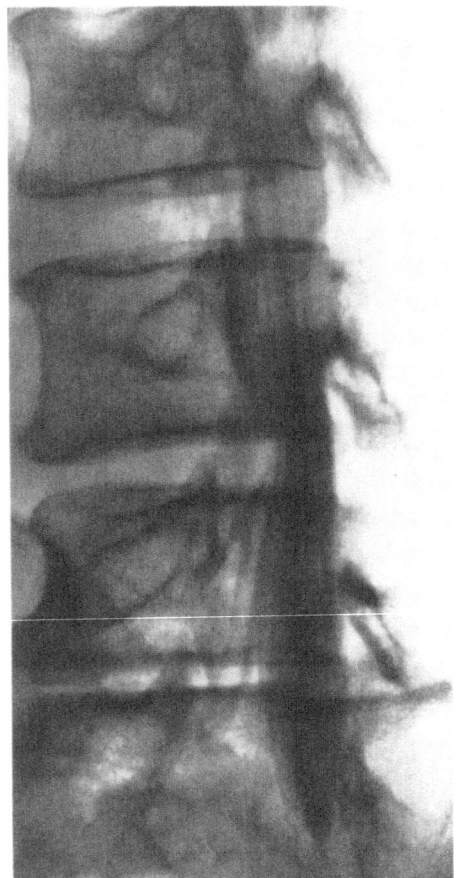
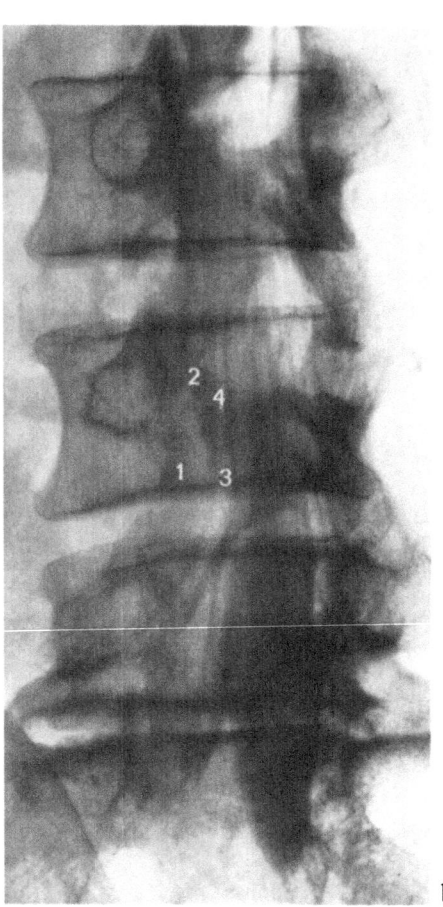

a   b

Fig. VI,5. **Supraradicular Herniation.** The low origin of the L5 roots, i.e., below the L4–5 interspace, makes a supraradicular compression possible and consequently an imprint on the anterolateral aspect of the dural sac (*1*), a compression and a deviation of both L5 (*2*) and S1 (*3*) roots before their emergence, and an accumulation of the contrast in the axillary region of the L5 root (*4*). Note that on the 45° oblique projection (a), the hernial imprint is more marked whereas the radicular courses are shown better on a 25° oblique projection (b)

b) Median herniations seem to be frequently associated with a narrow lumbar canal. They appear on frontal projections as a localized blurring of the margins and of the radicular sheaths on either side. However, these "median" herniations are always slightly paramedian, which goes along with the unequal degree of deviation of the roots on oblique projections. This slight predominance on one side usually corresponds to the side of the sciatic pain. This arises from the differential diagnosis between the above-described entity and bilateral herniation, which could produce a localized stenosis of the dural sac and bilateral radicular compression signs. The latter are, however, very rare [31] (Fig. VI,6).

c. Lateral herniations are negatively characterized in so far as they have little or no repercussion on the dural sac [1, 24], mainly on the lateral views (Fig. VI,7), and few specific radicular signs. Usually they deviate medially to a low extent the corresponding root and may even completely spare it at the L5 S1 level. This type of herniation thus represents a cause of "false

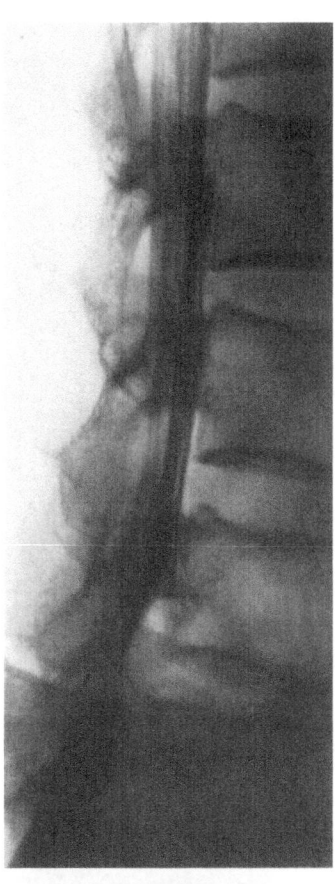

Fig. VI,6. **Median Herniation in a Narrow Lumbar Canal.** (a) On the lateral view, the whole dural sac is pushed backward; it shows a desaxation and a blurred pattern at the level of the L4–5 disc. (b, c, d) Frontal view and right and left posterior oblique projections; there is a segmental lack of opacification at the same level with blurred pattern and blunted anterolateral margins and root emergences on both sides. Note the associated signs of narrow lumbar canal, i.e., the intrasaccular roots are too clearly displayed, stasis above the herniation, behind the vertebral bodies as well as in the immediately overlying axillary regions

a

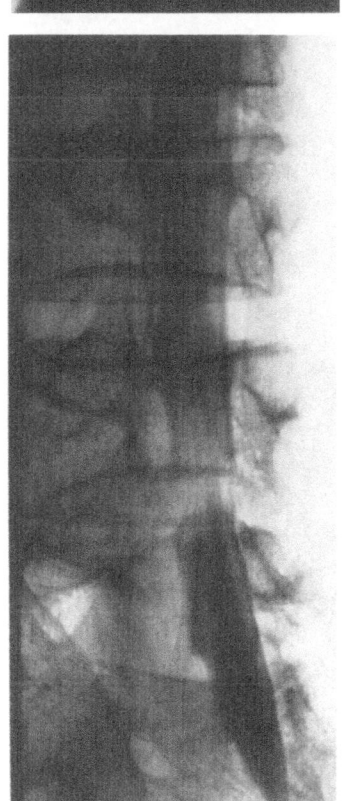

b

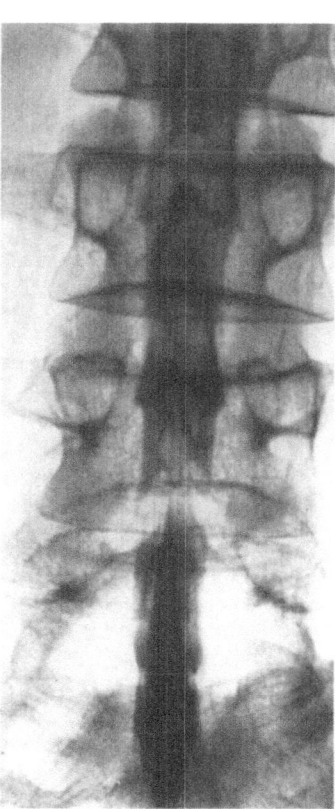

c

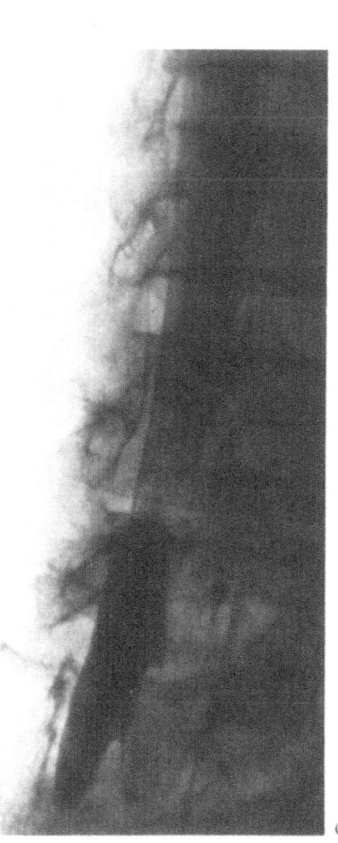

d

81

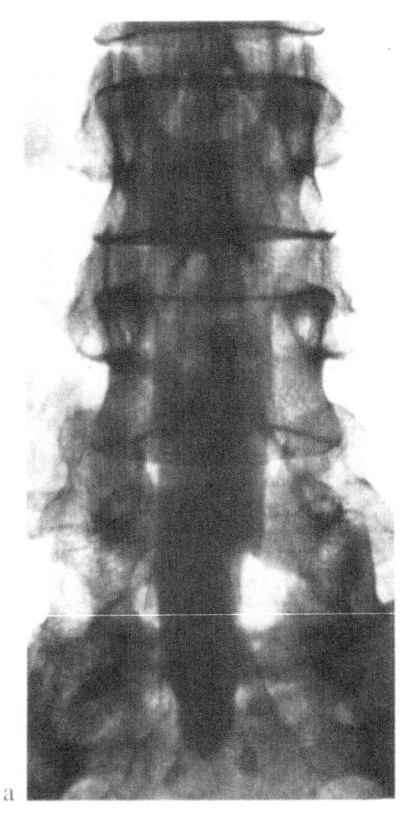

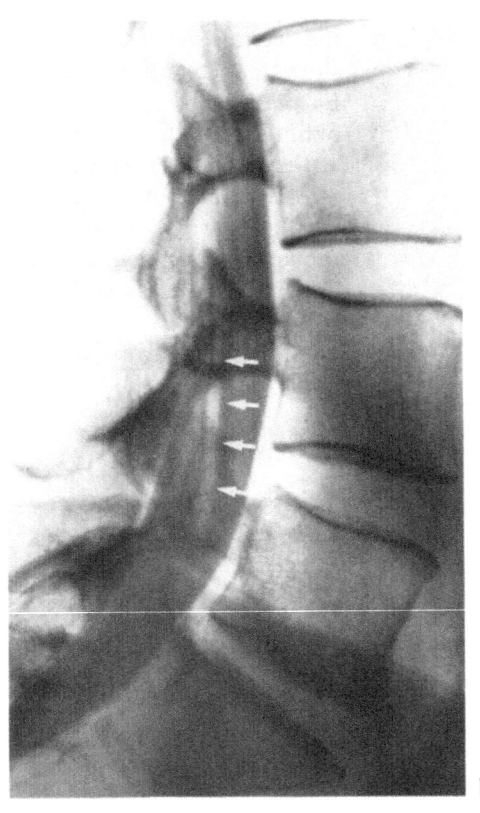

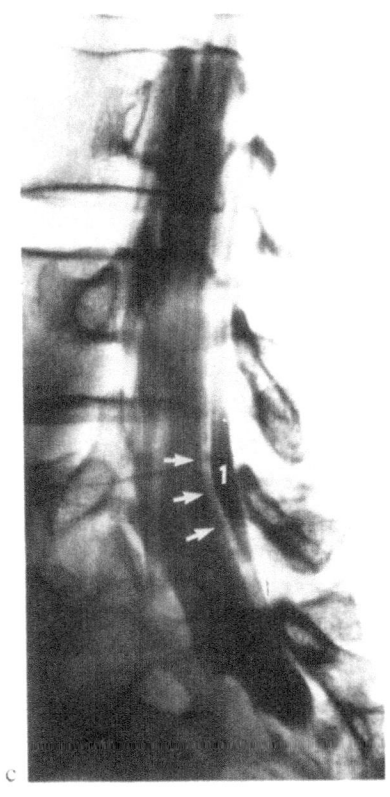

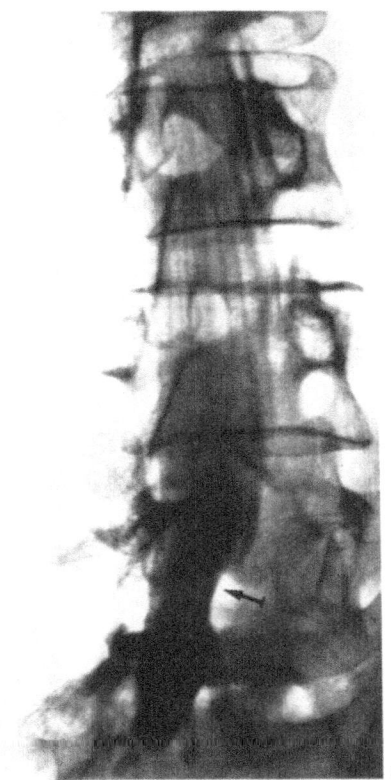

82

Fig. VI,8. **Absence of a Root Sheath as Only** ▷
Sign of Disc Herniation. The right S1 root is
not visible, but there is no clear imprint on
the dural sac. This is a frequent occurrence at
the L5–S1 interspace and in lateral herniations

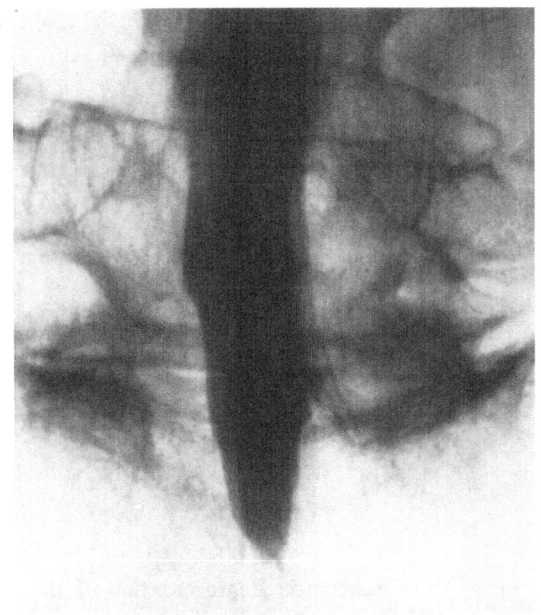

negatives" in RSG. They are the most able
to provide an isolated radicular sign which
is difficult to interpret; for example, simple
nonfilling or proximal opacification with
a distal filling defect of a sheath (Fig. VI,8).

B. Migrating Herniations

We distinguish three circumstances, depending on whether the herniation migrates
cranially, caudally, or anteroposteriorly.
The semiology of these — frequent — varieties of herniations is to be kept in mind
since it provides eminent information for
the surgeon concerning the intervertebral
space to be operated upon as well as the
surgical technique, and aids in the search
for free fragments which may sometimes
be located quite far from their discs [7, 23].

1. The Conditions of Hernial Migrations

Possibilities of migration depend on the
anatomical variety of the dural sac, and
more particularly on the radicular emergence pattern (Fig. VI,9).

In cases with low emergence of the roots,
the herniation is situated laterally to the
corresponding root and will migrate either
cranially and toward the midline (*ascending
retrovertebral herniation*) or cranially to-

ward the axilla of the overlying root which
it then compresses at the point of its entrance into the intervertebral foramen.

Conversely, in cases of high emergence
of the roots, the herniation is located immediately between the root and the dural sac,
near the axilla which checks an upward migration, so that it migrates caudally in two
possible ways, i.e.:

a. Either it runs along the radicular
course rather vertically and laterally and
may then be located at the entrance of the
intervertebral foramen, or even penetrate
into it in the form of a small free fragment
(*retrovertebral and preradicular herniation*).
This variety of herniation may also be encountered when the radicular emergences
are of the common type. A herniation may

◁ Fig. VI,7. **Lateral Herniation.** (a) Frontal view.
(b) Lateral view. (c) Right posterior oblique view.
(d) Left posterior oblique view. The lateral
location of the herniation with regard to the
dural sac is suggested by a more marked imprint
on the frontal view (a) than on the lateral view
(b). The lack of opacification and the postero-

medial deviation of the left S1 root at its emergence point are visible on the left posterior
oblique projection (*crossed arrow*), whereas the
intrasaccular edema of the root appears on the
lateral view and on the right posterior oblique
projection as a more marked linear translucency
(*arrows*) outlined by the stasis (*1*)

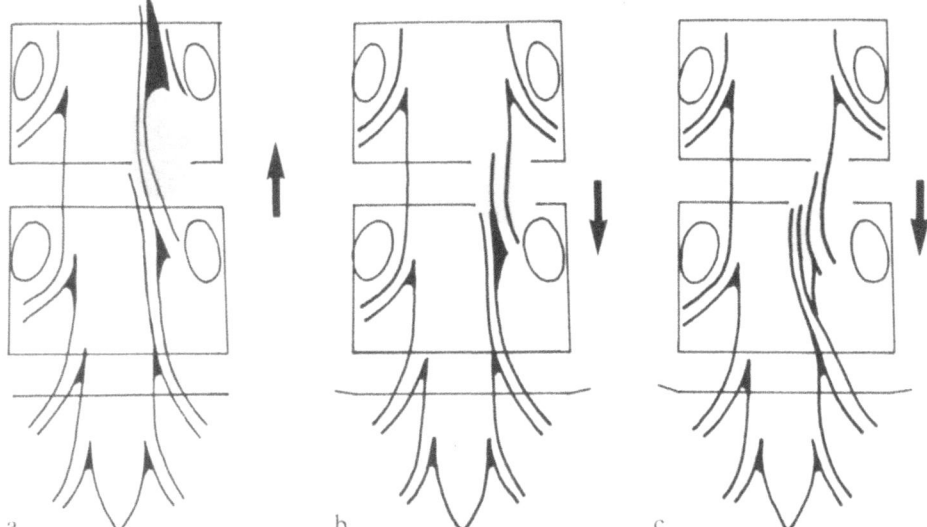

a

b

c

Fig. VI,9. **Schematic Representation of the Upward and Downward Possibilities of Hernial Migration.** (a) An upward migrating hernia may compress the corresponding root, and additionally compress the overlying one near its entrance into the intervertebral foramen. The axillary pouch of this latter is then deformed. This condition is more frequent in cases of low originating roots. (b) Moderately descending hernia located at the entrance of the corresponding root into its intervertebral foramen. (c) Descending retrovertebral herniation, which compresses the corresponding root at its emergence point and the intrasaccular roots. These herniae are generally voluminous

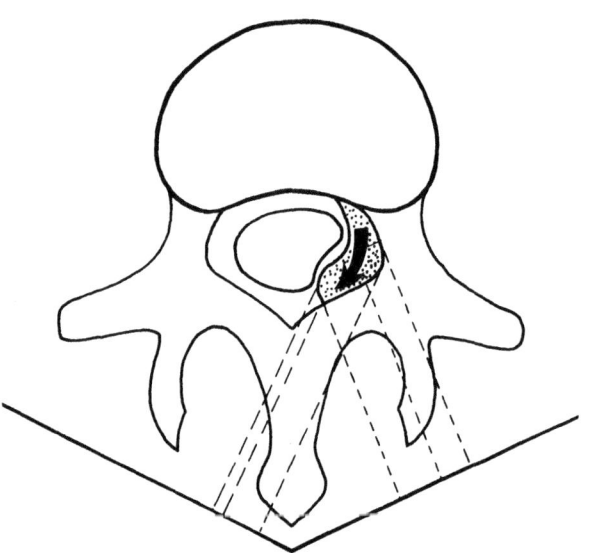

Fig. VI,10. **Horizontal Migration of a Discal Herniation.** The small caliber of the dural sac at the L5–S1 interspace allows the herniation to turn it laterally by passing above or below the root; thus it produces a posterolateral compression on the dural sac

84

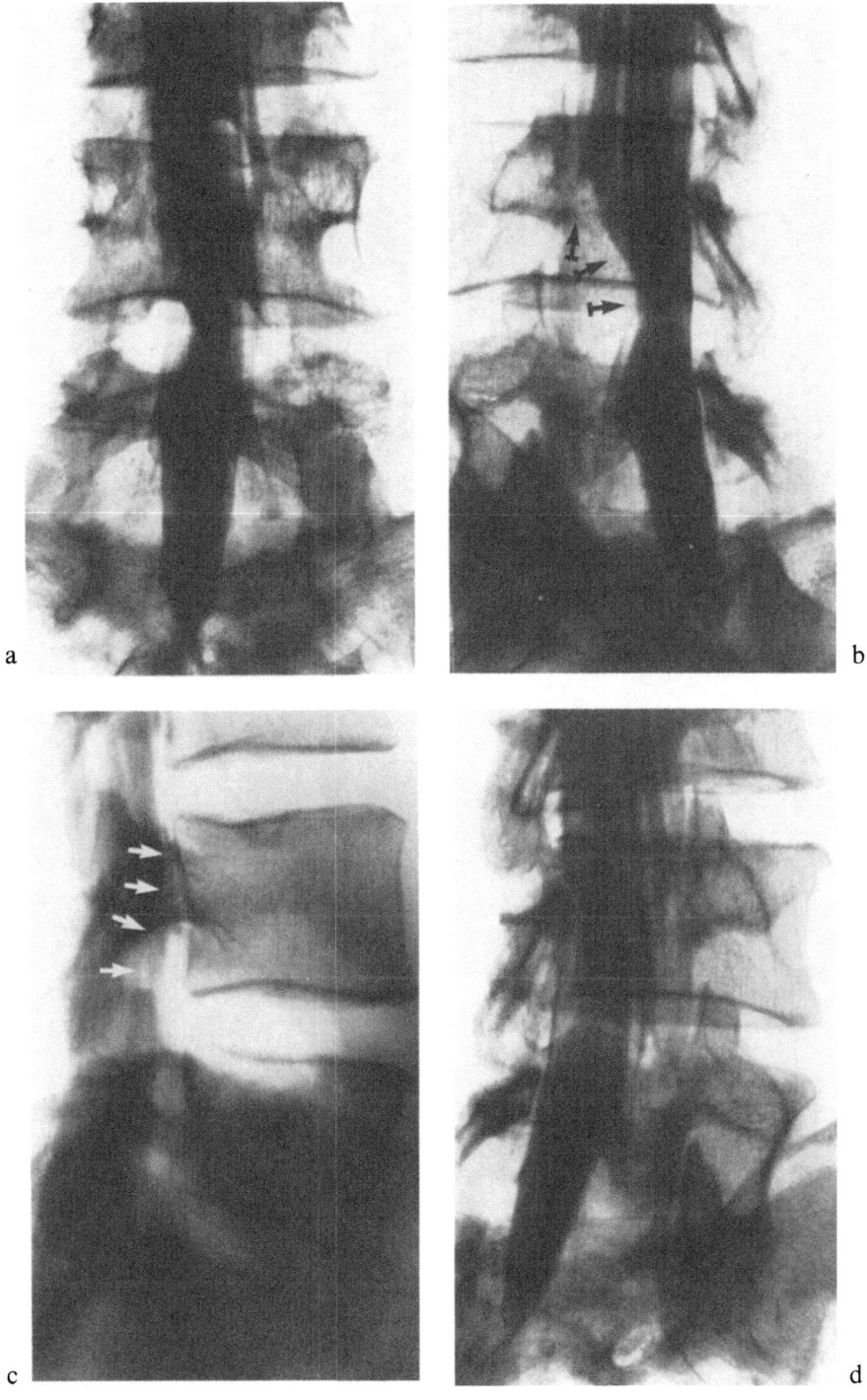

a

b

c

d

Fig. VI,11. **Herniation Ascending Toward the Intervertebral Foramen.** Lateral L4–5 herniation, with a well-visible imprint on frontal view (a) and on the right posterior oblique projection (b). Its double contour prolonging upward is visible on lateral view (c) (*arrows*) and witnesses its ascending character. The divergence of the L4 and L5 roots and the compression of the L4 axillary region (b) (*crossed arrows*) indicates that the herniation is prolonged up to the L4 intervertebral foramen. The contralateral oblique projection is normal (d)

85

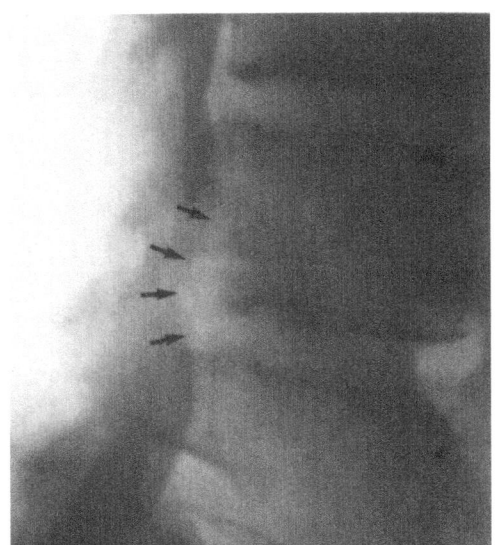

a

Fig. VI,12. **Ascending Retrovertebral Herniation.**
The ascending type and the paramedian location

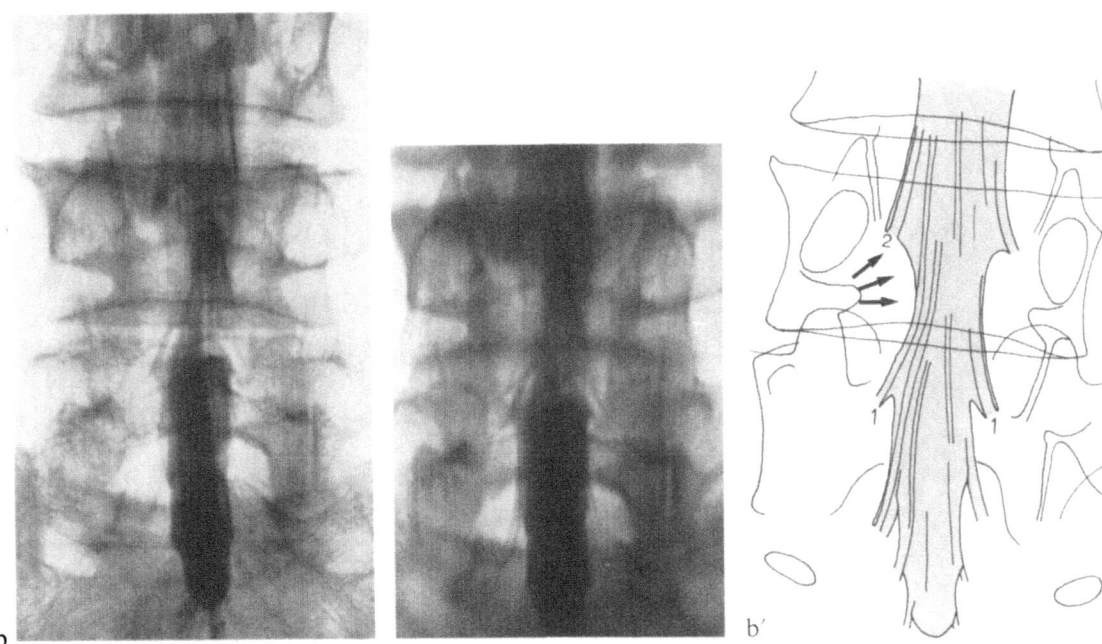

b

b′

be predicted to be situated within the intervertebral foramen when only radicular signs are disclosed, in the absence of signs of pressure on the dural sac.

b. Or it migrates caudally and toward the midline, and thus becomes a descending *retrovertebral herniation.*

Finally, there exists a rare possibility of anteroposterior migration at the level of the L5–S1 interspace due to a small caliber dural sac which allows the herniation to turn it and locate between this dural sac and the lamina (*retroradicular and prelaminar herniation*) [23] (Fig. VI,10).

86

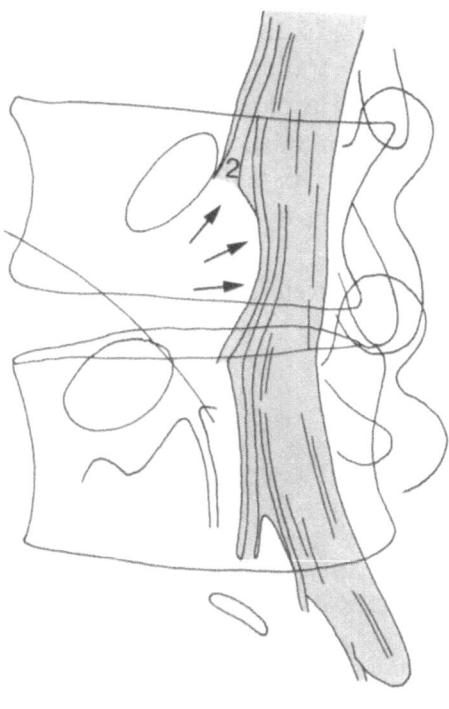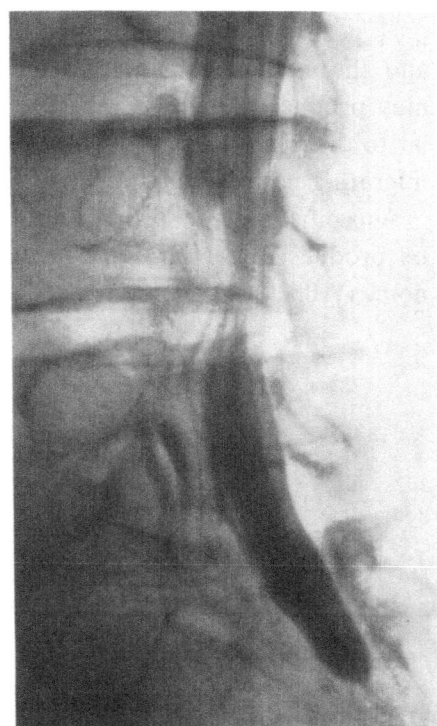

Fig. VI,12 (cont.). Legend see opposite page   c

2. Radiculosaccographic Signs of Migrating Herniations

The saccular anomalies consist mainly in elongated imprints overlapping the intervertebral space caudally or cranially. This is always readily shown on the lateral projection, where the upward detachments are more reliably in favor of migrating herniations than downward detachments.

These elongated imprints are less reliable on frontal views, so that at least incidences are to be performed taking the lordosis into account.

Moreover, these imprints should be localized with regard to the axis of the spinal canal based on the synthetic interpretation of the different views (see Chap. 5) (Fig. VI,11–VI,17).

The radicular signs reinforce the previous data due to the anatomical type of emergence of the roots and the elementary radicular anomalies; for instance, in a case of ascending L5–S1 herniation and of low originating roots, the concerned L5 root fails to opacify and is laterally deviated.

III. Differential Diagnosis of Discal Herniations as They Are Displayed by RSG

An indentation on the dural sac does not always correspond to a herniation. As a matter of fact, other pathologic entities may be diagnosed though they are more rarely encountered:

Bone hypertrophy, chiefly the one due to degenerative changes of the facetal joints, gives rise to elongated imprints similar to those of upward or downward migrating herniations. The differential diagnosis is based on a frontal zonography which shows the relations between the imprint and the bone structures [9].

87

Hypertrophy of the ligamenta flava [28] and the extradural ganglion cysts [6, 19] may produce posterolateral imprints similar to those of horizontally and posteriorly migrating herniations.

Aspecific imprints on the dural sac may be produced by rare extrasaccular neurinomas [10, 30], tuberculous abcesses [4, 20, 26, 29], vascular malformations such as extradural varices [11, 14, 17, 25, 30], and hematomas [13, 27, 29, 32], for example related to a lumbar puncture practiced in a patient with hemopathy or in a patient receiving anticoagulant therapy.

References of Chapter 6 see page 151.

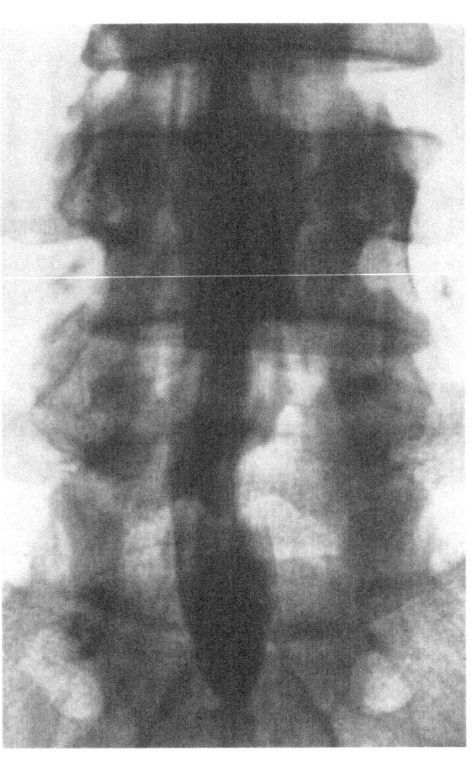
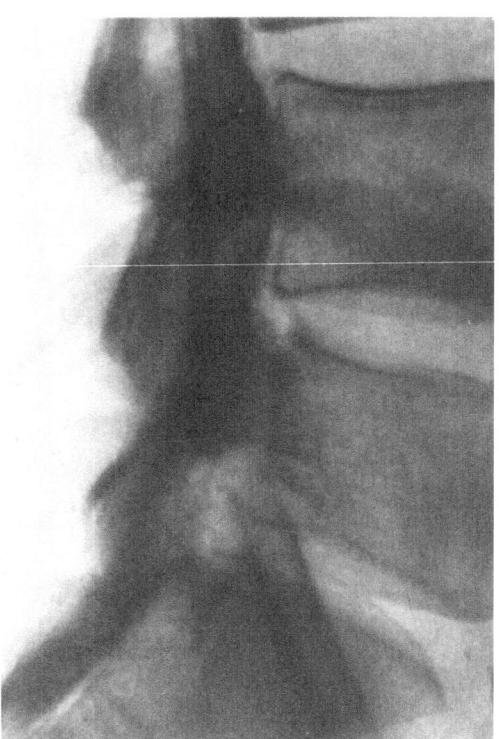

a

b

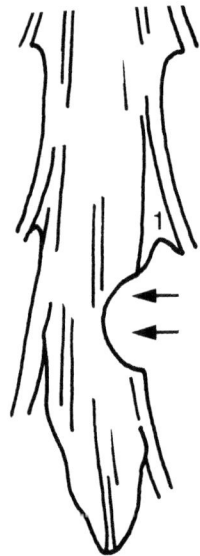

Fig. VI,13. Legend see opposite page

88

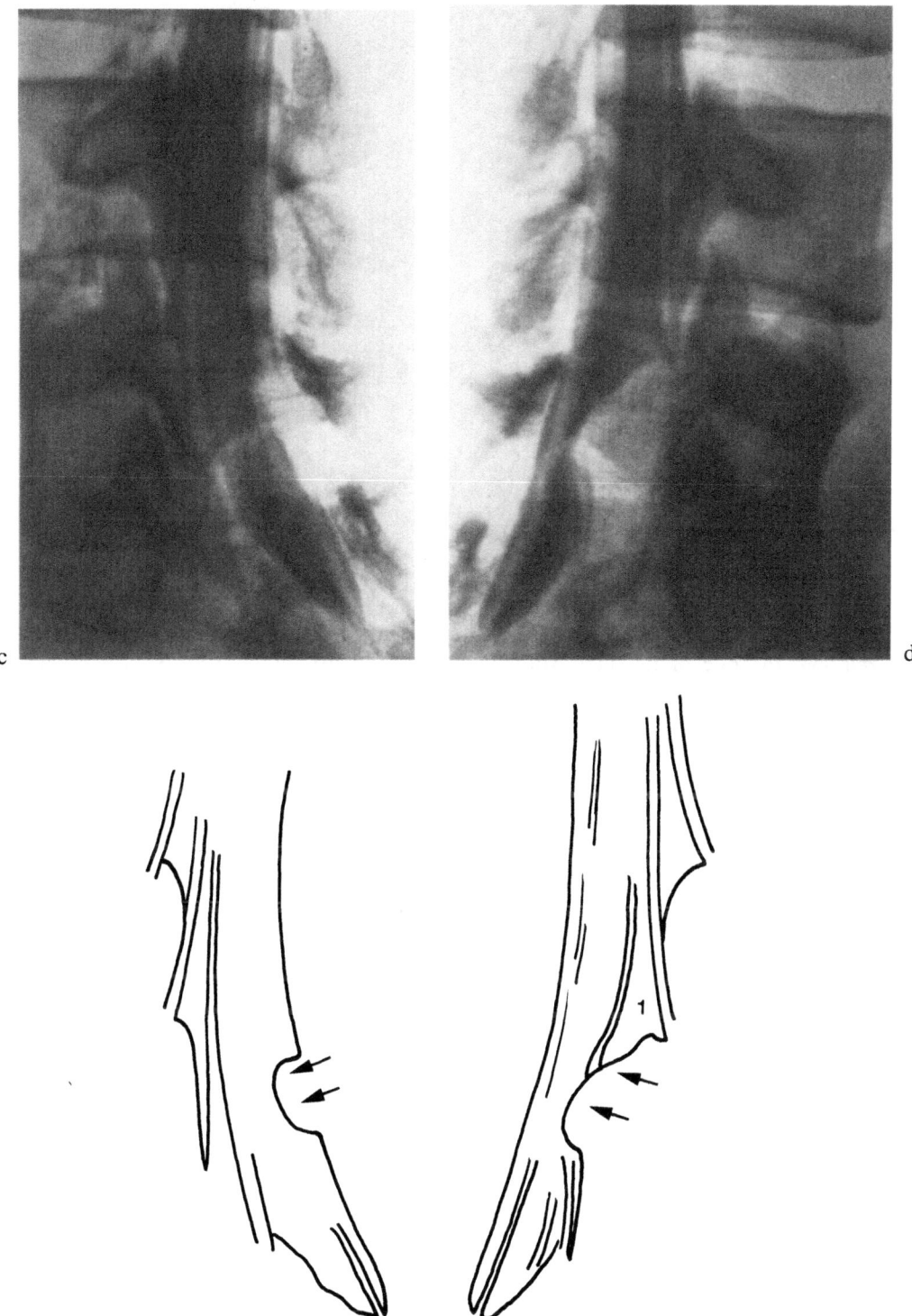

c   d

Fig. VI,13. **Lateral and Ascending Extraligamentous Herniation.** The imprint (*arrows*) visible on the frontal view (a) and on the two oblique projections (c, d) — located on the anterior margin on the corresponding one and on the posterior margin on the contralateral one — and not visible on the lateral projection (b) bares witness to the lateral location of this extraligamentous herniation. The imprint prolongs up to the L5 axillary region (*1*) which becomes wider

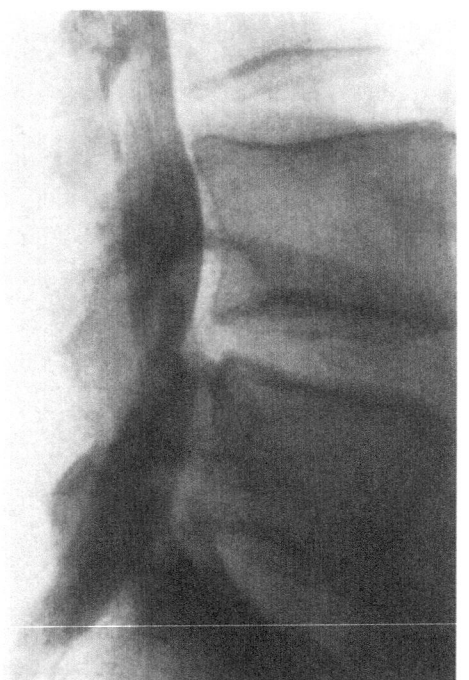
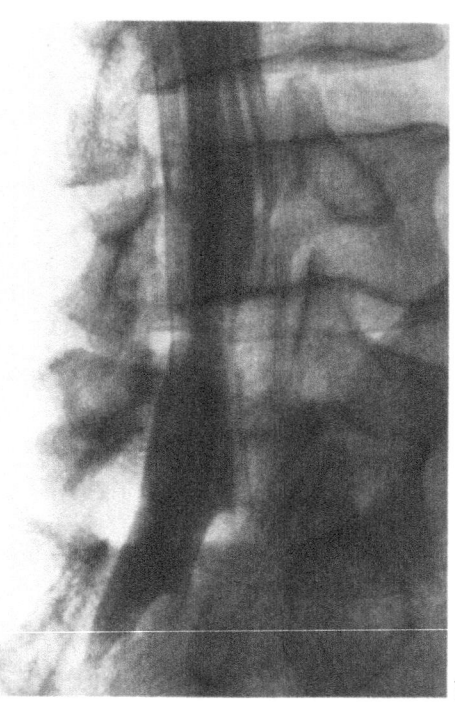

a   b

Fig. VI,14. **Retrovertebral and Subligamentous Herniation.** In spite of its small volume, this herniation is the more compressive for the left L5 root since it is located just before its entrance into the intervertebral foramen. Just before its interruption, the root is pushed backwards and the imprint on the dural sac is minimal. (a) Lateral view. (b) Left posterior oblique view

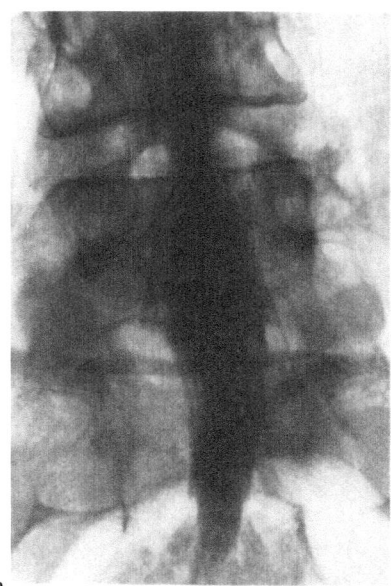
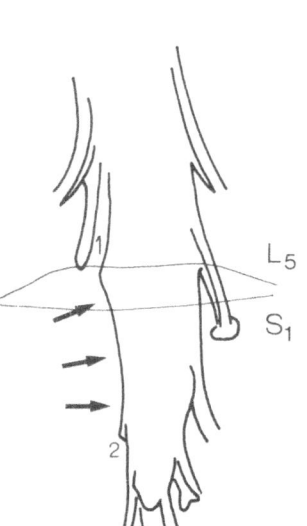
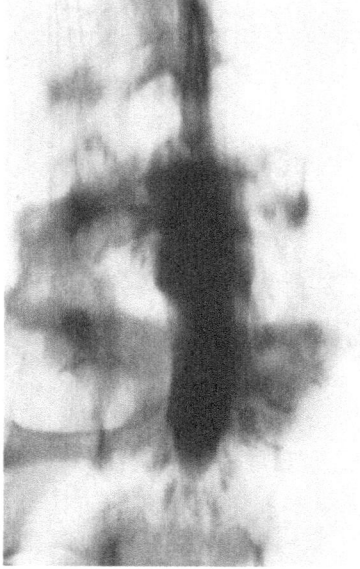

a   a′

Fig. VI,15. **Retrosacral Herniation.** The right S1 root (*1*) is interrupted at the level of the lumbosacral interspace (a, a′) The right anterolateral imprint (*arrows*) is maximum below the L5–S1 interspace in frontal (a, a′) as well as in oblique (b) and lateral views (c). The S2 (*2*) root is also interrupted (a and c)

90

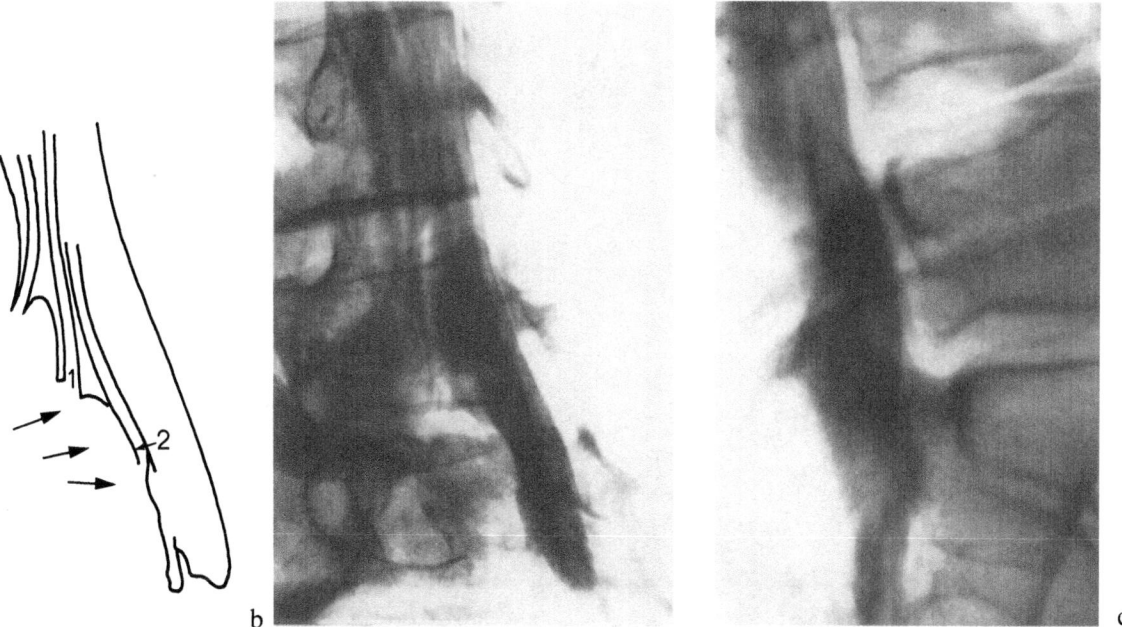

b

c

Fig. VI,15 (cont.). Legend see page 90

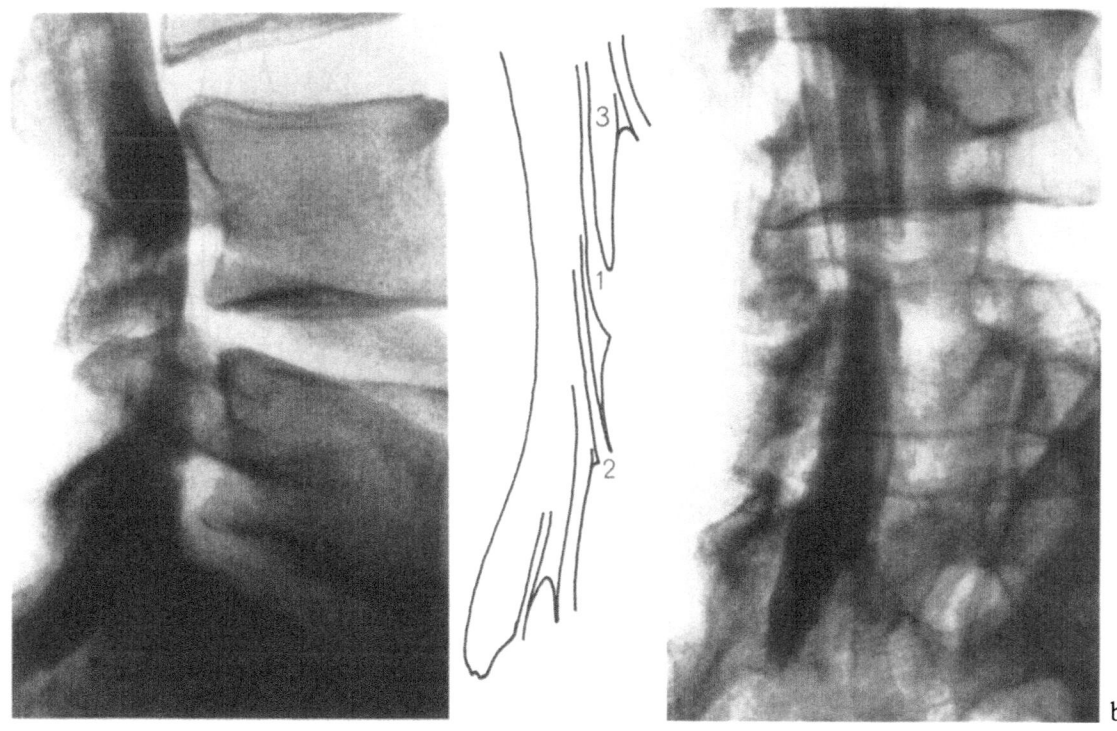

a

b

Fig. VI,16. **Descending L4–5 Herniation.** The descending type is visible on a lateral view (a) by the retrovertebral L5 detachment and on the oblique projection (b) by the increased distance between the dural sac and the L5 pedicle. Both the L5 (*1*) and the S1 (*2*) sheaths are interrupted and there is an area of accumulated contrast in the L4 axillary region (*3*)

91

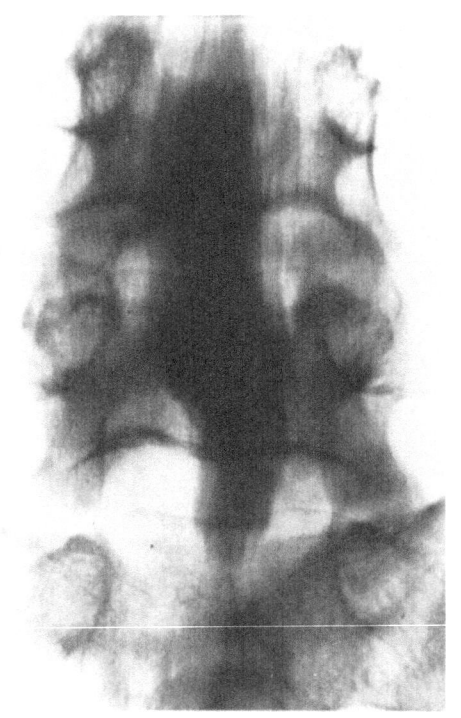
a

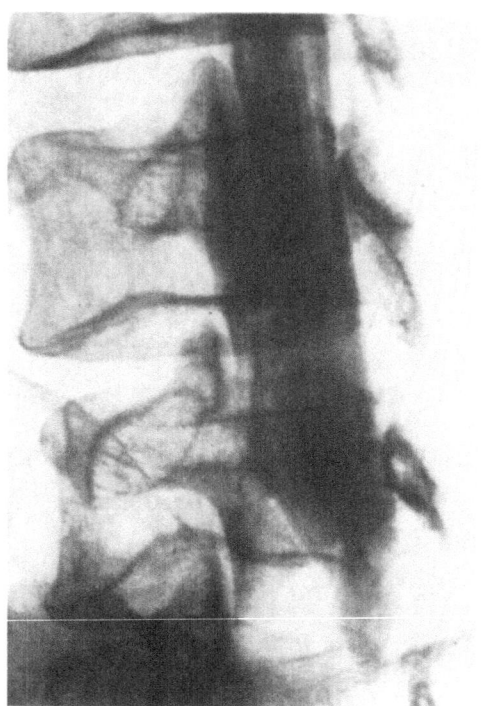
b

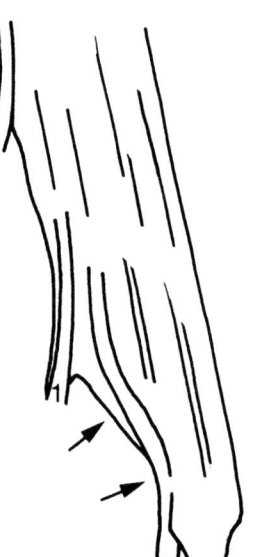

Fig. VI,17. Legend see opposite page

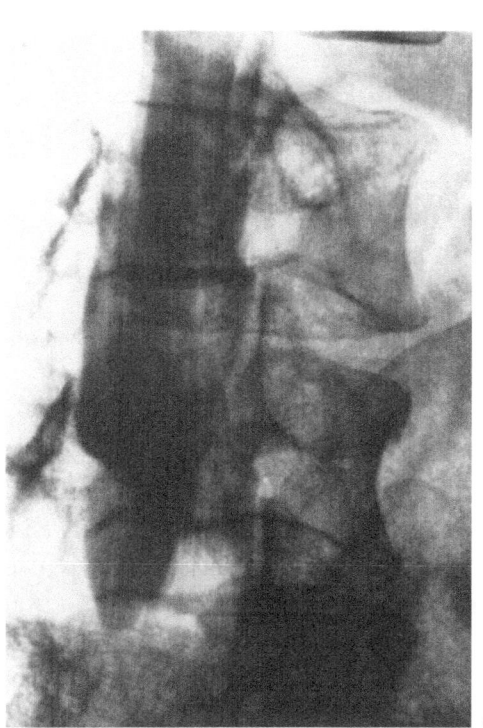

Fig. VI,17. **Prelaminar and Retroradicular Herniation.**
(a) Frontal zonography. (b) Right posterior oblique
projection. (c) Left posterior oblique projection. The
posterolateral compression of the dural sac (*arrows*)
by the right L5–S1 herniation is characterized by a
marked posterior imprint on the contralateral oblique
projection (c). The right S1 root (*1*) is visible when
it passes along the herniation. The S2 (*2*) root is
strongly pushed medially

c

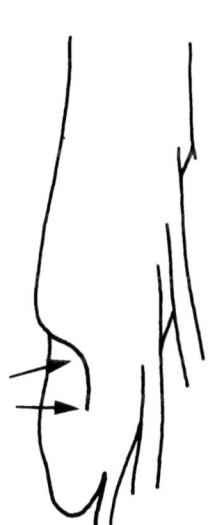

Chapter 7. Postoperative RSG*

I. Clinical Circumstances

In most cases, the patient is referred for RSG some months or some years after the operation, either because of persistent pain or recurrent symptomatology — similar to that preceding the operation —, because of the development of another lumbar radiculitis, or, finally, because of the occurrence of a very painful cauda equina syndrome. We have never been asked to perform RSG in the early postoperative period.

The causes of failure or of postoperative aggravation are numerous, and it is difficult to document these bad results [5, 18]. Apart from the psychic and professional intricacies resulting from lumbar radiculalgiae, some precise circumstances may be considered, which could at least partly explain the failure of the disc operation, i.e.:

1. Error in the diagnosis concerning the disc responsible or concerning the mere discal origin of the compression (associated narrow lumbar or radicular canal) [8, 18].

2. Faulty technique such as the microbic contamination of the operating field, a rupture of the dura mater with subsequent constitution of an arachnoidal diverticulum [9, 14, 15], insufficiently careful hemostasis [16] with secondary hematoma evolving toward hardened scarring tissue [11].

3. The presence of a herniation at a level other than the one operated may correspond to a second herniation neglected at

* This chapter has been written with the collaboration of D. Maitrot, M.D.

the operation time, or to a herniation which has appeared in between.

4. The presence of a forgotten fragment [13].

5. The occurrence of postoperative arachnoiditis raises doubt as to its origin , i.e., is it due to RSG or the operation itself [1, 10, 12]?

6. The scarring processes vary with individuals, and even after the most careful hemostasis, a hypertrophic scar may be found, the relation of which to a painful symptomatology is then discussed. In favor of this hypothesis is the fact that the patient improves after the excision of the scarring tissue. These pathologic scarring processes might be due to the use of spongel as an hemostatic.

The bony stenoses after laminectomy or after posterior arthrodesis [2, 3] are dealt with in Chapter 9.

II. Radiologic Features

A. Normal Postoperative Findings

1. A very localized bulge of the dura mater close to the interlaminar approach [16] is commonly seen on the contralateral posterior oblique view (Fig. VII,1 b) with regard to the side operated upon. On the frontal view, this bulge is less visible, and there is only a moderate hump along the lateral margin of the dural sac (Fig. VII,1 a).

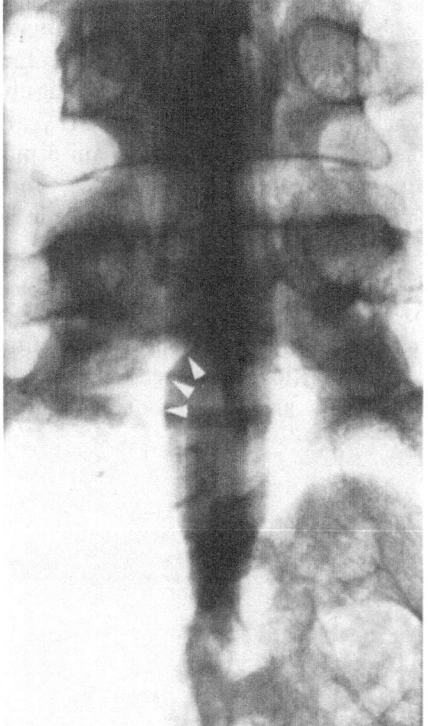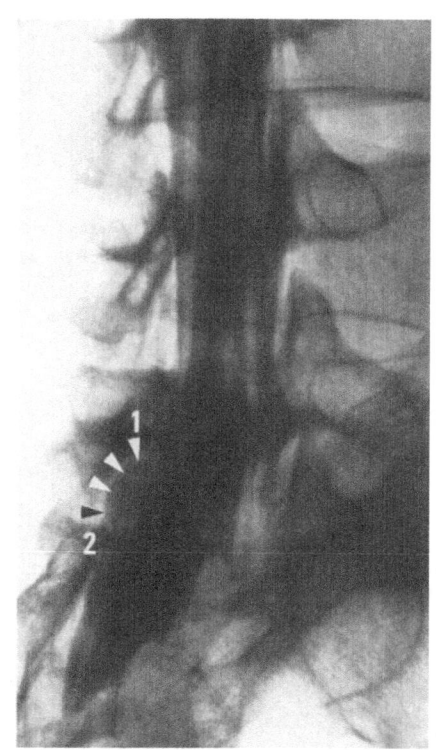

a   b

Fig. VII,1. **Postoperative RSG** (Right L5–S1 discal hernia operation). Bulge of the dural sac close to the laminar fenestration. (a) Frontal view: Slight bump of the lateral margin of the dural sac at the level of the laminar fenestration (*arrowheads*). The right L5 and S1 radicular sheaths are not opacified. (b) Left posterior oblique view. The additional image of the posterolateral aspect of the dural sac (*arrowheads*) is situated between the projections of the L5 (*1*) and S1 (*2*) laminae. A thin translucent band separates this bulge from the laminar cortices

2. The lack of opacification of the root concerned by the operation has, in the absence of other discal herniation signs, no pathologic value (Fig. VII,1 a).

B. The Hypertrophic Extradural Scar

According to Cronqvist [4] an indentation related to a hyperplastic scar may be differentiated from a hernial indentation by some features, i.e.:

1. It is situated on one of the posterolateral aspects of the dural sac.

2. It is located between two intervertebral levels.

3. It is elongated and has clear-cut and irregular margins (Fig. VII,2).

As a matter of fact, the differential diagnosis between hypertrophic scar and hernial recurrence is very difficult [7], taking into account the fact that free herniations produce indentations with irregular margins, and that herniations may migrate — i.e., leave the intervertebral space — and become retrovertebral (Fig. VII,3).

C. Recurrence of Discal Herniation

This is a condition we have encountered more often than the previous one.

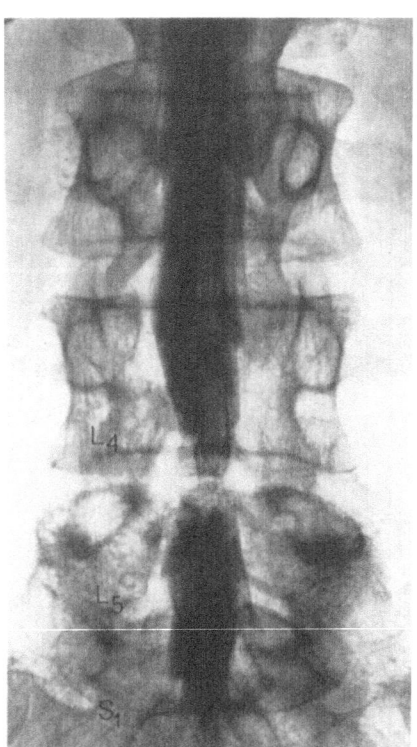

Fig. VII,2. **Elongated Lateral Indentation Due to Extradural Scar Tissue With Residual Fragments of the Disc.** 47-year-old male operated upon for the first time 15 years before for right discal hernia (double L4–5 and L5–S1 fenestration), operated again 1 year before in L4–5 at the right. Pains appeared again 6 months later with paralyzing L4 and L5 radiculitis, prompting a RSG. The irregular stenosis of the dural sac is the most marked at the level of the L4–5 disc, and on the right side, the L4 radicular sheath is not opacified, but the two L5 and S1 sheaths are also lacking (epidural scar tissue, ascending herniation?) After the third intervention (L5 hemilaminectomy, ablation of a free fragment ascending up to the L4 axillary area) the L4 deficit regressed

D. Postoperative Arachnoiditis

The more peculiar postoperative features of lumbar arachnoiditis are difficult to isolate since almost all patients underwent a preoperative RSG (see Chap. 2, Sect. VIC).

By and large, postoperative arachnoiditis [20] and mixed postoperative and post-RSG arachnoiditis [1, 10, 12] have more pronounced radiculosaccographic signs than a mere post-RSG arachnoiditis. Jorgensen et al. [12] have been the only ones to differentiate between these two types of arachnoiditis from the radiologic point of view, i.e., they termed *type I or post-RSG* a homogeneous intrasaccular contrast pattern, without root shadows and with a rounded shortening of the root pockets, and *type II or "postoperative and mixed"* a pattern made of some proliferation added inside the dural sac diffused or localized at the site of the operation. These postoperative RSG images consist of: (Fig. VII,4) (Fig. VII,5)

1. Localized or diffuse irregularities of the dural sac margins.

2. Irregular, diffuse, or localized narrowing, possibly with shortening of the dural sac.

3. The saccular area may become either abnormally homogeneous and loose its normal radicular striation [19], or become heterogeneous with dense areas and juxtaposed translucent areas. Abnormal ribbon-shaped translucencies [17] suggesting the bunching of the roots may appear within the saccular area. These abnormal translucencies are prolonged high in the dural sac, and at the most become a unique, central elongated translucency underlined by the surrounding contrast medium.

4. Diverticula of the fundus [22] may have different sizes and irregular shapes. When they are large, they show a horizontal

96

Fig. VII,3. **Lateral Indentation of the Dural Sac Due to a Scarring Process.** 37-year-old male, who suffered from lumbalgiae for 15 years, operated upon for a left S1 sciatica due to a L5–S1 extraligamentous hernia. (a) Frontal view of the preoperative RSG. Indentation in the lateral margin of the dural sac and lack of opacification of the left S1 sheath. Recurrence of left S1 radicular pain 1 year after the operation. On the RSG then carried out (b and c), persistence of a clear-cut indentation in the lateral aspect of the dural sac, better visible on the oblique projection (c), with a lack of opacification of the left S1 radicular sheath. The RSG features differ little from the preoperative ones. The second operation shows the presence of cicatricial tissue without disc material

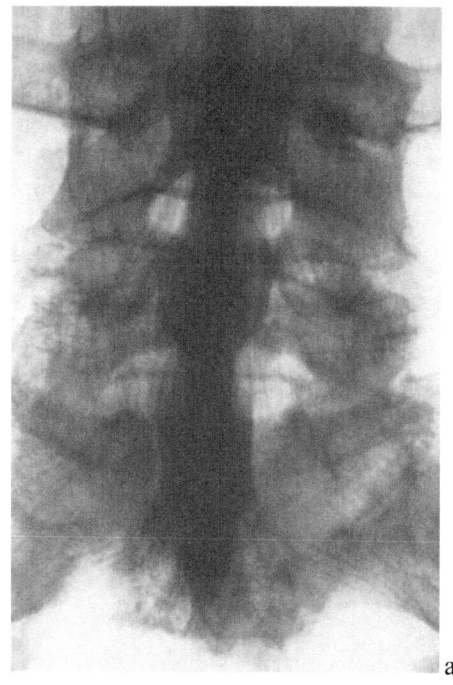

a

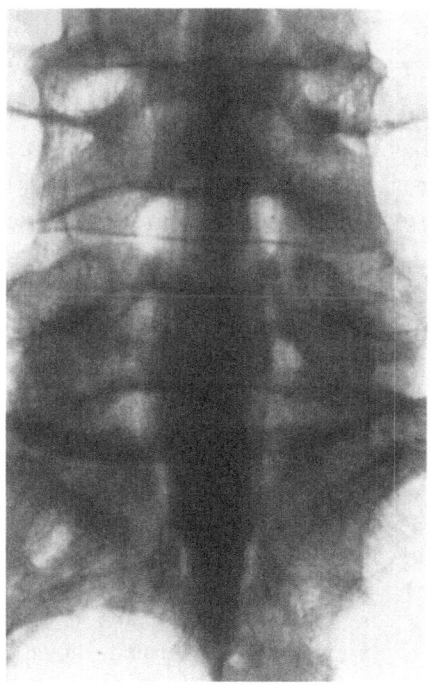

b

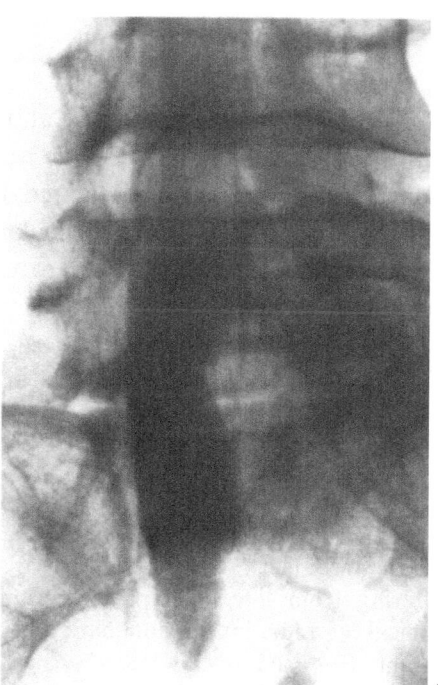

c

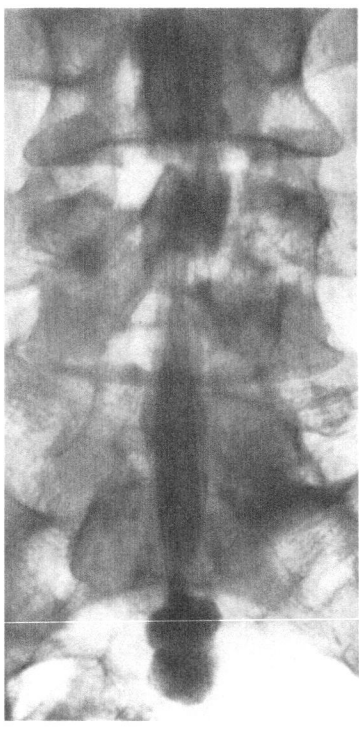

Fig. VII,4. **Arachnoiditis of the Dural Sac.** 41-year-old male operated 9 years previously for a left L5–S1 discal hernia, operated again 1 year previously for a right L5–S1 hernia, referred for a right L4 radiculitis. RSG shows an irregular stenosis of the cul-de-sac from L5 on and lack of opacification of the root sleeves. The saccular area has a heterogeneous appearance, and the opacification of an uneven medial diverticulum attached to the bottom of the dural sac by a narrow pedicle can be noted

level due to incomplete filling; at the reverse, they may be reduced to a small, rounded, more or less pediculated image. Note that, contrary to giant radicular cysts of the cauda equina [21], they are unique, medial, and readily opacified.

5. At the utmost, there may exist a lack of filling of the bottom of the dural sac which may show various features (Fig. VII,6). When the stop is not situated at the level of a disc (Fig. VII,7), it is more likely to be of arachnoiditic than hernial origin.

References of Chapter 7 see page 152.

Fig. VII,5. **Postoperative Arachnoiditis in a Case of Narrow Lumbar Canal.** 39-year-old female suffering from low back pain with bilateral atypical leg radiation predominant on the left. (a) and (b) Frontal and lateral views of the preoperative RSG. The diagnosis of a L4–5 discal herniation was made on the view of these x-rays, and the signs, though quite obvious, of narrow lumbar canal were overlooked, i.e., multiple anterior imprints of discal origin, intrasaccular hypertranslucency due to the bunching of the roots. The L4–5 stenosis with nonfilling of both L4 radicular sheaths is due to the occurrence of a slightly more important protrusion at that level in a narrow canal. The operation ▷ consisted of bilateral excision of the L4–5 disc. Two years later the patient complains of recurrence of the same pains. (c) and (d) The RSG x-rays then performed showed, on a frontal view (c), that the cul-de-sac is bare from roots from the L3–4 disc on, its margins are irregular, and the contrast pattern of the saccular area diminishes progressively toward the bottom. On a lateral view (d), the centrosaccular translucency is accentuated and surrounded by strips of high grade opacity. Thus, there exist signs of arachnoiditis added to those of a narrow canal

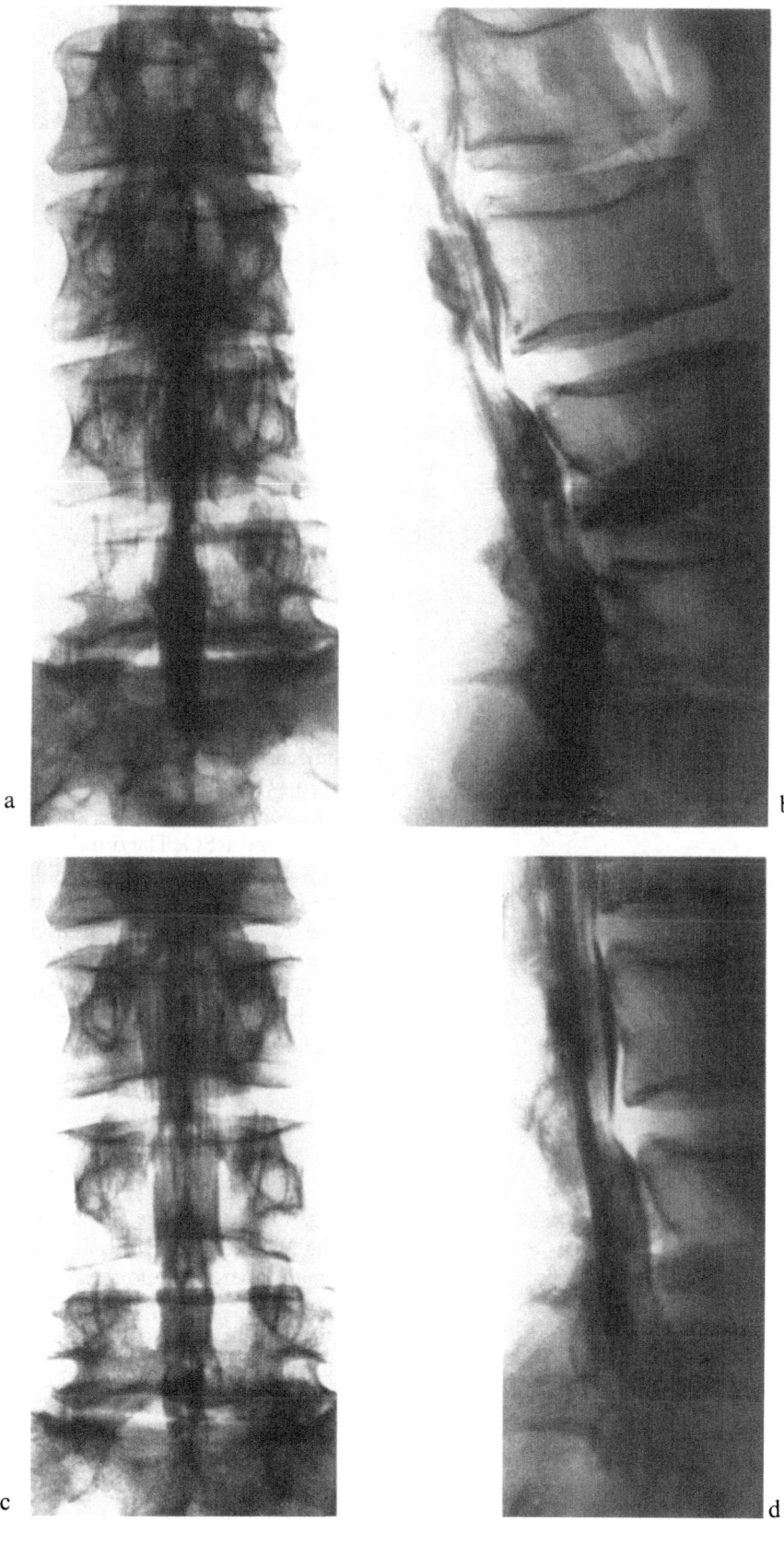

a

b

c

d

99

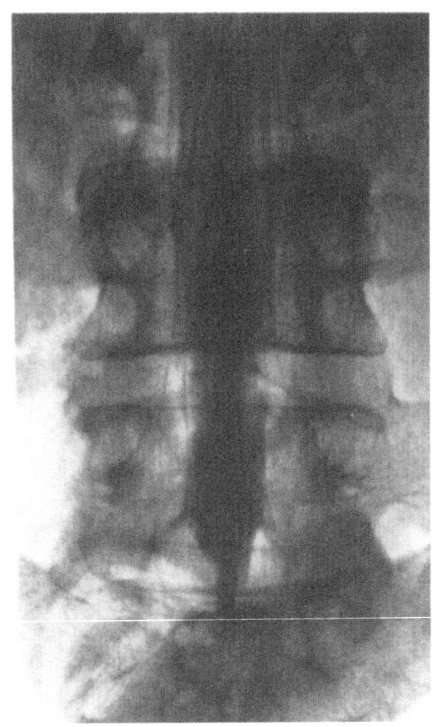
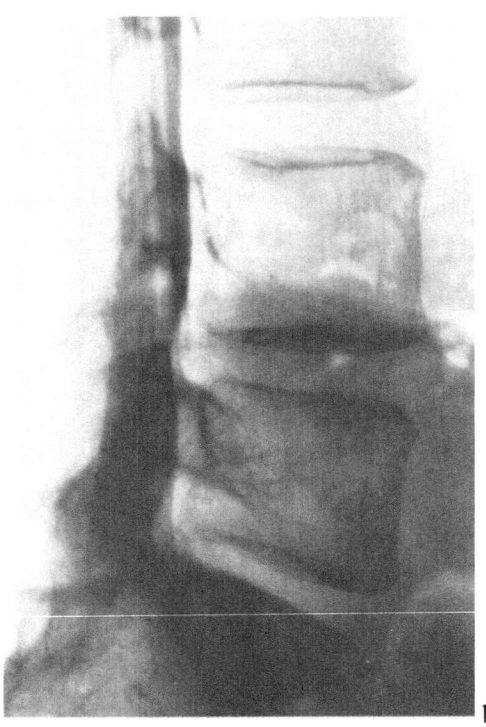

a

b

Fig. VII,6. **Amputation of the Cul-de-sac Due to Associated Arachnoiditis and Epidural Scar Formation.** 44-year-old female presenting a cauda equina syndrome from S1 downward, who already underwent RSG in another department (a) Frontal view of the second RSG. (b) Lateral view of the second RSG. The dural sac is stenosed in an asymmetric way and markedly detached from the posterior aspect of the L5–S1 disc. Operation is performed, consisting in excision of the L5–S1 herniation and showing the presence of a marked calcified epiduritis associated to arachnoiditis of the whole of sacral roots. This inflammatory process is felt to be the consequence of a bleeding lumbar puncture, in the absence of another known etiology

Fig. VII,7. **Complete Block Due to Arachnoiditis in a Patient who Underwent Multiple Disc Operations.** 60-year-old female operated upon twice on the L4–5 disc. A frontal view of the RSG performed 1 year after the second operation shows the lack of the posterior arch of L4, as well as a complete block of the contrast at the half-height of a vertebral body with well-filled overlying root sleeves. The level of the complete block at once suggests a nondiscal origin. As a matter of fact, a further operation shows signs of adhesive arachnoiditis when the dura mater is opened. No recurrence of herniation is then seen

Chapter 8. Dilatations of the Lumbosacral Nerve Root Sleeves and Megacauda

In this Chapter, we shall attempt to establish the radiologic diagnosis of such varied anomalies as megacauda, cystic dilatations of the root sleeves, and intrasacral cysts.

These anomalies are felt to be responsible for very various clinical signs, though they are often chance findings and therefore considered asymptomatic.

Their pathogeny is not well-known and the histologic examination of their walls helps very little in the precise diagnosis of their origin. The only cases in which the origin is proved are the uncommon post-traumatic or postoperative pseudocysts and those which occur—very rarely—in the course of an ankylosing spondylitis or spinal echinococcosis.

I. The Megacauda

We quote it here since it is often encountered associated with cystic and diverticular deformations of the lumbosacral nerve roots [41]. Megacauda is usually admitted to be of congenital origin, due to a growth disharmony between the bony canal and the dural sac.

Three main hypotheses were made, i.e.: (1) the lack of closure of the bony sacral canal [13] in favor of which is the frequent association of transitional anomalies and spina bifida, (2) the failure of ascent of the meningeal sac [20], which in the fetus reaches the coccyx; while the neural tube retracts upward, this meningeal sac ascends progressively up to S2 and remains attached to the coccyx by the filum terminale, and (3) a disturbance in the CSF resorption [15, 16, 26, 31, 38] producing a dilatation of the dural sac and a subsequent erosion of the vertebrae.

The main clinical signs attributed to those abnormal dilatations [40] consist in atypical lumbalgiae and lumbosacralgiae increased by the standing position, pains radiating to the legs, and sphincter disturbances. The onset of the symptoms occurs usually in adult life, often after a trauma or delivery.

Hanraets [32] proposed the following mechanical explanation for the occurrence of the radicular pains, viz., the roots are confined between the dural sac and the bony canal and show an angulation before their entrance into the intervertebral foramina. The operation consisting in longitudinal columnization which this author proposes should restore a normal course to the roots. Others perform laminectomies at several levels [40].

Vivid descriptions of the morphology of these megacauda have been given, such as "queen-bee-belly" or "leper's hand-shaped" [21, 22]. The only major difficulty consists in the decision from what size on a large dural sac becomes a megacauda. It is rather a global and morphologic appreciation than the result of a measurement (Fig. VIII,1). Let us quote both methods, i.e., Chaouat's, who says [15, 16] that this diagnosis can be established when the anteroposterior diameter of the dural sac at a

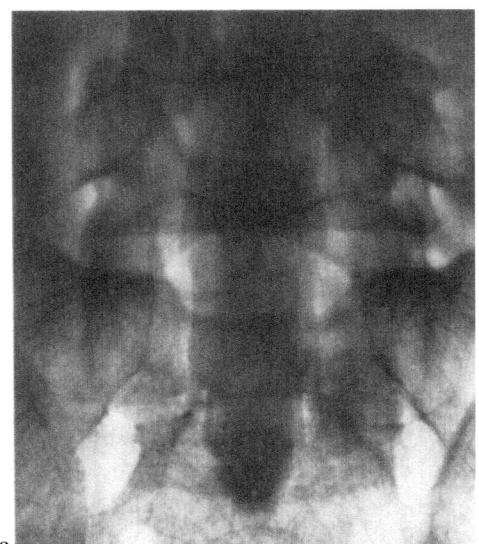

Fig. VIII,1. **Megacauda.** (a) Frontal view centered at the L5–S1 interspace. (b) Lateral view. (c) Posterior oblique view. Note the associated "muff-shaped" dilatations of the sacral root sleeves

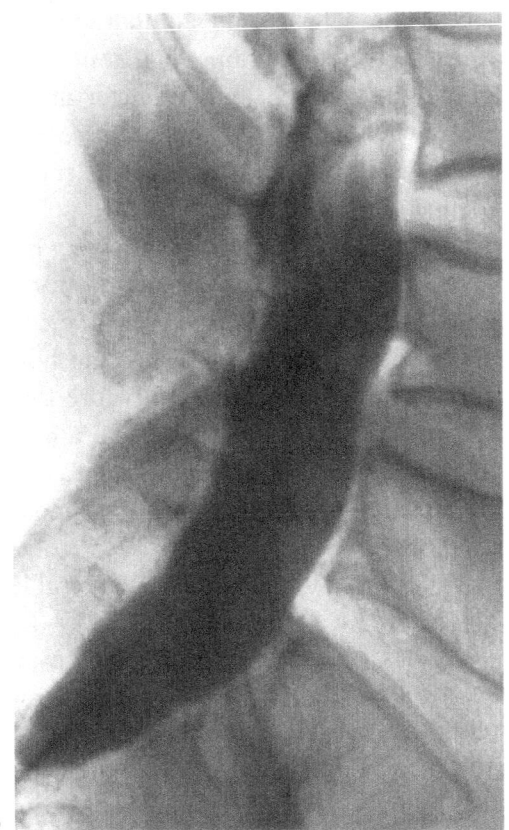

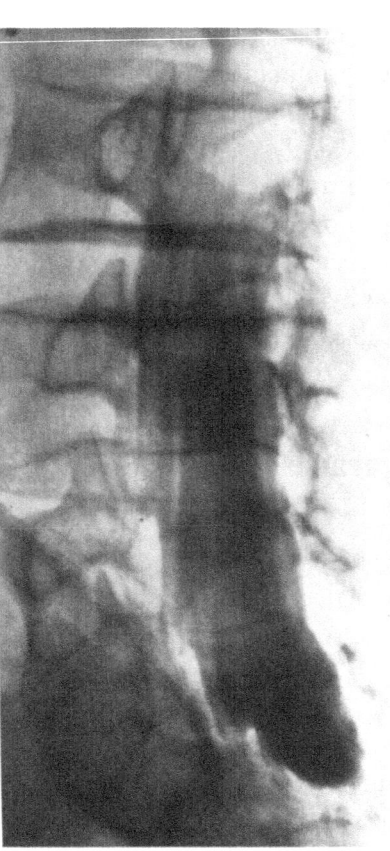

b

c

given level is greater than the hemidiameter of the corresponding vertebra and Komminoth et al. [40], who evaluate on a frontal view of the RSG the ratio between the interpedicular width and the width of the contrast columns as being approximately one at the L5 level.

Besides the increased anteroposterior and transverse diameters of the dural sac, other radiculosaccographic signs have been retained, viz., either a broad and short "mega cul-de-sac" with rounded fundus, or an overly long one protruding into the sacral canal with an ampulla-shaped dilatation [18]; the poor visualization of the radicular sheaths [40], or conversely the coexistence of cyst-like dilatations of the radicular sheaths which then become more apparent [49]; an intrasacral terminal dilatation, or even a bifid termination; an opacification of only a small height due to the increase of volume as well as to the excessive length of the megacauda [49]. Moreover, it has been pointed out [40] that the diagnosis of discal herniation is very difficult in the case of mega cul-de-sac, i.e., the imprint is not very obvious on a frontal view and may poorly appear with a double contour on the corresponding oblique projection; there is a lack of radicular signs owing to the nonvisualization of the root sleeves, so that in the end effect the lateral view proves to be the most informative.

Let us point out that the reverse condition of a narrow or "skimpy" thecal sac has also been reported [22]. It has been related to signs of neurologic claudication; but it seems quite rare that this narrowness is exclusively due to the dural sac itself whereas the bony canal has normal diameters. To our knowledge, the only case was reported by Hanraets [32].

II. Cyst-like Conditions and Dilatations of the Lumbosacral Nerve Root Sleeves

They are observed in varying degrees in 5–10% of the patients who underwent RSG. They usually involve several nerve roots and preferably the low lumbar and sacral roots. We usually call them "cystic dilatations" though their opacification demonstrates that they are communicating with the subarachnoid space.

The type most often described is the perineurial cyst of Tarlov, but other types of abnormally long arachnoidal prolongations over nerve roots have been reported (Fig. VIII,2). We shall try to specify their radiologic differential signs.

The pathologic significance of these different types of meningeal dilatations is discussed [6, 17, 59, 63].

A. Perineurial — or Periradicular — Cysts

They have been described in 1938 by Tarlov on postmortem examinations [67–70]. They are electively located on the sacral roots and may thus cause erosions of the sacral canalar walls. They are dilatations of the perineural sheaths, that is to say, at the level of the posterior root ganglion. Their wall is transparent, constituted by meningeal tissue with some nervous fibers within it.

Their clinical significance is discussed and their discovery is very often a chance finding during a positive contrast examination of the subarachnoidal space. However, they could be correlated with sacral radiculalgiae and genitourinary disturbances. Tarlov reports some cases of clinical recovery due to excision of the cysts [70], and proposes three criteria for their differentiation from other meningeal diverticula, i.e.:

1. Delayed opacification by the oily contrast medium after myelography [60]
2. Location on the course of a nerve root
3. Typical histologic pattern of their walls

Their radiculosaccographic aspect may be considered characteristic when supplementary, more or less rounded cystic dilatations suspended to the sacral nerve roots,

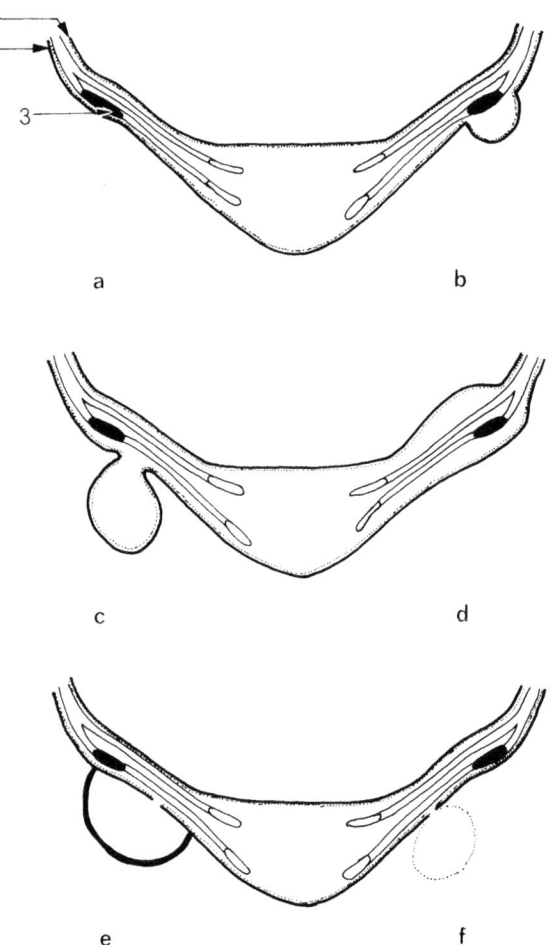

Fig. VIII,2. **Schematic Drawing of the Different Types of Dilatations and Diverticula of the Lumbosacral Root Sleeves.** (a) *Normal anatomical conditions.* (1) dura mater, (2) arachnoid, (3) nerve root ganglion. (b) *Tarlov's cyst.* The cystic dilatation is located close to the nerve root ganglion and has the histologic peculiarity of containing nervous fibers and ganglionic cells within its wall. (c) *Meningeal diverticle.* Localized dilatation of the radicular meningeal layerings. (d) *Diffuse dilatation of the radicular sheath.* (e) *False cyst.* This has a nonmeningeal wall and develops through a—possibly traumatic—breach in the meningeal layerings. (f) *Arachnoidal diverticle.* Its wall has an arachnoidal wall and it is evaginated through a dural breach

bilateral and more or less symmetric, are belatedly opacified—30–60 min after injection. On x-rays taken immediately after the injection, one may suspect their presence at the sight of poorly contrasted opacities with blurred margins superimposed on the sacrum (Fig. VIII,3). In oily myelography, Tarlov's cysts are opacified only several days—or even weeks—later; the earliest was observed 24 h postmyelography [4].

B. Other Types of Diverticula and Dilatations of the Lumbosacral Nerve Root Sleeves

An unusually long arachnoidal prolongation over nerve roots causes them to be better visualized. They may show several bulges along their course and more or less proximal dilatations.

The histologic pattern of the diverticular walls is variable: they are constituted either

Fig. VIII,4. **Multiple and Symmetric Dilatations** ▷ **of the Radicular Sheaths.** (a) Rounded and exclusively distal dilatations (*arrows*) projecting under the pedicular shadows. The incomplete opacification of the distal dilatation of L5 sheaths (*arrowheads*) may be related to the hypertrophied facetal joints L4–5 (*asterisks*) causing narrow radicular canals. (b) Diffuse dilatations proximal as well as distal of the L5 and S1 sheaths (*arrows*). The delayed opacification of the right L5 radicular sheath (*arrowheads*) is consistent with a compression by a discal herniation of the root emergence (*crossed arrow*)

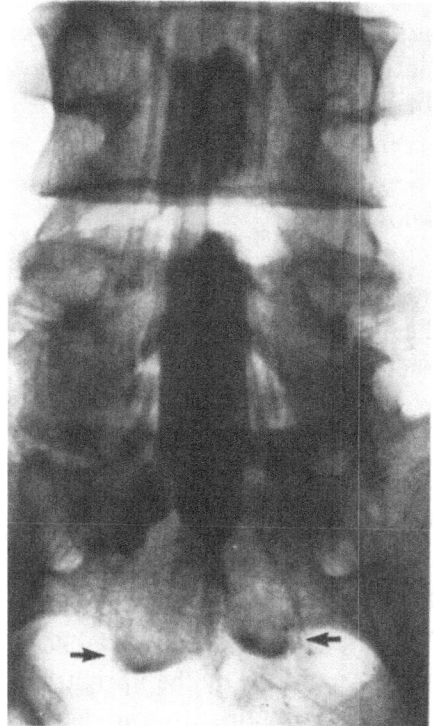 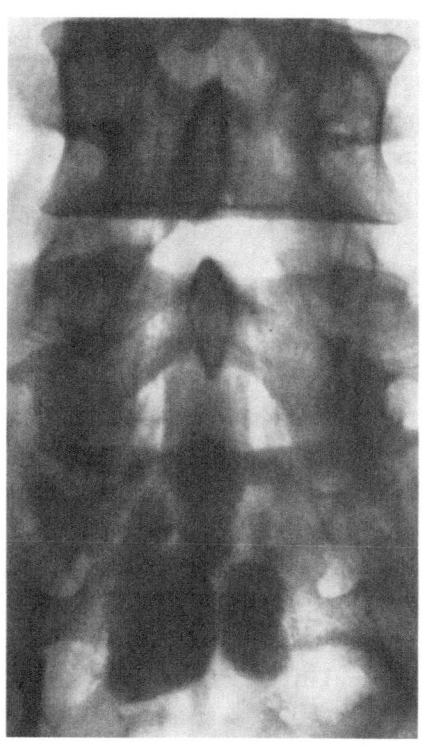

a   b

Fig. VIII,3. **Periradicular Cystic Dilatations (Perineurial Cysts of Tarlov).** (a) Early film. (b) Delayed film (1 hour later). The early view (a) shows a diffuse "muff-shaped" dilatation of the S1 and S2 radicular sheaths. Late views have been undertaken because abnormal cystic pouches had been seen (*arrow*) projecting on the sacrum. One hour later (b), these cystic pouches are well-opacified, almost symmetric, suspended at the bottom of the dural sac, and located at the place of the inferior sacral roots

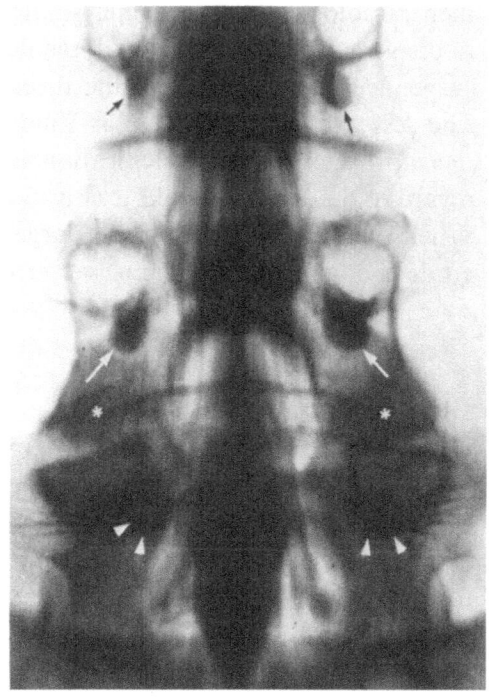 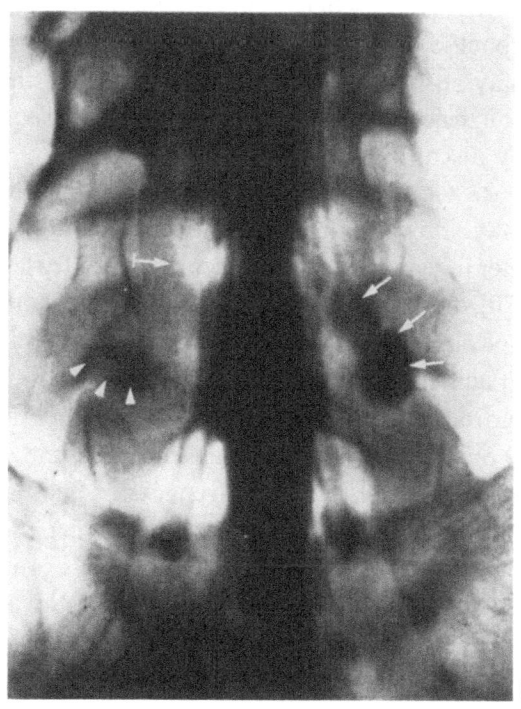

a   b

by a meningeal layer—i.e., dura mater lined with arachnoid—or only by an arachnoidal one, presumingly due to an evagination mechanism through a dural breach. In any case, the absence of nervous fibers seems to be constant.

We shall describe three morphologic types:

1. The first is a variety with diffuse and symmetric dilatations of the nerve sheaths all along the lumbosacral spine characterized by their smooth pattern and the constant presence of terminal dilatations situated at the entrance of the intervertebral foramina. This is only a variant of the normal pattern, as a rather large increase of the caliber of the sheaths, resulting in a more distal opacification (Fig. VIII,4). The terminal diverticula may be found isolated, as rounded or semilunar opacities projecting along the inferior margin of the pedicular cortex, chiefly in the upper lumbar region, where the opacity of slender sheaths may fail to appear on plain films. The constant occurrence and the symmetry of these dilatations may be used for diagnostic purposes, viz., when one of them is not opacified or had delayed opacification, one may suspect a mechanical obstacle on the course of the root, such as a compression by discal herniation.

2. Contrariwise, the radicular sheaths may show localized dilatations resembling meningeal diverticula. According to Tarlov [70], these diverticula differ from the perineurial cysts in that they are readily opacified and their site along the root is more proximal. According to the same author, such a diverticulum may become a cyst and thus be pathogeneous when an inflammatory process obstrudes its neck (a postmyelographic arachnoiditis, for example).

3. Finally, one can observe in cases of megacauda irregular or bumpy dilatations of the lumbosacral root sleeves, which seem to be common and without significance.

C. Intrasacral Cyst

These lesions have been termed differently, viz., occult intrasacral meningocoele [2, 3, 25, 35, 36, 53, 73], sacral extradural cyst [61], caudal diverticulum of the thecal sac or giant intrasacral cyst [64], and expansion of the subarachnoid space in the lumbosacral region [34], which causes some confusion. A peculiar variety is described as anterior sacral meningocoele [10–12, 19, 39, 43, 45, 58, 62, 71].

The related clinical picture is very variable, i.e., low backache possibly accentuated by the upright position and possibly radiating to the legs, micturition disturbances, tenderness on firm pressure over the sacrum.

Even with the help of a histologic examination of the cystic wall, it is not always possible to differentiate meningeal diverticula from true meningocoeles. Moreover, their radiologic aspect is rather similar and is displayed as a unique and medial sac suspended at the bottom of the thecal sac. The less the contrast agent is fluid, then the more delayed its opacification is with regard to that of the dural sac (Fig. VIII,5). When the cystic formations are large, they erode the walls of the spinal sacral canal.

D. Rare Varieties of Meningeal Dilatations in the Lumbosacral Area

Multiple etiological circumstances may be accompanied or followed by epidural cyst formations in the sacral or lumbar spinal canal—intradural arachnoidal cysts are exceptional in the lumbar area [5, 51, 72, 74].

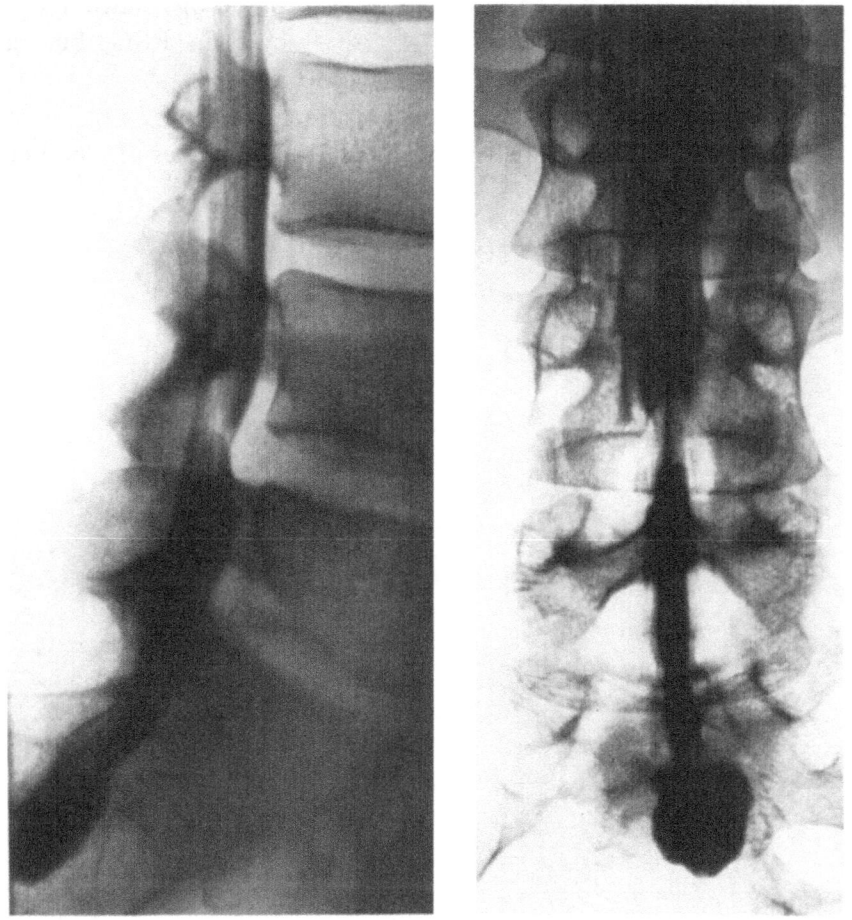

Fig. VIII,5. **Medially Located Intrasacral Cyst.** (a) Lateral view. (b) Frontal view. This patient additionally presents a right L4–5 discal herniation and an atypical narrowing of the lower part of the dural sac

1. *Posttraumatic meningeal diverticula* may occur after a fall [1, 14, 24, 27, 48, 50] or an operation [8, 23, 29, 30, 44, 55, 56, 65]. They consist either in arachnoidal evagination through a breach in the dura mater or in false cysts surrounded by a fibrous capsule. Those cystic elements may increase their volume by two types of mechanisms, i.e., either by the constitution of a valve mechanism retaining the CSF or by a wide communication with the subarachnoid space which causes them to be submitted to the hydrostatic pressure. Their volume causes them to compress the neigh-boring structures which accounts for the fact that their clinical signs are accentuated by the standing position.

2. *Extradural Cysts Associated with Rheumatoid Spondylitis.* A cauda equina syndrome [7, 28, 33] may occur in the late and nonevolutive stages—"burned out stages"—of a rheumatoid spondylitis. The most commonly encountered myelographic picture consists of multiple arachnoidal cysts [42, 46, 47, 57], which may erode the posterior walls of the lumbar spinal canal. It has been postulated that these arachnoidal cysts are probably a late result of the

arachnoiditis which existed in the early inflammatory stages of the disease.

3. *Extradural Ganglion Cysts* of synovial origin [9, 37, 54, 66] do not belong to this pathology since they do not behave like cysts in RSG, but rather like extradural masses.

References of Chapter 8 see page 153.

Chapter 9. Lumbar Spinal Stenosis

I. Introduction

Under the heading of lumbar spinal stenosis we deal with all circumstances in which one or several cauda equina roots are involved by an osteoligamentous narrowing [3, 61, 66, 104, 105], whether by a stenosis of the spinal canal on the whole or by a deformation of the radicular canal [67], i.e., stenosis of the lateral part of the spinal canal [39, 85] up to the intervertebral foramen (see Chap. 3) [38, 50].

Two types of stenosis may be schematically opposed, one related to a congenital dysplasia of the spine itself (*developmental stenosis*) [82, 102, 103] and the other to degenerative changes of the posterior arch (*spondylotic degenerative stenosis*) [17, 27, 33, 34, 92, 97].

Bone dysplasia combines in varying degrees narrowness of the posterior arch and hypertrophy of its constituting elements (Fig. IX,1 b) [31, 32, 84]. The narrowness is chiefly related to short pedicles and to verticalization of the laminae with location close to the midline (Fig. IX,1 c) [43, 78], whereas the hypertrophy predominates in the facetal joints, which moreover have an abnormally medial location [35]. The resulting canalar stenosis is concentric, anteroposteriorly predominant, with a possible trefoil-shaped deformation of the canalar lumen, and constitution of two lateral recesses and a posterior one [62, 84].

The canalar narrowing related to spondylosis is caused more by the hypertrophy and the deformation of the facetal joints than by a posterior hypertrophic spur formation of the vertebral end-plates. The deformation of the canalar lumen is similar to the previous one but mainly concerns the radicular canals [17, 38, 67], since the arthrosic changes of the facetal joints accentuate the lateral recesses and create a posterior recess. It is thus an acquired deformation of a congenitally normal or subnormal canal (Fig. IX,1 d).

The developmental stenoses are often diffuse, whereas the degenerative stenoses involve one or several segments and often develop on an spine already dysplastic. The condition is even more complicated when a discal herniation occurs, the clinical signs of which are earlier the narrower the lumbar canal is [86, 98].

The diverse clinical features [20] are due to the fact that the radicular compression is located either outside the dural sac in the lateral part of the spinal canal — neurogenic intermittent claudication with sensory motor deficit of one or two roots [67] — or inside the dural sac that is compressed on the whole — neurogenic claudication of the cauda equina (see Chap. 3) [41, 81, 109, 110].

II. Bony Radiologic Signs

The examination of the x-rays of the lumbar spine provides, on the one hand, a number of morphologic anomalies suggest-

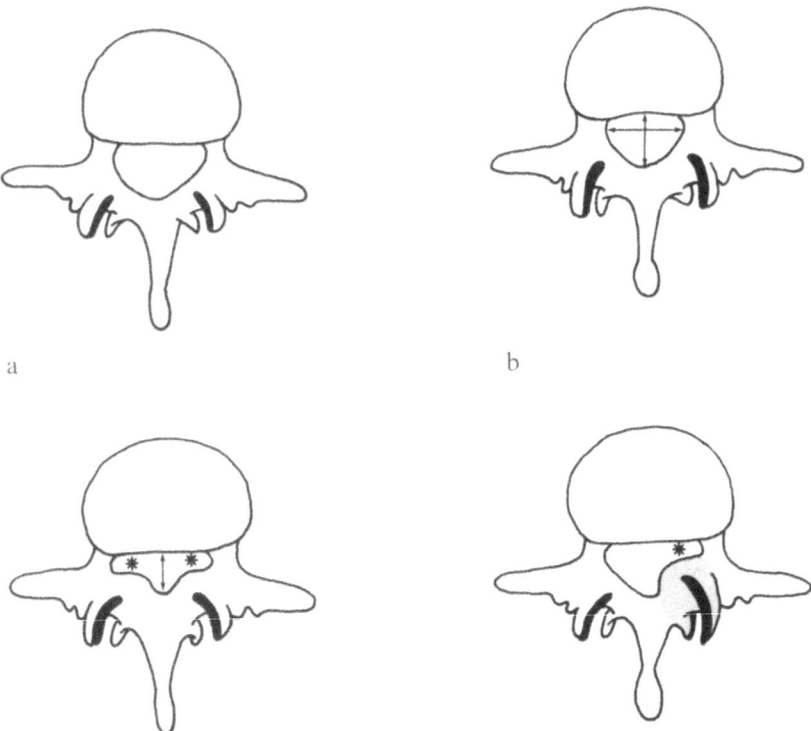

a   b

c   d

Fig. IX,1. **Schematic Drawing of the Different Types of Bony Stenoses in Axial View.** (a) *Normal anatomical conditions*. The canalar area is approximately triangular in shape. Note the normal obliquity of the facetal joint spaces with regard to the midsagittal axis and the cylindric section of the facets. (b) *Concentric stenosis* of the canal. The canalar area is narrowed in all its dimensions but keeps its triangular shape. Pedicles are short and the dysplastic posterior arch renders facetal joint spaces more sagittal, more flat, and more medially located. (c) *Trefoil-shaped deformation* of the canal. The hypertrophic facetal joints bulge into the canalar lumen and are responsible for the narrowing of the lateral recesses (*asterisks*) (narrow radicular canals). Moreover, the midsagittal diameter is the most narrowed. (d) *Asymmetric deformation* of the canalar lumen due to arthrosic changes involving the facetal joints. The transverse and midsagittal diameters of the canal are normal, though the canalar area is deformed by the bulging of an hypertrophied arthrosic facetal joint, which narrows the lateral recess (*asterisk*) (narrow radicular canal) and creates a posterior recess

ing the presence of stenosis and, on the other hand, objective features derived from the canalar measurements.

A. Elementary Morphologic Anomalies [5]

They are already visible on plain x-rays, but the tomography allows a better analysis of the anomalies of the posterior arch.

1. Abnormal features suggesting *the spinal dysplasia* to be possibly related to a stenosis are:

a. On lateral views: The anteroposterior diameter of the intervertebral foramina is reduced and they may show biloculate deformation (it is necessary to keep in mind that the L5–S1 intervertebral foramen is normally smaller). The decreased anteroposterior diameter of an intervertebral foramen is related to short pedicles, whereas

110

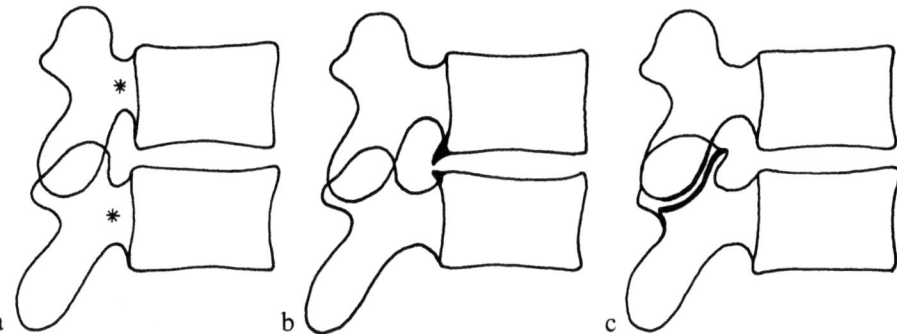

Fig. IX,2. **Biloculated Deformation of the Inter-vertebral Foramina.** (a) Related to short pedicles (*asterisks*). (b) Related to an osteophytic spur formation of the vertebral end-plate or of the superior articular facet (c)

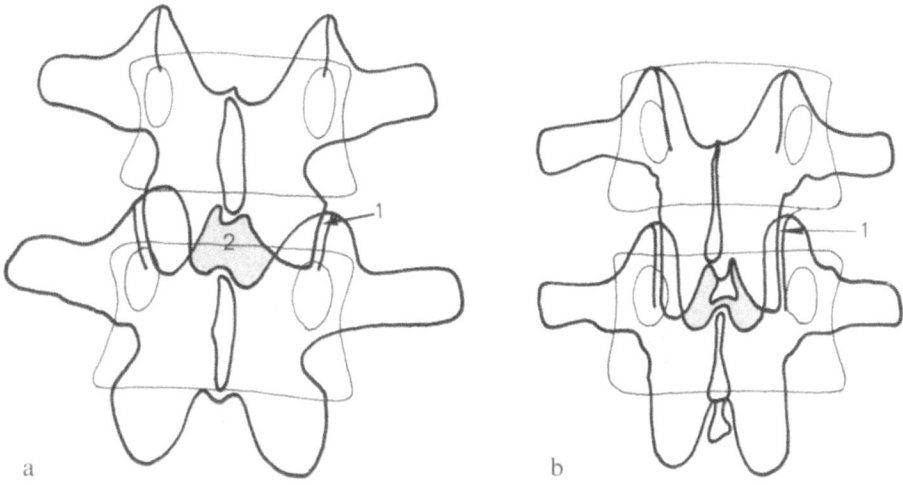

Fig. IX,3. **Schematic Representation of the Structures of the Posterior Arch in Frontal Projection.** (a) Under normal conditions. (b) In the case of narrow lumbar canal of developmental origin. The facetal joint spaces (*1*) are too vertical and more visible than normally due to their sagittalization. The closure of the interlaminar angle (*2*) with reduction of the interapophysola-minar radiolucent area passes through the ab-normally medial location of the facetal joints

the biloculated deformation is due either to the presence of a vertebral spur forma-tion or the degenerative hypertrophy of a superior articular process (Fig. IX,2).

b. On frontal views and on tomograms: Hypervisibility of the radiolucencies of the facetal joint spaces is related to the abnor-mal orientation of the facets (Fig. IX,3). The laminae appear to be higher, partly because they are really higher and partly because they are too vertical. Since the an-gle they form posteriorly by joining each other closes, this leads to the occlusion of the losange-shaped laminar interspace (Fig. IX,4) [5].

2. In cases of *degenerative stenosis,* the striking features are, on the one hand, a marginal condensation of the posterior in-terapophyseal interspaces—especially vis-ible on oblique projections—and, on the other hand, the hypertrophy of the corre-sponding facetal joints—especially visible on frontal views as abnormal, rounded, uni-or bilateral bony opacities at one or several

111

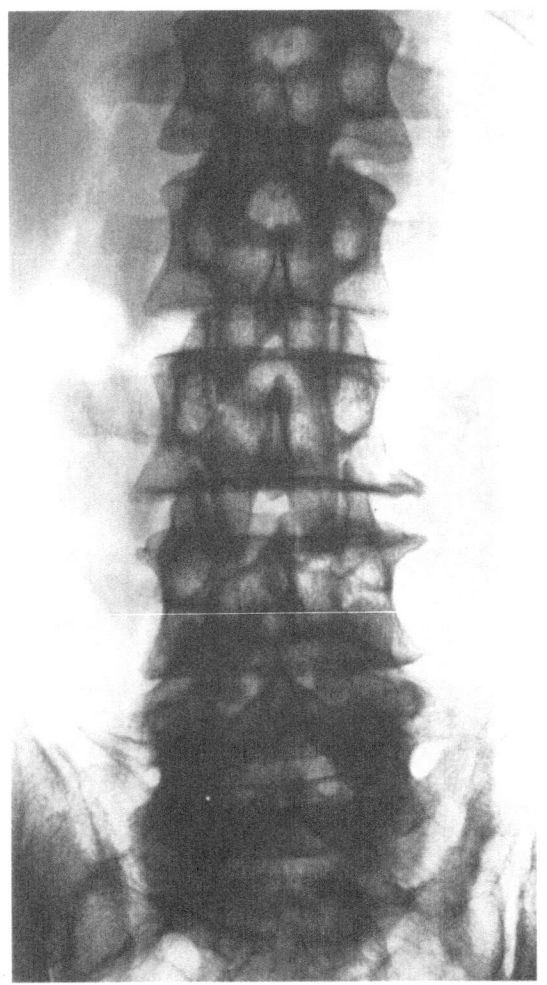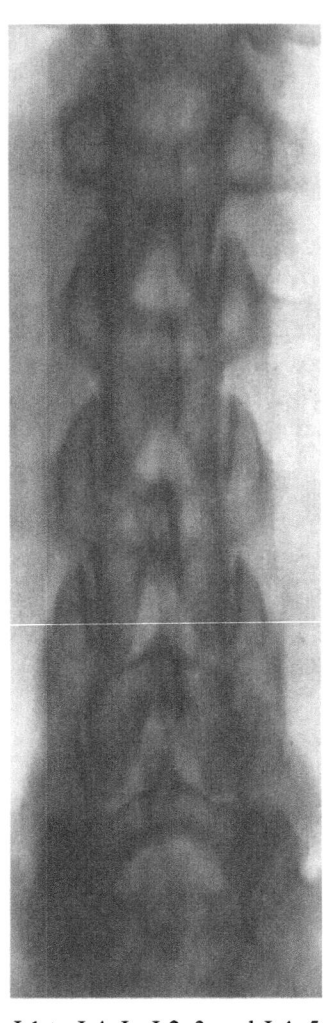

a b

Fig. IX,4. **Signs of Dysplastic Posterior Arch in a Case of Narrow Lumbar Canal.** (a) Frontal view. (b) Frontal tomography in the plane of the facetal joints. The facetal joint spaces are sagittal and more visible than normally from L1 to L4. In L2–3 and L4–5, the interapophysolaminar space is markedly reduced, and in L4–5, it is at once reduced and deformed by the hypertrophic left L4–5 facetal joint

levels (Fig. IX,5) [12, 79, 90]. More rarely, the above-described anomalies are associated with a spondylolisthesis with intact neural arch, which makes canalar stenosis more important.

B. Appreciation of the Morphology of the Canal and Measurements

Conventional (44, 57) and computerized (48, 51) tomography are the only types which provide information about the shape of the canal at each level, i.e., retrovertebral (intraosseous segment) and retrodiscal (articular segment) [58, 91]. Verbiest (1976) [105] points out the lack of precision of measurements made on tomographic x-rays, viz., on midsagittal tomograms performed with a complex motion, the posterior limit of the canal is ill-defined; conversely, in conventional transverse axial tomography, it is the anterior limit of the canal

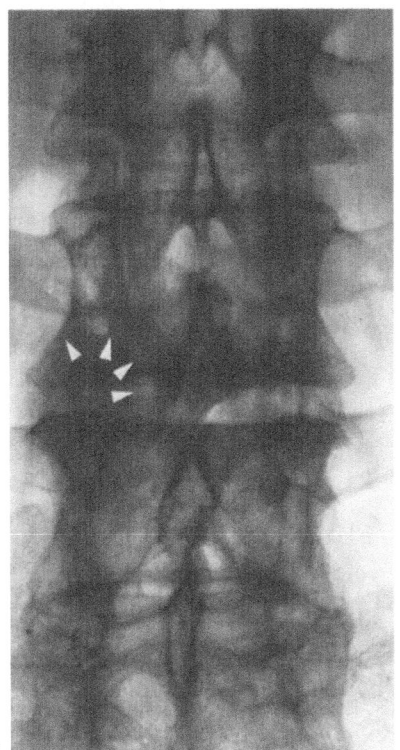

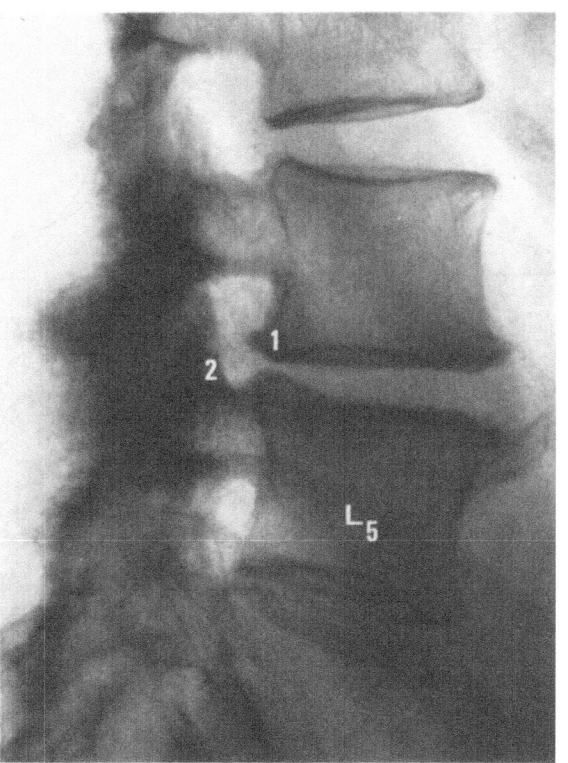

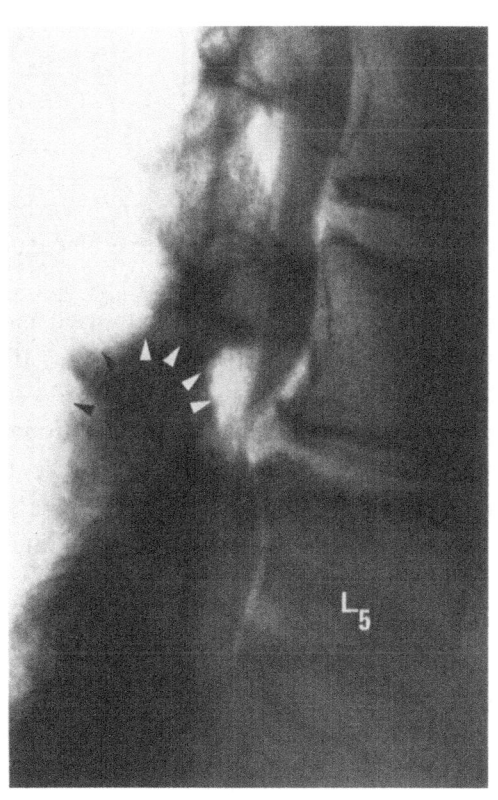

Fig. IX,5. **Degenerative Stenosis.** (a) Plain frontal view. (b) Lateral plain film. (c) Lateral view of RSG. Hypertrophy and densification of the facetal joints are predominant on the right (*arrowheads*). It is such that the corresponding interapophysolaminar space has disappeared. The intervertebral foramen is narrowed at the same level by a posterior vertebral osteophyte (*1*) and a hypertrophied superior articular facet of L5 (*2*). RSG confirms the canalar stenosis to be predominant in L4–5, i.e., marked disturbances of the intrasaccular contrast distribution and anterior indentation facing the osteophyte

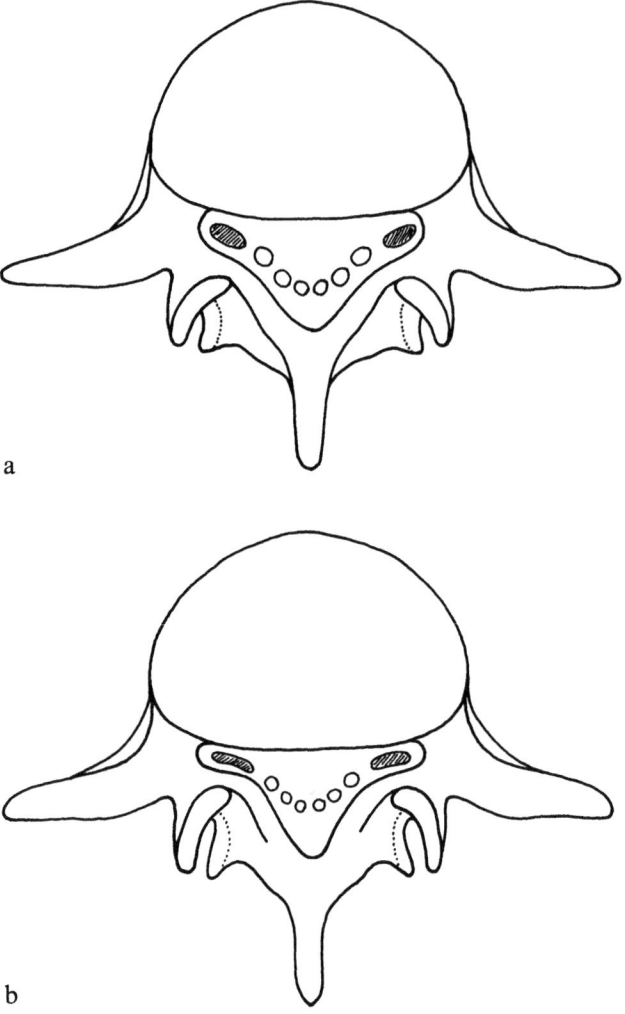

a

b

Fig. IX,6. **The Limits of the Canalar Measurements.** Theoretically, a narrow canal may show a typical trefoil deformation and have normal anteroposterior and transverse diameters. (a) Schematic representation of a normal lumbar vertebra. (b) Representation of a lumbar vertebra with narrow canal

which is ill-defined. Therefore, Verbiest took into account peroperatory measurements for his studies.

The radiologic measurements used most frequently [22, 23, 30, 54, 106, 107], i.e., anteroposterior diameter — APD — and transverse diameter — TD — are additionally criticizable because they do not take the possibility of a trefoil-shaped deformation of the canal and/or of the presence of lateral and posterior recesses into account (Fig. IX,6).

The measurement of the APD — on midsagittal tomograms — proves, however, to be the most useful in current practice for the detection of predominantly antero-

posterior stenoses, which are the most common.

Jones and Thomson's index [59] is also a quite useful method of approach by providing an approximate ratio between the surface of the canalar section and the surface of the vertebral body section.

III. Radiculosaccographic Signs

RSG provides a supplementary number of arguments for the diagnosis of stenosis [11] and contributes to determine its upward extent.

114

A. RSG Signs of Diffuse Stenosis

The dural sac which does not have enough space is molded against the canalar walls and assumes its internal reliefs [11]. This is mainly seen on the lateral projections, i.e.:

1. Its anterior margin is undulated by the successive concavities due to the discs and the convexities related to the concave posterior aspects of the vertebral bodies.

2. Its posterior margin is also undulated because of its alternating contact with the bony and the ligamentous structures of the posterior arch.

Thus, the dural sac takes on a narrow, even moniliform appearance, which is still accentuated in the extension position [111]. The ascent of the contrast medium column is commonly observed as well as the appearance of segmental lacks of opacification at the level of the narrowed "articular segments" of the canal (Fig. IX,7).

Within the dural sac, the roots appear too clearly [11, 105] and may moreover be bunched together to form a unique, central translucency. The contrast medium is then distributed around these roots and appears as opaque areas, either multileveled and retrovertebral or as double-track on either — anterior or posterior — side of the cauda equina (Fig. IX,8).

It should be noted that intrasaccular lacunar defects displayed through positive myelography with oily contrast media have been felt by some authors to be due to hypertrophied and sinuous roots — "redundant or knotted nerve roots" — [42, 49, 87, 94] and would be chiefly encountered in narrow lumbar canals [21, 29, 75, 79, 101]. We would like to suggest [11] that these images are to be compared with images of hypervisible and bunched roots in RSG [62] and that they are more striking in oil myelography due to the absence of penetration

of the less fluid contrast between the roots that are encased in a narrow dural sac.

The radicular sheaths are poorly visible and on a course which is too short; several among them may be nonfilled as soon as their emergence.

The frontal views of RSG are the least valuable for the diagnosis of stenosis. Indeed, the low contrast pattern of the saccular area with blunted contours are rather evocative signs, but they are easily overlooked since they are considered to be the result of poor technique (Fig. IX,9).

B. RSG Signs of Localized Stenosis

They are mainly related to a discal herniation or to hypertrophic degenerative changes developing in a narrow canal.

In cases of narrow canal, the herniated disc often causes a stop of the water-soluble contrast medium (Fig. IX,10). Besides, there may be multiple herniations which give rise to localized stenoses of the dural sac rather than to exclusively radicular signs or indentations of the lateral margins of the dural sac (Fig. IX,11).

Spondylotic changes in the posterior facets produce more or less symmetric anatomical changes, due to their bilaterality. In RSG, frontal tomography permits a precise determination of the bony origin of the compression by demonstrating on the same section the close contact of the lateral aspect of the dural sac and the hypertrophic facetal joint. This type of compression, exerting on the posterolateral aspects of the dural sac, most often spares the roots (Fig. IX,12) [10–12].

Localized stenoses may be anteroposterior when a large facetal joint is at the same level as a hypertrophic vertebral bar. At this precise narrowed level, an abnormal increase of the root translucencies may be

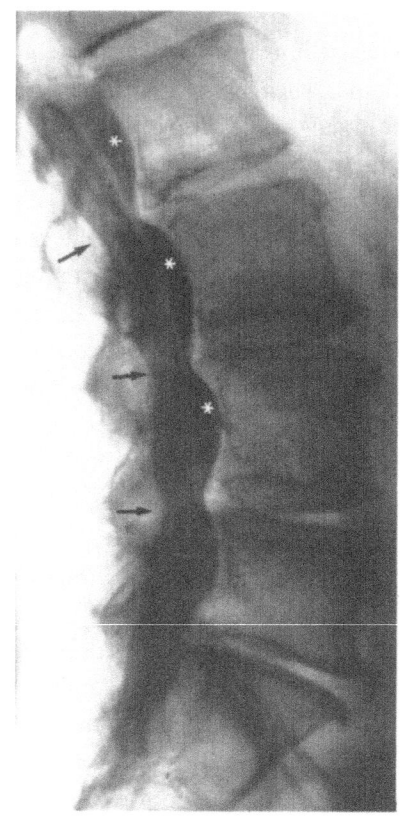

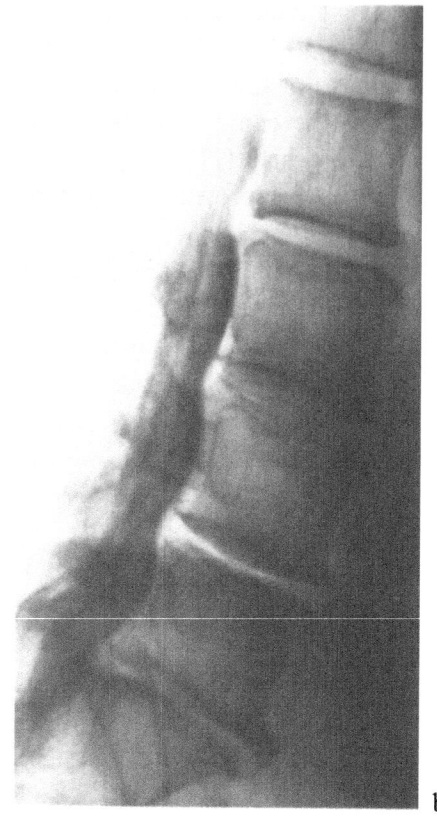

a

b

Fig. IX,7. **Increase of the RSG Signs of Narrow Canal During the Extension** (a), and with regard to the flexion position (b). The extension chiefly accentuates the multileveled posterior indentations (*arrows*) and the retrovertebral stasis (*asterisks*)

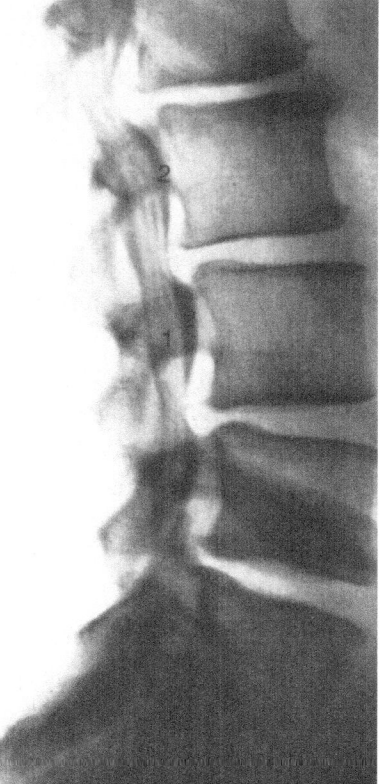

Fig. IX,8. **Signs of Intrasaccular Constraint in a Case of Diffuse Degenerative Narrowing.** The signs of intrasaccular constraint are marked, i.e., centrocanalar translucency (*1*) and multileveled stasis (*2*). The posterior vertebral osteophytosis and the thickening of the retrovertebral soft tissues is a sign of degenerative involvement

116

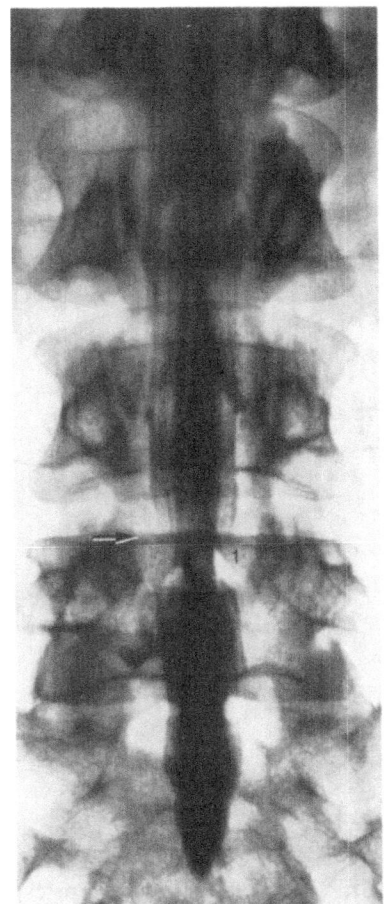

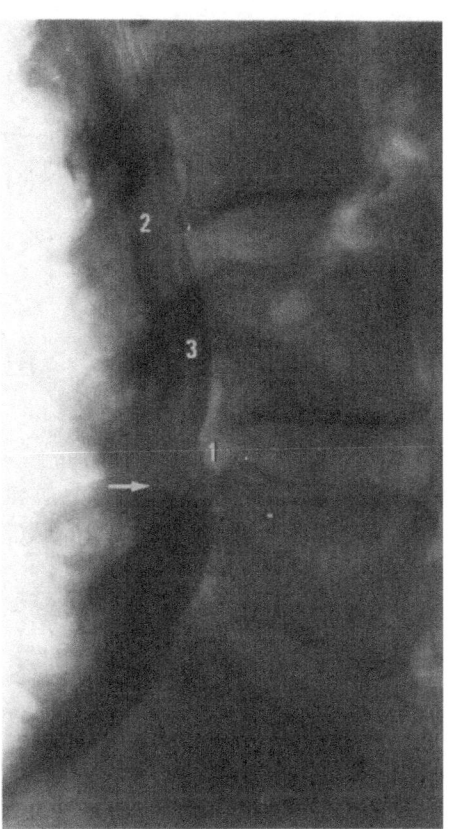

a

b

Fig. IX,9. **Discal Herniation in a Narrow Canal.** (a) Radiculo-saccographic frontal projection. (b) Lateral projection. (c) Left posterior oblique projection. The coexistence of a left antero-lateral compression due to a hernia (*1*) and a right postero-lateral one due to an enlarged facetal joint (*arrow*) accounts for the L4–5 stenosis. The intrasaccular roots above the stenosis are hyperlucent (*2*) and there is a retrovertebral image of "stasis" above the hernia (*3*)

c

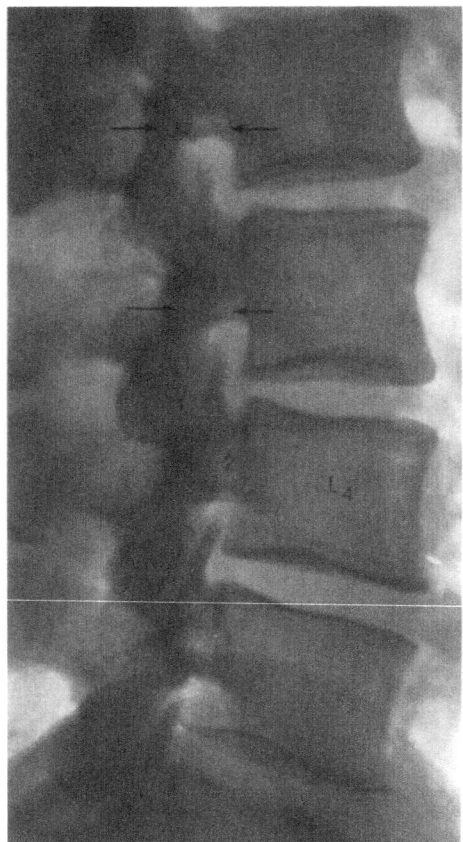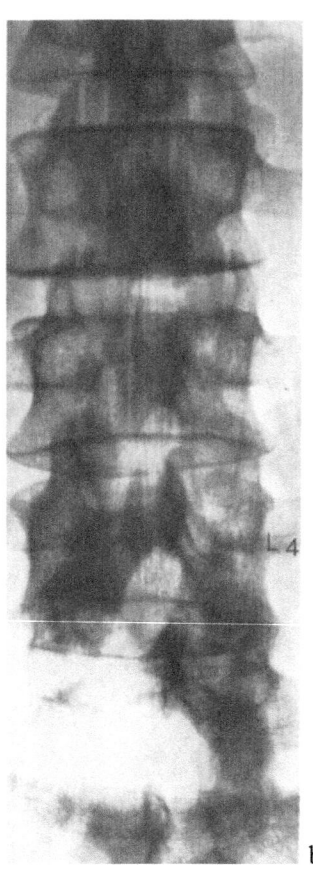

a
b

Fig. IX,10. **Developmental Lumbar Spinal Stenosis With Complete Stop Due to Discal Herniation.** (a) Plain lateral projection of the lumbar spine: marked sagittal narrowing of the three last intervertebral foramina, obstructed by the superimposition of the upper articular processes (*1*). The pedicles are especially short (*2*). The anteroposterior diameter can be evaluated in L2 and L3 to be about 15 mm (*facing arrows*). (b) RSG shows the stop to be located at L4–5

seen, and above this level, retrovertebral areas of contrast medium accumulation, which also point out the very size of the stenosis.

IV. Value of RSG With Regard to Other Contrast Examinations for the Investigation of Narrow Lumbar Canals

In this field, RSG seems to be the method of choice [11, 12, 70, 74, 83, 105] because of the fluidity of the contrast medium used and of the possibility of its dilution in CSF. The water-soluble contrast is more able to opacify homogeneously the whole of the lumbar subarachnoid space, thus allowing the study of its entire content and inside morphology. Moreover, it permits one to display the heterogeneous features witnessing the intrasaccular contraint of the roots inside the dural sac. Thanks to its fluidity, the contrast medium reaches the lowermost segments of the narrowest dural sacs, thus providing indispensable indications as to the vertical extent of the stenosis. Finally,

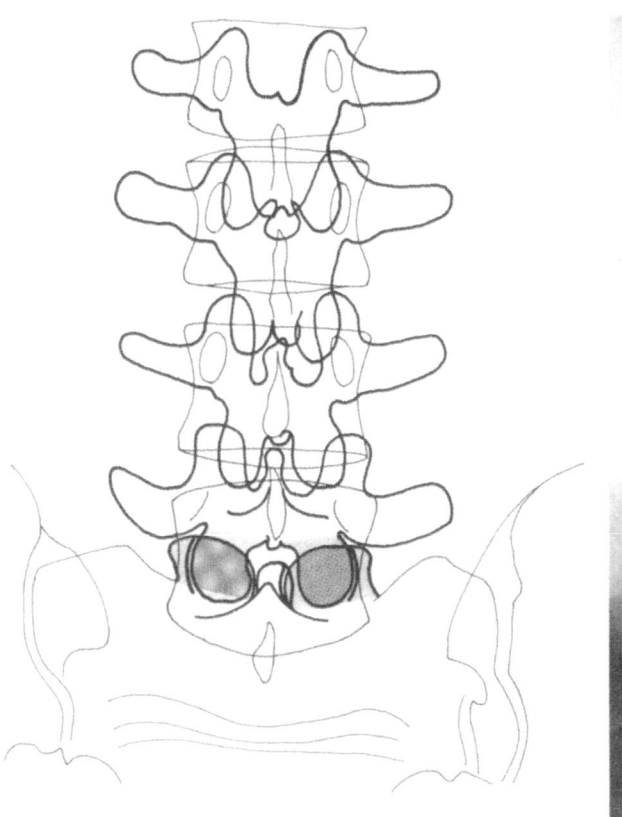

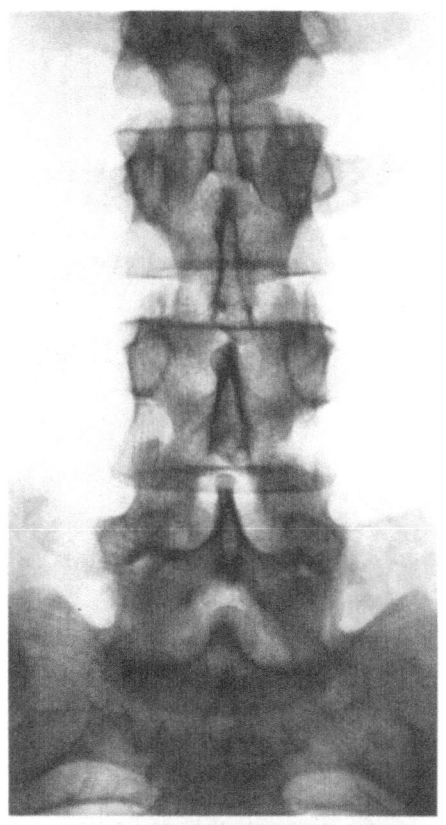
a

Fig. IX,11. **Lumbar Spinal Stenosis Localized in L5–S1 Due to Dysplastic Facetal Joints.** (a) Plain frontal view. (b) Plain lateral view. (c) Frontal zonogram. The facetal joints are abnormally bulky and densified, especially the left one. This is displayed on the lateral projection by a deformation of the translucency of the corresponding intervertebral foramen which is in contrast with the particularly large appearance of the overlying foramina. The L5–S1 stenosis is striking with regard to the rather wide appearance of the dural sac situated above

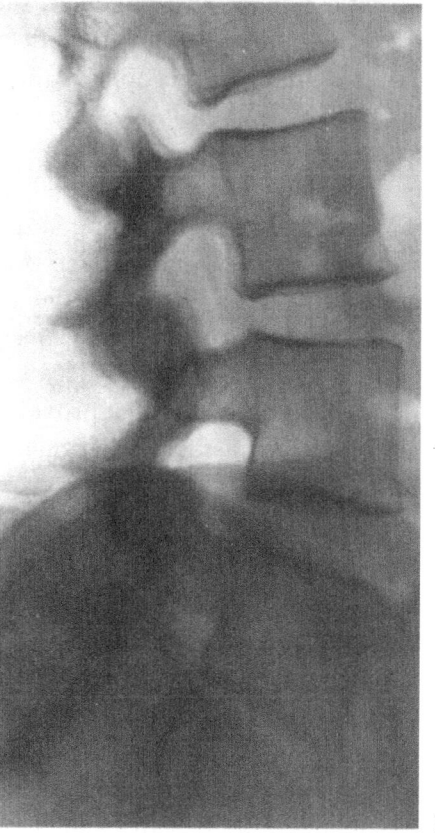
b

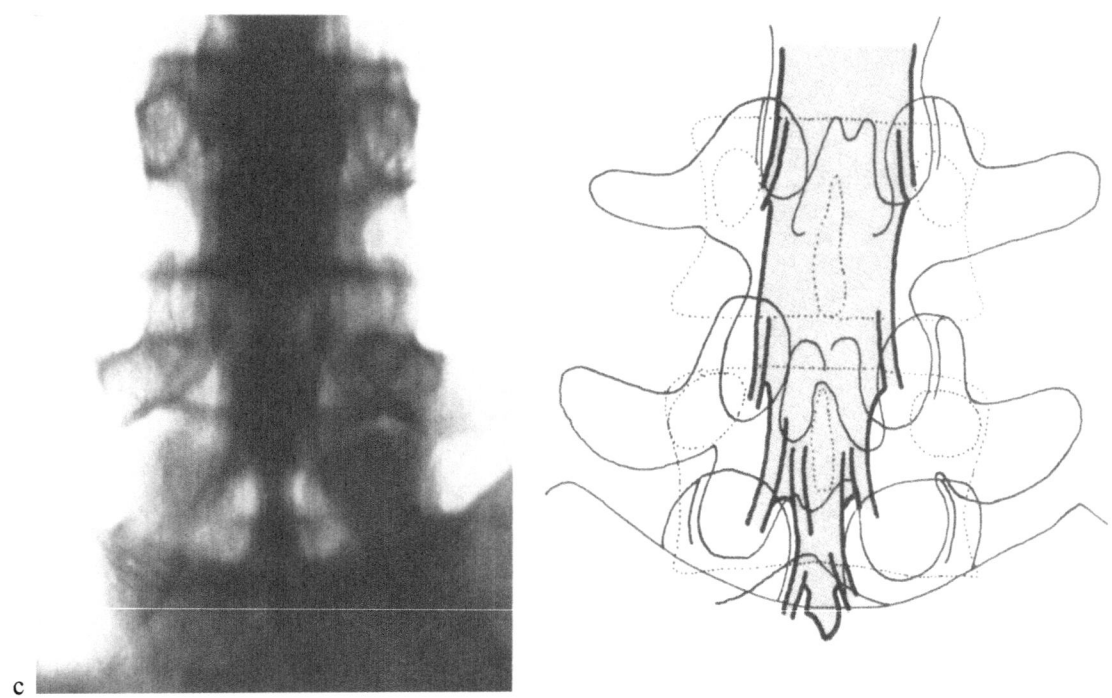

Fig. IX,11 (cont.). Legend see page 119

opacification of the radicular sheaths by a water-soluble agent allows detection of extrasaccular compressions of the roots belonging to the pathology of the narrow radicular canals.

Fat-soluble agents [28, 79, 90, 111] have the drawback of undergoing stops [53, 59, 73, 79] in the stenotic areas and thus providing a caricatural image of the thecal sac due to nonfilling of the narrow recesses [66]. Similar to gas myelography [4, 19, 24], positive myelography does not provide any data about the extra-saccular segments of the roots.

Due to its ready performance and simplicity, RSG is particularly suited for the exploration of degenerative stenoses in aged patients.

It become insufficient in cases of stenosis with neurogenic intermittent claudication related to a pathology of the conus, for which gas myelography, possibly completed by angiography, is better suited.

V. Miscellaneous Etiologies

Most of the lumbar spinal stenoses are either of developmental or of degenerative origin. Sometimes, the clinical picture and the radiologic investigations enable one to find evidence of a less common cause.

Thus, a diffuse lumbar stenosis has been described in cases of achondroplasia [2, 26, 40, 46, 64, 76, 95, 96] or in Paget's disease [13, 25, 47, 52, 55, 56, 63, 80], in acromegaly [45, 60], in cases of tabetic osteoarthropathy [9, 88, 89, 93, 99], and in rare cases of lumbar hyperlordosis associated with a dorsal kyphosis [71] or with a severe scoliosis [36].

A localized lumbar spinal stenosis may be related to a spondylolisthesis with intact neural arch [14–16, 37, 68, 72] or with sequelae of arthrodesis or laminectomy [6, 7, 18].

Usually, stenosis is caused mainly by the bones, but it may also be due to the hypertrophied soft tissues which make up the

120

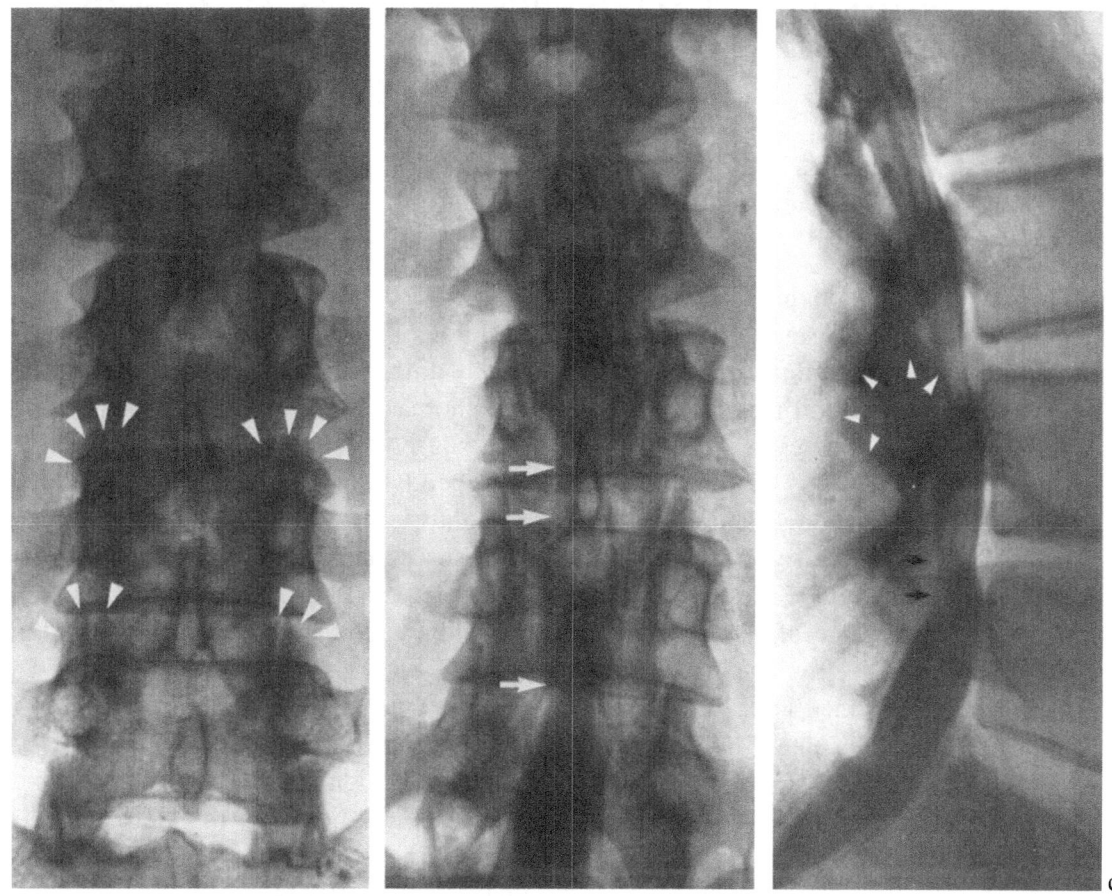

a
b
c

Fig. IX,12. **Posterior Imprints Due to Hypertrophied Facetal Joints.** (a) Plain frontal view. Signs of degenerative hypertrophic changes of the facetal joints predominant in L3–4 and L4–5 (*arrowheads*). (b) Frontal RSG views (c) Lateral RSG view. Elongated posterolateral imprints are displayed at the two previous levels (*arrows*) witnessing the bony and nonhernial origin of the compression

canalar walls, such as the ligamenta flava [1, 8, 60, 69, 77, 100]. In cases of severe proliferating arachnoiditis, the hypertrophy and the fibrotic changes of the soft tissues may be such that the term "fibrous spinal stenosis" has been used [65, 108].

References of Chapter 9 see page 156.

Chapter 10. Miscellaneous (Tumors, Osteoarticular Diseases, etc.)

RSG may provide valuable data, either by demonstrating the deformation of the dural sac by dural and extradural masses or by delineating an intradural mass.

It is not useful in cases of giant tumors of the cauda equina [28, 47, 54], the diagnosis of which is based on plain x-ray findings, i.e., marked increase of the diameters of the spinal canal with scalloped vertebrae and polycyclic lacunae of the sacrum [29, 53].

It is rarely performed in cases with bone tumors of the lumbar spine (Fig. X,4). However, it is intersisting in other osteoarticular diseases.

I. Intradural Tumors

They are clinically characterized by low back pain radiating in the legs clearly increased by bed rest and associated to a marked stiffness of the spine [45, 67, 70, 71, 78].

The laboratory tests in the CSF show a disproportion between cell count and protein content, i.e., high protein content without excess of cells. Plain films and tomograms of the lumbar spine are often silent [69]. Only the isolated widening of an intervertebral canal or an increased interpedicular distance at a single level may draw one's attention. Note that the vertebral scalloping is sometimes seen, but the proof of its topographic relation with the tumor is still to be found: Recklingshausen's disease

may indeed have different and associated radiologic signs.

The intradural tumors are most often neurinomas [71] of the cauda equina roots, more rarely filum terminale tumors [13], i.e., ependymomas, lipomas [18, 26, 39, 60], vascular tumors [23], and, exceptionally, cholesteatomas related to a previous lumbar puncture [30]. Lipomas occur mainly in children and belong to a complex malformation of the lumbosacral region. The same is true for dermoid cysts [3, 16, 51].

These intradural masses are more or less rounded, benign tumors, the type of which cannot be predicted on the view of the x-rays. Moreover, their radiculosaccographic images are similar [45].

Among these tumors, the neurinoma is the most commonly encountered, so that we shall describe its features. It is usually found at a stage when it obstrudes the dural sac where it causes a cupula-formed stop [15, 33]. If this stop is incomplete, x-rays carried out later permit visualization of the inferior pole of the mass and delineation of the whole contour of the tumor [8]. The dural sac may be slightly widened cranially [15]; the cupula-formed limit is often outlined by a thin, dense line of contrast [15] and seen on several projections to be symmetric with regard to the canalar axis [8]. A sinuous vascular-type translucency may rise above the highest point of the cupula-formed limit [15], but this does not allow a prediction of the type of the tumor (Fig. X,1 and X,2).

An intradural tumor is very rarely dis-

Fig. X,1. **Intradural Neurinoma of the Cauda Equina.** Cupula-formed, regular, and symmetric stop, located at the half-height of the L3 vertebra. Above its pole lies a sinuous translucency of very likely vascular origin ▷

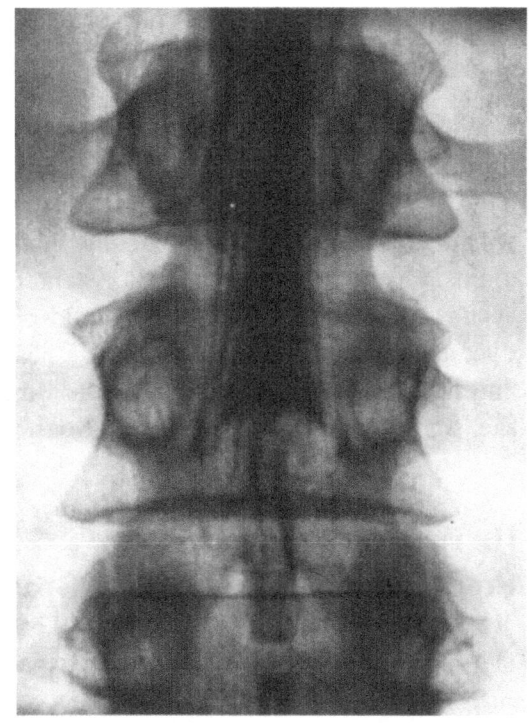

Fig. X,2. **Ependymoma of the Filum Terminale.** (a) Frontal view. (b) Lateral view. (c) Oblique view. The cupula-formed stop located behind the L4 vertebral body is seen on all projections. Its margin is bumpy and delineated by a thin, dense, and regular line. Above the stop, the dural sac is slightly widened. A very small amount of contrast reaches the fundus ▽

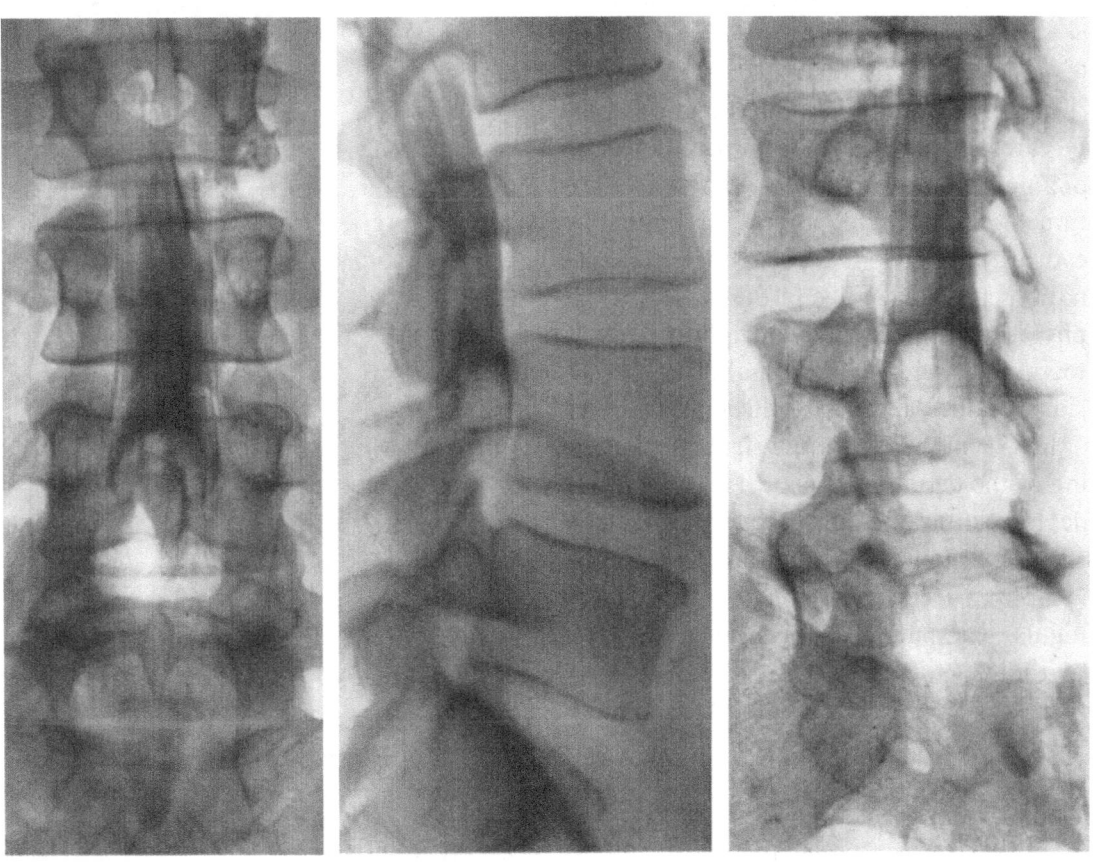

a
b
c

covered before the obstruction stage, then it is displayed as an intrasaccular rounded lacuna [31, 72].

We reported an exceptional case of intradural-extrasaccular neurinoma, growing in a cystic dilatation of a first sacral root and which gave rise to an ovalar lacunar image amidst the cystic dilatation [2, 8]. Normally, such extrasaccular neurinomas should produce a nonfilling of the concerned sheath and a corresponding imprint on the dural sac, signs consistent with discal herniation.

II. Tumoral and Infectious Processes of the Extradural Space

The extradural conjunctivovascular space may be a fixation site for neoplastic cells or, more rarely, a site for the development of an infectious process (abcess).

The clinical symptomatology of these conditions is equivocal since it may merely be consistent with a trivial root pain.

The plain radiologic investigation must be carefully performed, it permits detection of an osteolytic or densifying bone localization of a malignant process or anomalies evocative of spondylodiscitis. This examination can be negative in the case of a staphylococcus abcess or lymphoplasmocytosis, and moreover, minimal osteolytic lesions of the sacrum are difficult to elicit.

RSG will then show the signs of thickening of the extradural space, i.e., a localized detachment of the dural sac and/or its progressive thinning out due to an all-around invading process. There may also be an irregular amputated appearance of the fundus.

A. Tumoral Etiologies

Malignant tumors of the lumbosacral spine (bone sarcomas, malignant giant-cell tu-

mors) may be accompanied by infiltration of the epidural space at the same level (Fig. X,3 and X,4). Vertebral metastases of osteophilic carcinomas and, more rarely, bone localizations of malignant or benign hemopathies behave in the same way [32, 38].

Neoplastic infiltrations of the epidural space may also be found in the absence of bone involvement, due to dissemination of malignant cells via the blood or the lymph, most often in hemopathies, but also in cases of neoplasms (Fig. X,5). Such a neoplastic dissemination to the cauda equina may produce, on contrast examination of the dural sac, irregularities of the saccular contours and small intrasaccular lacunae [6, 19, 46].

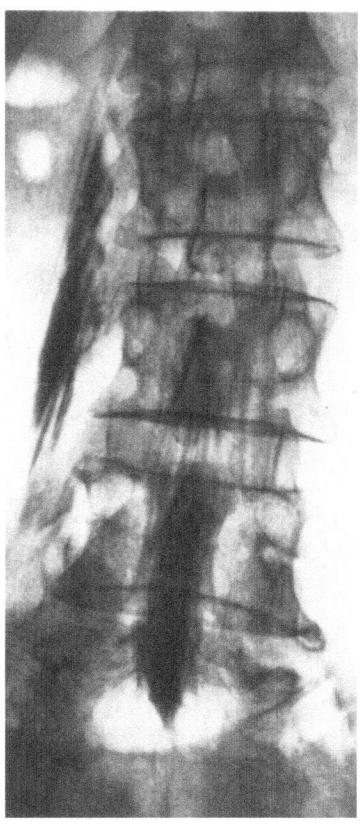

Fig. X,3. **Epidural Sarcoma.** The fundus is amputated and irregularly tapered. Note the presence of trails of contrast medium, projected laterally to the spine

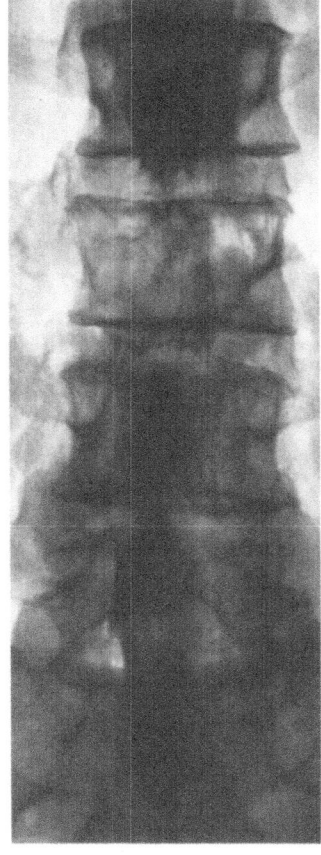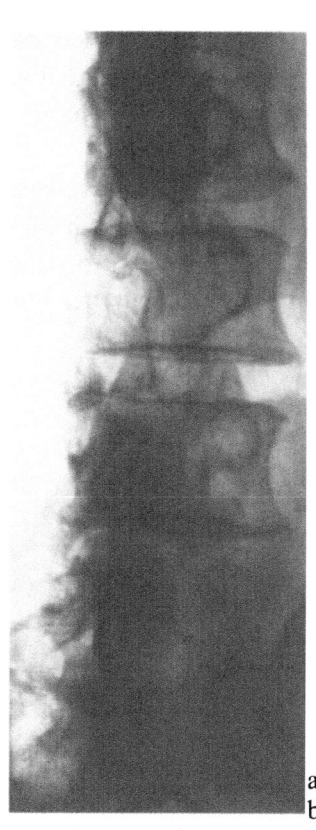

Fig. X,4. **Giant-Cell Tumor of the L3 Posterior Arch.** (a) Frontal view. (b) Left posterior oblique view. Diffuse osteolytic bone changes of L3 mainly involving the right half of the posterior arch. The posterolateral compression of the dural sac becomes evident by an important detachment seen on the frontal and left oblique projections. Note the partial subdural injection of the contrast medium producing a double contrast pattern in the fundus

B. Extradural Infectious Processes

The extradural space may be the site of an abcess of hematic origin, either in case of septicemia or in patients predisposed to infections such as the diabetics.

It may also be invaded by the infectious process of a spondylodiscitis, for instance Pott's disease [14, 35] (Fig. X,6). These extradural localizations give rise to a clinical symptomatology similar to discal herniation [4, 5, 12, 17, 36, 57].

III. Various Osteoarticular Involvements of the Lumbar Spine

A. Tabetic Osteoarthropathy

The tabetic osteoarthropathy of the lumbar spine may compress the cauda equina roots by means of bone deformations and structural changes, i.e., angulation of the spine [37, 66], deformations of the intervertebral canals [59, 62, 66], collapse of the vertebrae [27], vertebral displacements [7, 58], and exuberant osteophytic proliferations.

Root pains have to be differentiated from the lightning pains of the tabes dorsalis, and the clinical examination has to separate the tabetic neurologic signs and the radicular signs.

125

RSG and gas or oil myelographs may show more or less complete blocks, localized or multileveled narrowings, and indentations related to disc protrusions or osteohypertrophic changes of the vertebrae (Fig. X,7).

Symptoms are relieved by extensive laminectomies, which allow one to consider tabetic osteoarthropathies to be a possible etiology for narrow lumbar canal [43, 56, 66, 68, 73, 76].

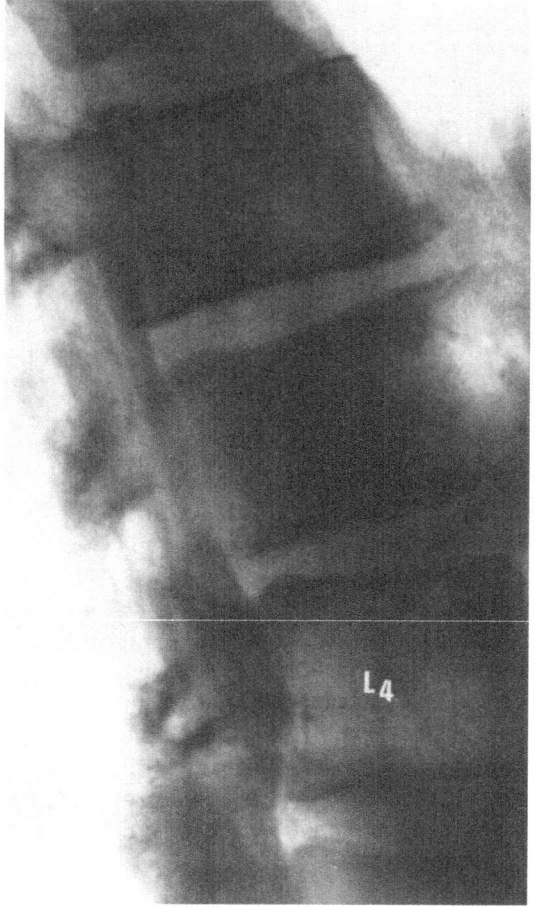

Fig. X,5. **Metastatic epiduritis.** Osteolysis of the L3 body and detachment of the anterior aspect of the dural sac facing an osteolytic area in the posterior part of the vertebral body

Fig. X,6. **Tuberculous Epiduritis.** Right sensory motor involvement of the L4 root evolving for 3 months in a 52-year-old male of North African origin. The tomograms of the lumbar spine (a) show a lacunar appearance of the anterior L3–4 osteophytosis and an extensive erosion of the upper L5 plate. The importance of the arthrosic changes and the absence of disc pinching led to an inadequate diagnosis. RSG (b, c) shows a segmental lack of opacification extending from the inferior third of L3 down to the upper end-plate of L5. Surgery confirmed the canalar invading by granulomatous tissue with disc fragments. Histology and bacteriologic tests confirmed its tuberculous origin

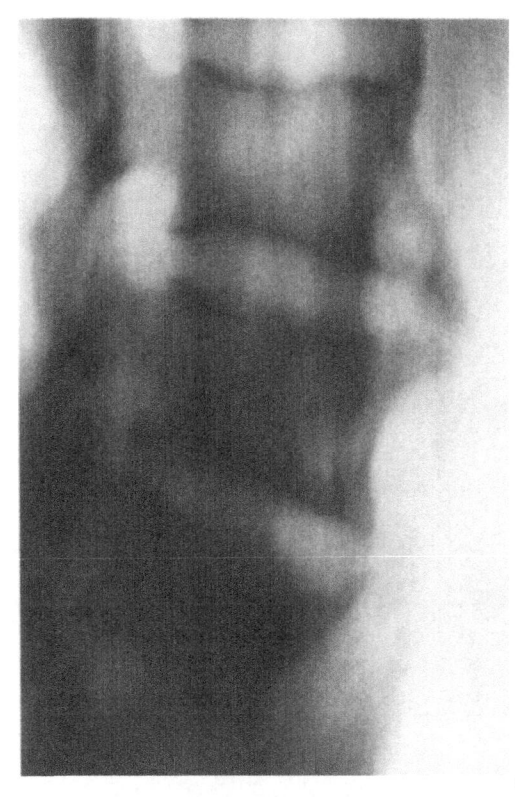

a

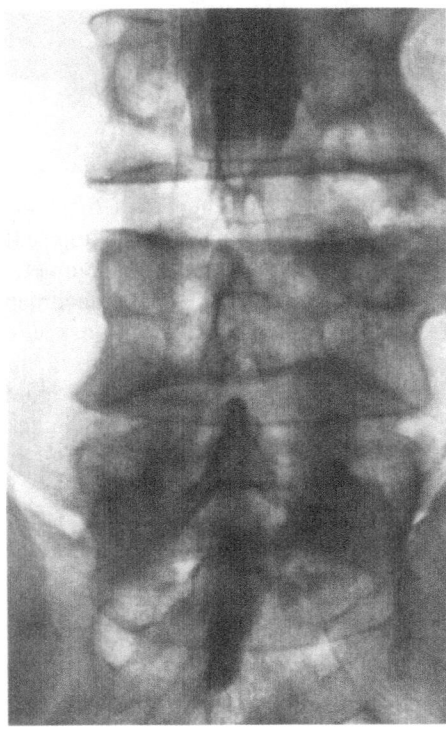

b

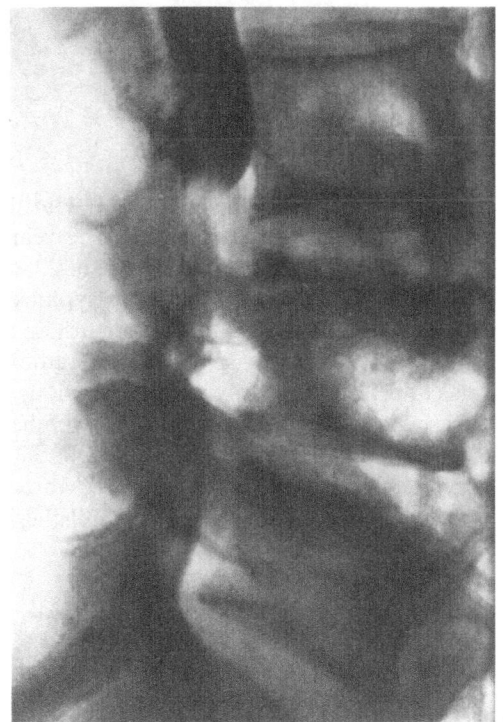

c

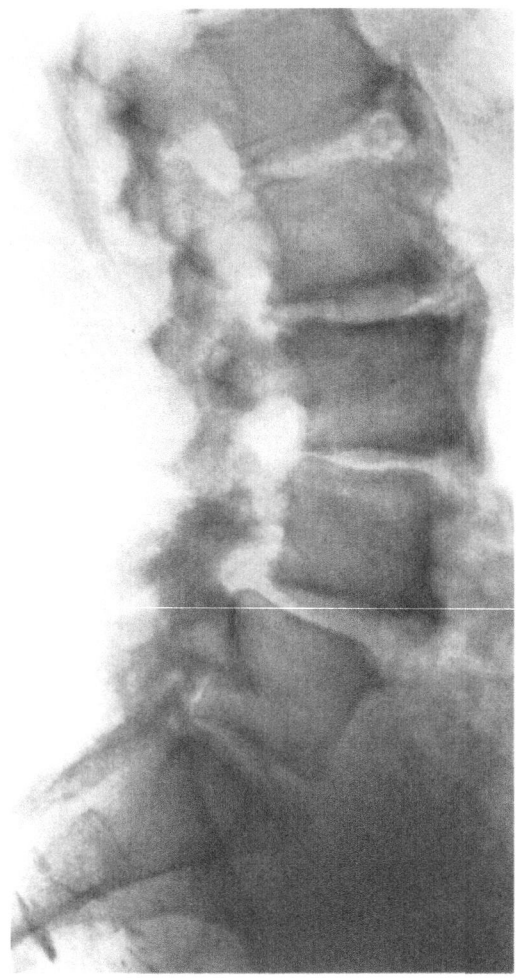 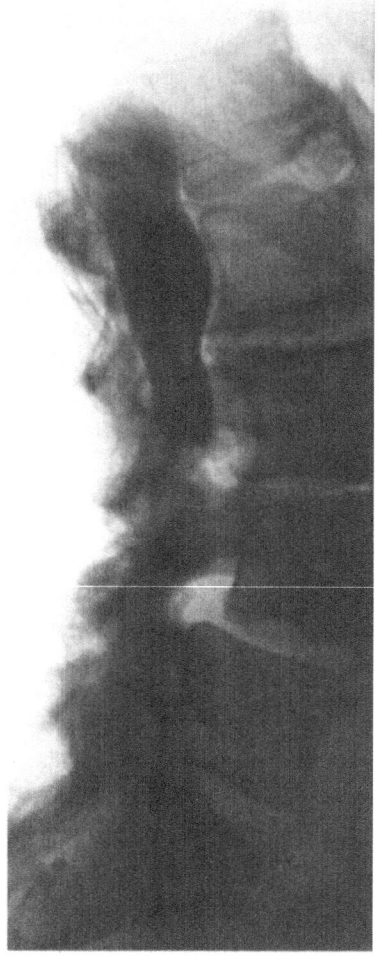

a
b

Fig. X,7. **Complete Stop Due to Epiduritis in a Case of Tabetic Osteoarthropathy.** 52-year-old hair dresser presenting, since the age of 22, clinical and biological signs of nervous syphilis. Bilateral sciatic pains led to the performance of an x-ray of the lumbar spine (a). The radiologic signs of osteoarthropathy are quite obvious, i.e., diffuse bone changes from L1–L4, exuberant osteophytosis of the vertebral end-plates, and prevertebral L1–L3 hyperostosis. Moreover, there is a moderate L4–5 spondylolisthesis, a reduction of the height of the L3–4 interspace, and densification of both adjacent L2–3 end-plates. RSG shows (b) a complete stop at the inferior third of L3 with detachment of the dural sac behind the posterior aspect of L3, which is scalloped. Above the stop, a linear translucency of very likely radicular origin is displayed. The enlarged L4 laminectomy indicated the excision of a lumbar epiduritis. After the operation the root pains disappeared

B. Spondylolisthesis

1. Definitions and Characteristics of the Different Types

Spondylolisthesis consists of a forward movement of one vertebral body with regard to the underlying vertebra or the sacrum. Two main anatomical types are encountered, whether the posterior arch remains connected to the sliding vertebral body or whether a rupture of the posterior arch separates it from the vertebral body [42, 48, 75].

128

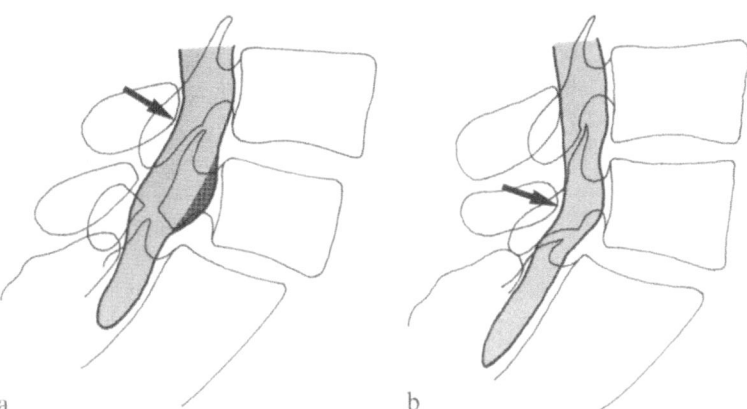

Fig. X,8. **Schematic Representation of the Dural Sac Deformation in Cases of Spondylolisthesis.** (a) *Spondylolisthesis due to spondylolysis.* The separation of the neural arch increases the anteroposterior canalar diameter. The anterior margin of the dural sac molds more or less closely the canalar deformation. A moderate posterior imprint may exist, due to the constraint exerted by the overlying neural arch. (b) *Spondylolisthesis with intact neural arch.* The posterior arch of the olisthetic vertebra compresses the posterior margin of the dural sac. This readily results in an anteroposterior shearing

In cases of *spondylolisthesis with intact neural arch,* the sliding movement is made possible by an anomaly in the facetal joints which may be congenitally hypoplastic or which may undergo a subluxation owing to degenerative changes. This variety has been described by Junghanns and termed pseudospondylolisthesis [34]; recently, Epstein stated that the exact denomination should be "degenerative spondylolisthesis with an intact neural arch [20]."

In cases of *spondylolisthesis with ruptured neural arch,* the rupture is bilateral and most often occurs in the isthmic area, i.e., the pedicles and the superior articular facets remain connected to the vertebral body and glide forward, while the inferior articular facets, the lamina, and the spinous process remain in situ [52].

These two types of spondylolisthesis differ in so far as in the first case, the lumbar spinal canal is rapidly narrowed at the site of the slipping, whereas in the second, the separation of the two parts of the neural arch causes a widening of the canal at the level of the slipping (Fig. X,8). This accounts for the rapid occurrence of cauda equina syndromes in cases of degenerative spondylolisthesis, whereas spondylolisthesis due to spondylolysis remains asymptomatic for a long time. These two entities will thus be studied separately.

2. Spondylolisthesis With Intact Neural Arch

It is most often of degenerative origin and related to the progressive subluxation of the articular facets involved in spondylotic changes [9–11, 20, 61]. More rarely it is due to a rheumatoid disease, for instance rheumatoid arthritis [24], or to a neurogenic arthropathy such as tabes [7, 58]. Only exceptionally, a spondylolisthesis of this type can be related to a congenital hypoplasia of the facetal joints [21] or to a traumatism that has caused luxation of the facets.

This anatomical condition is compulsorily accompagnied by segmental stenosis of the lumbar spinal canal, owing to a hori-

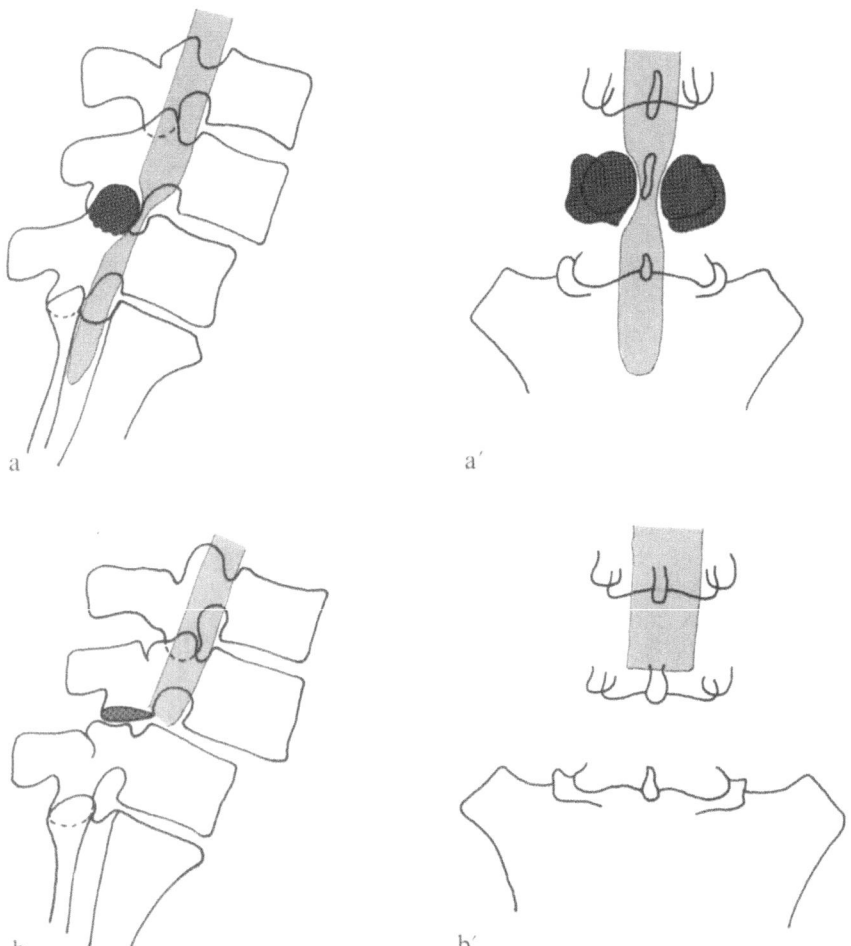

Fig. X,9. **Spondylolisthesis with Intact Neural Arch; Schematic Representation of Two Pathogenic Conditions.** (a, a') *Spondylolisthesis due to degenerative facetal changes.* The association of hypertrophy of the facetal joints and of moderate forward slipping causes a concentric narrowing of the dural sac. (b, b') *Spondylolisthesis due to facetal hypoplasia.* The hypoplasia favors the sliding and mainly provokes a shearing displayed by a stop with horizontal linear limit on a frontal projection

zontal shearing mechanism [44]. It is often associated with periarticular hypertrophic changes of the facetal joints (Fig. X,9), belonging to an important diffuse degenerative arthropathy which most of the patients present. These hypertrophic facetal joints bulge into the canalar lumen and contribute to its narrowing [20] and to the narrowing of the intervertebral canals [9–11].

Clinically, the onset may be trivial root pain or a more typical symptomatology of sensory motor intermittent claudication. The late stage results in a cauda equina syndrome.

The radiographs of the lumbar spine show the vertebral slipping, usually located in L4–5 [10, 61] and rather moderate—it does not reach the third of the underlying vertebral plate [20]. The changes in the morphology of the bone structures of the posterior arch accounts for the existence of a slipping. Above all, the facetal joints have

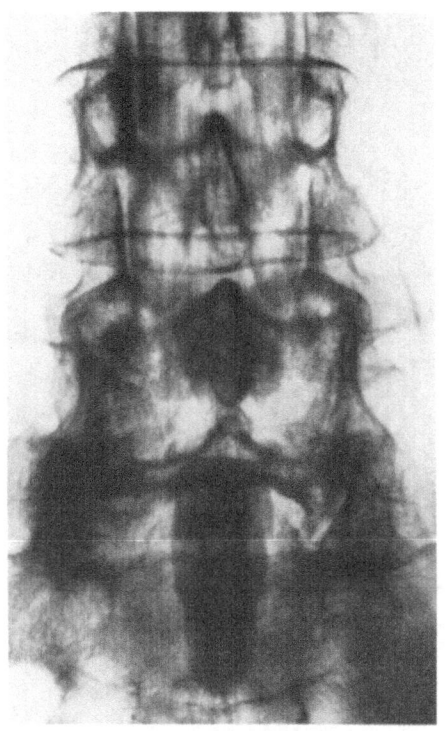

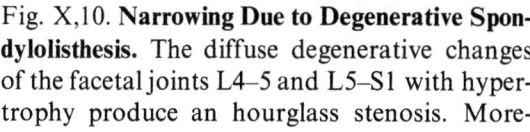

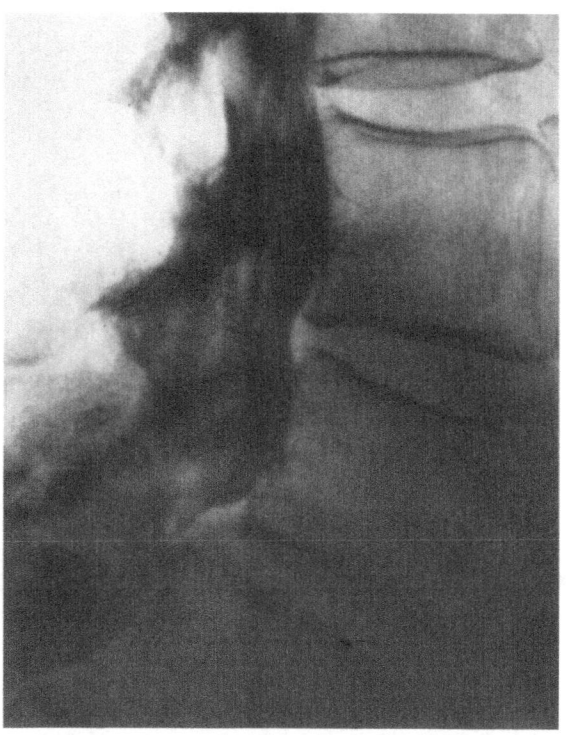

a   b

Fig. X,10. **Narrowing Due to Degenerative Spondylolisthesis.** The diffuse degenerative changes of the facetal joints L4–5 and L5–S1 with hypertrophy produce an hourglass stenosis. Moreover, a segmental lack of opacification with horizontal and clear-cut upper margin can be noted, explained by geometric reasons (see text). (a) Frontal view. (b) Lateral view of RSG

an abnormal density [20] and are massive, bulky, and there is a sclerosis of the margins of the interfacetal space. These are common signs of associated spondylarthrosis.

Tomograms will show, on the one hand, the narrowing of the spinal canal on midsagittal sections and, on the other hand, anomalies in the facets on lateral sections.

RSG objectivizes two types of dural sac deformations:

a. A concentric narrowing due to the predominant hypertrophy of the posterior arch with regard to the importance of the slipping [20]. On frontal projections the stenosis is displayed with an hourglass image. On the two oblique projections, there are anterior and posterior indentations facing each other and witnessing the concentric character of the stenosis. On the lateral projection, the deformation of the anterior margin of the sac is only mild with regard to the signs of the posteroanterior compression (Fig. X,10).

b. The bayonet-shaped deformation of the dural sac due to a horizontal shearing produces a linear horizontal and clear-cut obstruction to the flow of contrast medium on frontal views [44, 65] (Fig. X,11). The slight opacification of the fundus shows that the arrest is only partial. This horizontal image is due to the fact that the beam is tangent to the horizontal part of the bayonet-shaped cul-de-sac.

In this type of spondylolisthesis, the treatment aims to accomodate the cauda equina on the basis of a decompressive laminectomy with facetectomy [9–11, 20].

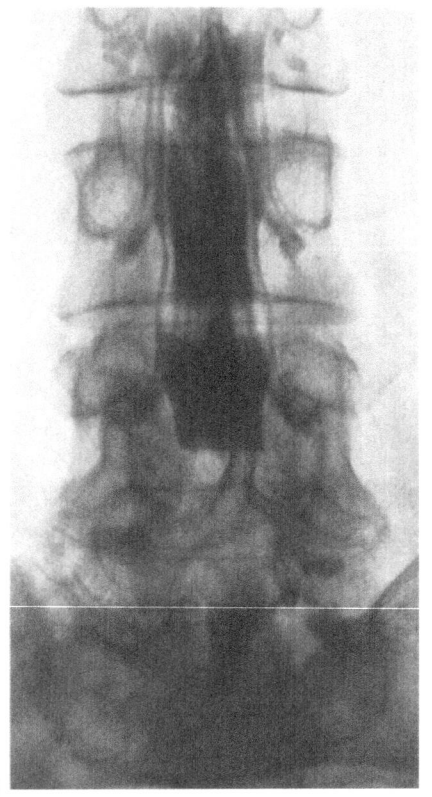

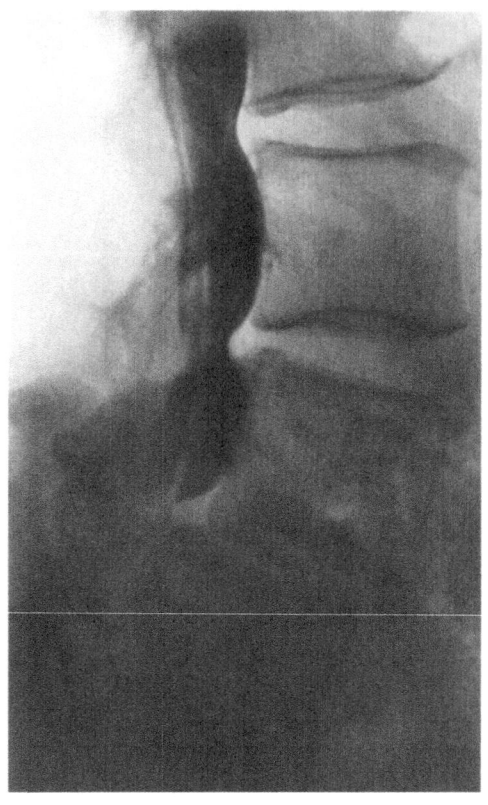

Fig. X,11. **Horizontal Stop Due to Spondylolisthesis With Intact Neural Arch*.** The horizontal stop with clear-cut margin is typical for this cause of compression. The overlying roots are too well-displayed and sinuous, which is a sign of narrow lumbar canal. Besides, there are diverticula of the radicular sheaths. (a) Frontal view. (b) Lateral view. (c) Right posterior oblique view

* courtesy of Dr. Dirheimer (Strasbourg).

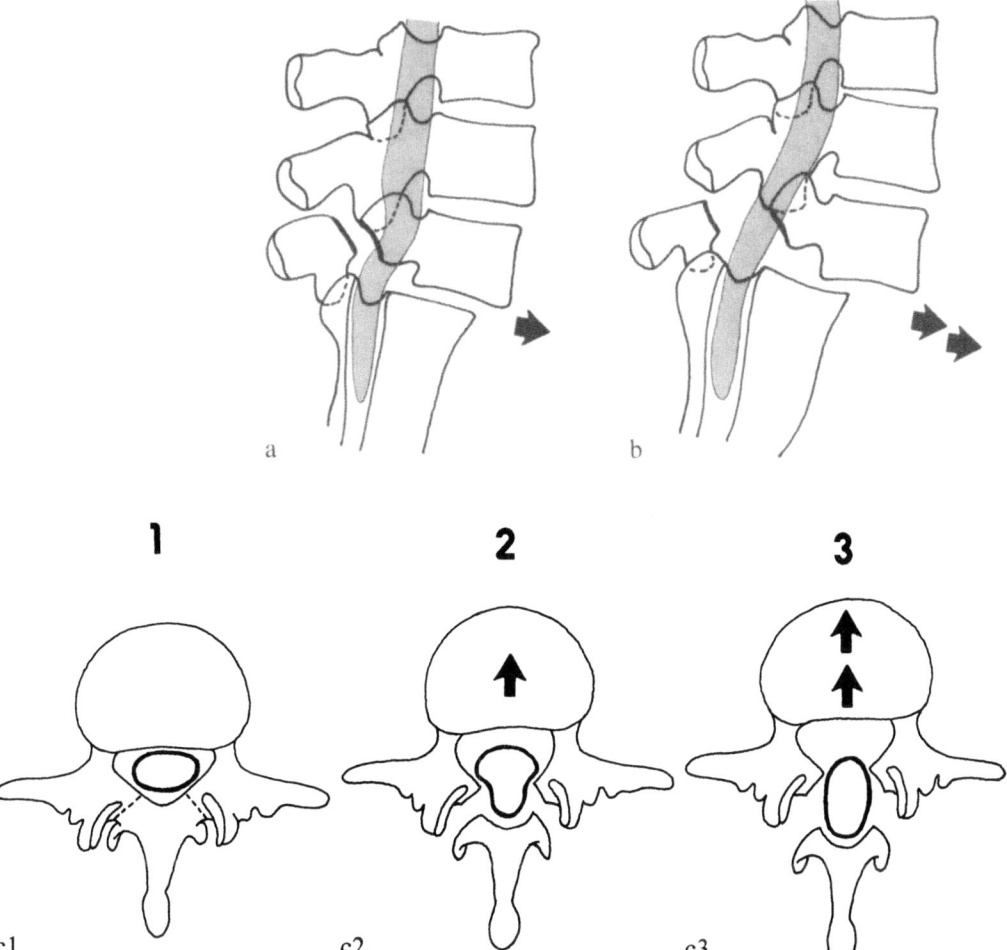

Fig. X,12. **Schematic Drawing of the Dural Sac Deformation at Different Stages of the Slipping Due to Spondylolysis.** (a) Moderate slipping. (b) More marked slipping. (c1, c2, c3) Axial representation of the normal situation with regard to these two slipping stages. Paradoxically, the moderate slipping (a) causes a posterior imprint which disappears later (b), and can be attributed to the temporary compression by the facetal joints before the dural sac has passed behind them (c3)

3. Spondylolisthesis Due to Spondylolysis

This is asymptomatic for a long time and becomes evident through low back pain, so that most of the cases do not justify RSG.

Bone radiographs show spondylolysis and allow evaluation of the degree of slipping. A functional test has to be performed in order to appreciate the possibility of reduction of the slipping. The forward movement is most often located at the L5–S1 interspace and may be associated to congenital anomalies of the lumbosacral posterior arches.

The discography [41] may be indicated to determine the degree of discal involvement and the number of discs concerned in order to perform a posterior arthrodesis.

RSG is only indicated in cases with root pain. The mechanisms of this root pain are numerous and already discussed [64, 74].. An associated discal herniation, usually lo-

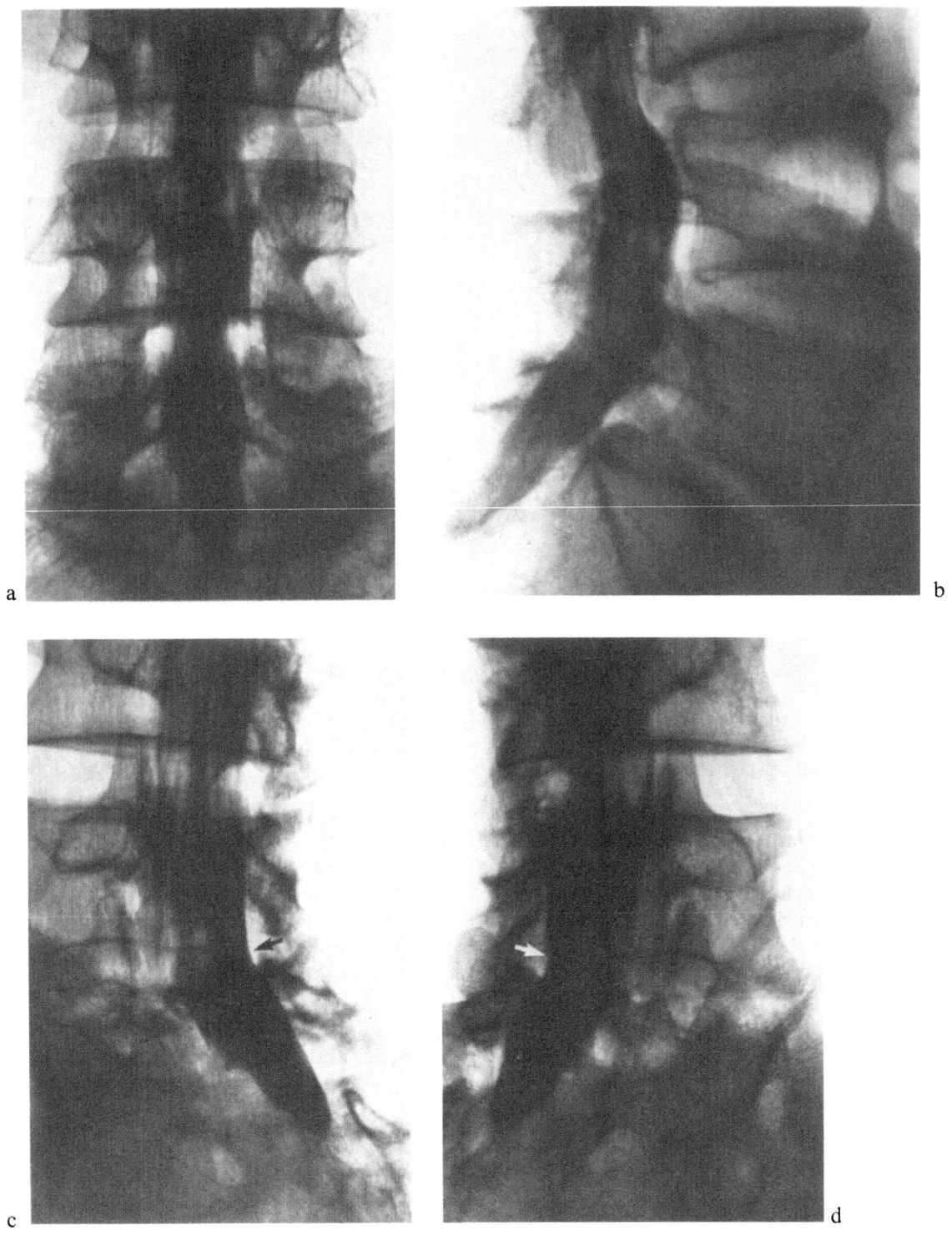

Fig. X,13. **Moderate Spondylolisthesis Due to Spondylolysis.** The posterolateral imprints on oblique projections (*arrows*) can be attributed to the constraint of the interapophyseal pass. (a) Frontal view. (b) Lateral view (c) and (d) Right and left posterior oblique views

134

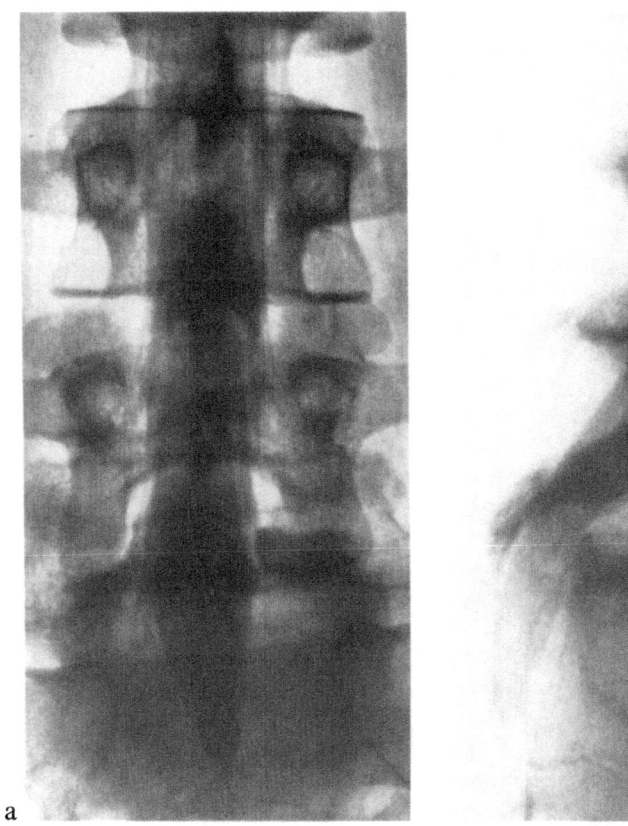
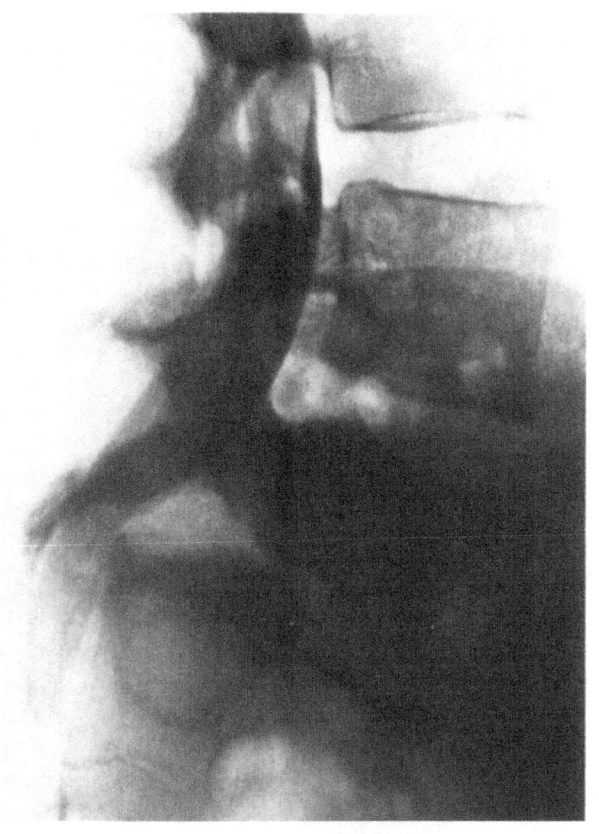

a

b

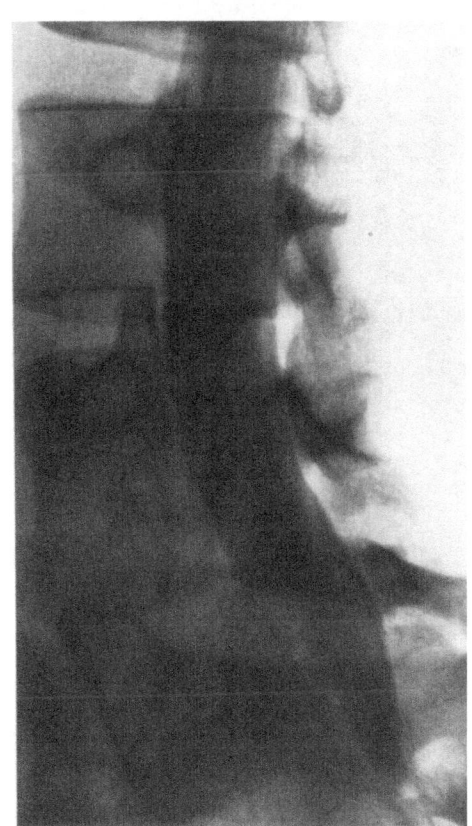

Fig. X,14. **Marked Spondylolisthesis Due to Spondylo-lysis.** The dural sac has passed behind the facetal joints, which accounts for the absence of imprints on the oblique projections. (a) Frontal view. (b) Lateral view. (c) Right posterior oblique view

c

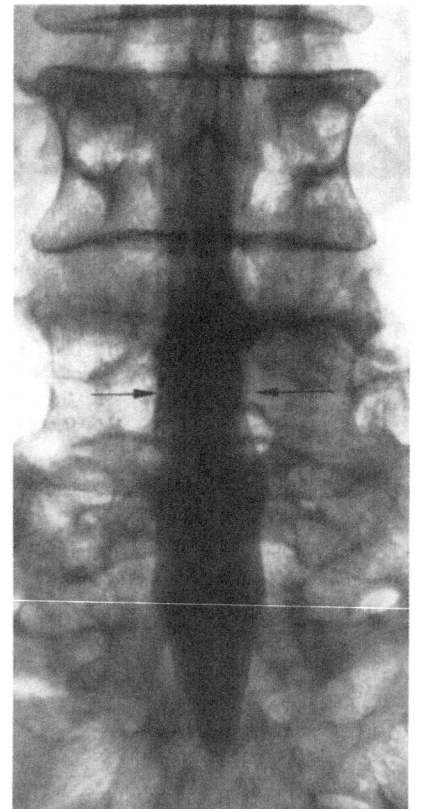

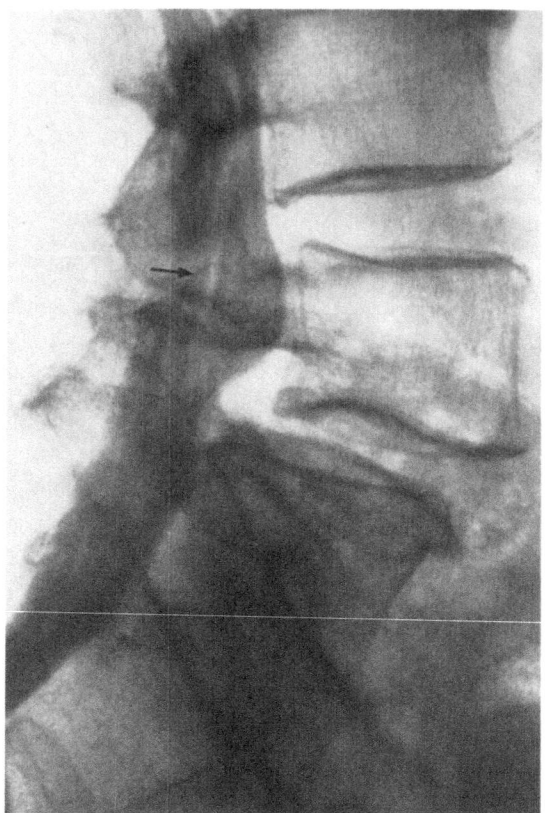

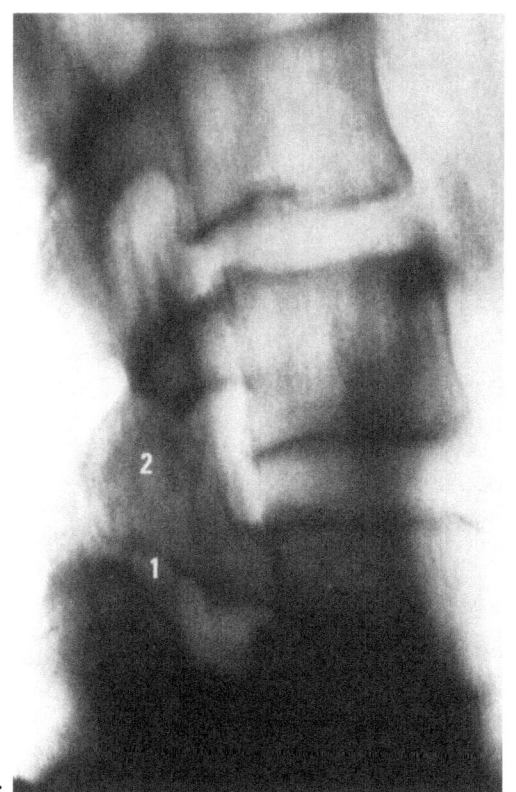

a

b

c

Fig. X,15. **Spondylolisthesis With Spondlyolysis (1) and Associated Facetal Degenerative Changes** (2). The degenerative facetal changes cause an hourglass stenosis (*arrow*) and a posterior indentation on the dural sac (*crossed arrow*). (a) Frontal view. (b) Lateral view of RSG. (c) Sagittal tomogram demonstrating the spondylolysis

cated at the space above the slipping is rare [41]. In cases with a severe degree of slip, the cauda equina roots and especially the first sacral roots are stretched in an elongated S bend between the neural arches of the last two lumbar vertebrae anteriorly and the knob of the back of the first sacral body posteriorly.

The development of a fibrocartilaginous isthmic nodule [1, 25, 40] may also compress the roots at the level of the intervertebral canals.

The RSG signs in these cases are limited to the deformations of the dural sac. The radicular signs fail to be displayed since the radicular sheaths are almost always poorly opacified in the area of the slipping. Thus, it is not always possible to rule out or to confirm the diagnosis of discal herniation at an overlying interspace. The deformation of the dural sac adapts imperfectly to the deformation of the bony canal [22, 48]; it passes from the lumbar canal to the sacral canal while forming a more or less angulated sigmoid curve (Fig. X,12). Its posterior margin remains close to the spared alignment of the interlaminal joining with the spinous process, whereas its anterior margin bridges the slipping and is thus either detached from the L5 body up to a variable height, or close to it, and thus has a marked anterior curvature. When the retrovertebral detachment extends more cranially [74], it constitutes an obstacle to the diagnosis of a possible discal herniation.

Let us point out that herniation do not exist at the level of the slipping since the disc is strongly laminated. In cases of moderate slipping, a symmetrical stenosis of the dural sac can be seen on frontal projections in the area of the slipping. It is related to posterior indentations just above the slipping on posterior oblique projections [74]. This condition has been explained by Ruprecht [63] to be due to a temporary compression of the lateral aspects of the dural sac between the facetal joints in cases of moderate slipping (Fig. X,13). Conversely, in more marked slippings, the dural sac would have passed behind the facetal joints and thus would no longer show these deformations. We could verify this in the cases which were available to us (Fig. X,14).

In elderly patients, with long-standing spondylolisthesis, the combined degenerative changes preferably involve L4–5 and may then provoke a narrowing due to hypertrophy of the facetal joints (Fig. X,15).

References of Chapter 10 see page 160.

137

References

Introduction

1. Abdullah, A.F., Ditto, E.W., Byrd, E.B., Williams, R.: Extreme-lateral lumbar disc herniations. Clinical syndrome and special problems of diagnosis. J. Neurosurg. **41**, 229–234 (1974)
2. Autio, E., Suolanen, J., Norrbäck, S., Slätis, P.: Adhesive arachnoiditis after lumbar myelography with meglumine iothalamate (Conray). Acta radiol. (Diagn.) **12**, 17–24 (1972)
3. Babin, E., Maitrot, D., Dirheimer, Y., Haller, M., Mugel, J.L., Buchheit, F.: L'intérêt de la zonographie frontale en sacco-radiculographie. Sem. Hôp. Paris **50**, 2081–2087 (1974)
4. Babin, E., Maitrot, D., Haller, M., Dirheimer, Y., Buchheit, F.: The value of frontal zonographic sections in saccoradiculography. Neuroradiology **7**, 161–166 (1974)
5. Bonte, G., Brenot, M., Trinez, B.: La tomographie axiale transverse. Paris: Doin Ed. 1955
6. Bonte, G., Decoulx, P., Waghemacker, R., Cecille, J.P., Huart, F.: La radiculographie lombo-sacrée au cours des lombalgies sans sciatique. J. Radiol. Électrol. **42**, 416–420 (1961)
7. Capesius, P.: Exploration radiologique d'une sciatique en 1975. J. méd. Strasbourg **7**, 289–290 (1976)
8. Capesius, P., Babin, E.: Tomographic exploration in radiculosaccography. Proceedings of the Symposium Actualitatis Tomographiae, Genoa, 11th–13th September 1975. Amsterdam: Excerpta Medica 1976
9. Capesius, P., Babin, E., Maitrot, D., Dupuis, M., Haller, M., Mancs, P.: Intérêt de la radiculosaccographie dans l'exploration radiologique d'une sciatique. Bull. Soc. Sci. méd. Luxemb. **113**, 169–177 (1976)
10. Cloward, R.B., Buzaid, L.L.: Discography. Technique, indications and evaluation of the normal and abnormal intervertebral disc. Amer. J. Roentgenol. **68**, 552–564 (1952)
11. Collis, J.S.: Lumbar discography. Springfield, Ill.: Charles C. Thomas 1963
12. Davatchi, F., Benoist, M., Massare, Cl., Helenon, Ch., Bloch-Michel, H.: Contribution à l'étude des canaux étroits à l'étage lombaire. Technique radiologique et valeur normale. Sem. Hôp. Paris **29**, 2008–2012 (1969)
13. Debeyre, J., Bernageau, J., Dorat, J.: Arthrodèses lombo-sacrées et discographies. Rev. Rhum. **36**, 203–211 (1969)
14. Di Chiro, G., Fisher, R.L.: Contrast radiography of the spinal cord. Arch. Neurol. **11**, 125–143 (1964)
15. Gargano, F.P., Jacobson, R.E., Rosomoff, H.L.: Transverse axial tomography of the spine. Neuroradiology **6**, 254–258 (1974)
16. Gargano, F.P., Meyer, J.D., Sheldon, J.J.: Transfemoral ascending lumbar catheterisation of the epidural veins in lumbar disc disease. Radiology **111**, 329–336 (1974)
17. Grossman, Z.D., Wistow, B.W., Wallinga, H.A., Heitzmann, E.R.: Recognition of vertebral abnormalities in computed tomography of the chest and abdomen. Radiology **121**, 369–373 (1976)
18. Hammerschlag, S.B., Wolpert, S.M., Carter, B.L.: Computed tomography of the spinal canal. Radiology **121**, 361–367 (1976)
19. Hinck, V.C., Hopkins, C.E., Clark, W.M.: Sagittal diameter of the lumbar spinal canal in children and adults. Radiology **85**, 929–937 (1965)
20. Hindmarsh, T.: Myelography with the non-ionic water-soluble contrast medium metrizamide. Acta radiol. (Diagn) **16**, 417–435 (1975)
21. Howland, W.J., Curry, J.L.: Experimental studies of pantopaque arachnoiditis. Radiology **87**, 253–261 (1966)
22. Hurteau, E.F., Baird, W.C., Sinclair, E.:

Arachnoiditis following the use of iodized oil. J. Bone Jt Surg. **36A**, 393–400 (1954)

23. Jacobson, R.E., Gargano, F.P., Rosomoff, H.L.: Transverse axial tomography of the spine. Trans. Amer. neurol. Ass. **98**, 5–7 (1973)
24. Jacobson, R.E., Gargano, F.P., Rosomoff, H.L.: Transverse axial tomography of the spine. Part 1. Axial anatomy of the normal lumbar spine. J. Neurosurg. **42**, 406–411 (1975)
25. Jacobson, R.E., Gargano, F.P., Rosomoff, H.L.: Transverse axial tomography of the spine. Part 2. The stenotic spinal canal. J. Neurosurg. **42**, 412–419 (1975)
26. Kistler, M.W., Pribram, H.W.: Epidural venography in the diagnosis of lumbar disc disease. Surg. Neurol. **5**, 287–291 (1976)
27. Krempen, J.F., Smith, B.S.: Nerve-root injection. A method for evaluating the etiology of sciatica. J. Bone Jt Surg. **56A**, 1435–1444 (1974)
28. Laplane, D.: Sciatiques. Conclusions pratiques. Rev. Prat. (Paris) **22**, 3185–3187 (1972)
29. Legré, J., Dufour, M., Debaene, A., Dalmas, J., Burrou, A.: La discorgraphie lombaire. Valeur et indications après 300 examens. Neuro-chirurgie **17**, 559–578 (1971)
30. Le Page, J.R.: Transfemoral ascending lumbar catheterization of the epidural veins. Exposition and technique. Radiology **111**, 337–339 (1974)
31. Massare, C., Bernageau, J.: Indications de la discographie. Bilan après 1200 discographies. J. Radiol. Électrol. **53**, 429–431 (1972)
32. Metrizamide, a non-ionic water-soluble contrast medium. Experimental and preliminary clinical investigations. Acta radiol. (Stockh.), Suppl. **335** (1973)
33. Patrick, B.S.: Lumbar discography: a five year study. Surg. Neurol. **1**, 267–273 (1973)
34. Patrick, B.S.: Extreme lateral ruptures of lumbar intervertebral discs. Surg. Neurol. **3**, 301–304 (1975)
35. Schobinger, R.A., Krueger, E.G., Sobel, G.L.: Comparison of intraosseous vertebral venography and Pantopaque myelography in the diagnosis of surgical conditions of the lumbar spine and nerve roots. Radiology **77**, 376–398 (1961)

36. Sèze, S., de, Levernieux, J., Cayla, G., Jurmand, S.: Les indications de la sacco-radiculographie au méthiodal. Presse méd. **73**, 1341–1344 (1965)
37. Sheldon, J.J., Russin, L.A., Gargano, F.P.: Lumbar spinal stenosis. Radiographic diagnosis with special reference to transverse axial tomography. Clin. Orthop. **115**, 53–67 (1976)
38. Takahashi, S.: Atlas of axial transverse tomography and its clinical applications. Berlin-Heidelberg-New York: Springer 1969
39. Tarlov, I.M.: Pantopaque meningitis disclosed at operation. J. Amer. med. Ass. **129**, 1014–1016 (1945)
40. Verbiest, H.: Neurogenic intermittent claudication – lesions of the spinal cord and cauda equina, stenosis of the vertebral canal, narrowing of intervertebral foramina and entrapment of peripheral nerves. In: Handbook of Clinical Neurology, Vol. XX, pp. 611–807. Amsterdam: North Holland Publishing Co. 1976
41. Vignon, G., Lespine, A., Calvel, V., Meunier, P., Vignon, E.: La mesure du canal lombaire. Lyon méd. **233**, 603–607 (1975)
42. Weinstein, M.A., Rothner, A.D., Duchesneau, P., Dohn, D.F.: Computed tomography in diastematomyelia. Radiology **117**, 609–611 (1975)

Chapter 1

1. Almen, T.: Contrast agent design. Some aspects on the synthesis of water-soluble contrast agents of low osmolarity. J. theor. Biol. **24**, 216–226 (1969)
2. Almen, T., Wiedeman, M.P.: Application of monomers and polymers to the external surface of the vasculature. Effects on microcirculation in the bat-wing. Invest. Radiol. **3**, 408 (1968)
3. Arcadio, F., Gacon, B., Roche, L.: Les complications neuroradiologiques sévères après méthiodal. Considérations médico-légales. Concours méd. **90**, 3599–3602 (1968)
4. Arnell, S.: Weitere Erfahrungen über Myelographie mit Abrodil. Acta radiol. (Stockh.) **25**, 408–413 (1944)
5. Arnell, S.: Myelography with water-soluble contrast with special regard to the normal

140

roentgen picture. Acta radiol. (Stockh.) Suppl. **75**, 1–85 (1948)

6. Arnell, S.: Discoradiculography with Skiodan. Amer. J. Roentgenol. **66**, 241–244 (1951)

7. Arnell, S., Lindström, F.: Myelography with Skiodan (Abrodil). Acta radiol. (Stockh.) **12**, 287–288 (1931)

8. Autio, E., Suolanen, J., Norrback, S., Slatis, P.: Adhesive arachnoiditis after lumbar myelography with meglumine iothalamate (Conray). Acta radiol. (Diagn.) **12**, 17–24 (1972)

9. Baumgartner, J., Bonte, G., Braun, J.P., Caron, J., Cécile, J.P., Fischgold, H., Gonsette, R., Hirsch, J.F., Legré, J., Metzger, J., Serre, H., Simon, L.: Confrontation critique de 847 examens radiculographiques lombo-sacrés à l'iothalamate de méthylglucamine. Neuro-chirurgie **15**, 503–507 (1969)

10. Baumgartner, J., Bonte, G., Braun, J.P., Caron, J., Cécile, J.P., Fischgold, H., Gonsette, R., Hirsch, J.F., Legré, J., Metzger, J., Serrre, H., Simon, J.: La radiculographie lombo-sacrée à l'iothalamate de méthyl-glucamine, (Contrix 28). Bilan de 847 examens. Rev. Rhum. **36**, 549–554 (1969)

11. Baumgartner, J., Braun, J.P., Caron, J., Cécile, J.P., Fischgold, H., Gonsette, R., Hirsch, J.F., Legré, J., Metzger, J.: Radiculographie au Dimer X. Premiers résultats après 630 examens. J. Radiol. Électrol. **51**, 557–559 (1970)

12. Björk, L.: The osmotic effects of Urografin 76 per cent and Isopaque 60 per cent in angiocardiography. Amer. J. Roentgenol. **98**, 922–926 (1966)

13. Boisen, E., Lindholmer, E.: Alvorlige myelografikomplikationer med jodtalaminmeglumin. Nord. Med. **85**, 520–524 (1971)

14. Bonte, G.: L'intraduragraphie au méthiodal dans le diagnostic des lombo-sciatiques. Presse méd. **65**, 1920 (1957)

15. Bonte, G., Trinez, G.: Radiculographie lombo-sacrée par contrastes hydrosolubles résorbables. Presse méd. (Atlas de radiologie clinique) **63**, 1–4 (1955)

16. Bonte, G., Trinez, G., Delandtsheer, J.M., Galibert, P.: Radiculographie lombo-sacrée aux organo-iodés résorbables. J. Radiol. Électrol. **38**, 72–78 (1957)

17. Bouchard, Ch., Tranier, J., Desgeorges, M.: Intérêt de la saccoradiculographie dans les indications chirurgicales des lombo-sciatiques (à propos de 600 cas). Lyon méd. **230**, 773–776 (1973)

18. Braband, H., Wenker, H., Lessmann, H.D.: Klinische Prüfung eines neuen wasserlöslichen Kontrastmittels zur lumbosakralen Myelographie. Fortschr. Röntgenstr. **115**, 609–614 (1971)

19. Buchheit, F., Maitrot, D., Philippides, D., Babin, E.: Les formes topographiques de hernies discales. Apports de la saccoradiculographie avec zonographie. Neuro-chirurgie **21**, 43–54 (1975)

20. Calabro, A., De Rosa, G., Palmieri, A., Pirolo, R.: Radicolografia con Dimer X. Esperienza su 314 casi. Radiol. med. (Torino) **61**, 49–52 (1975)

21. Calabro, A., Palmieri, A., De Rosa, G.: Un nuovo mezzo di contrasto idrosolubile per radicolographia lombare: Dimer X. Rass. int. Clin. Ter. **50**, 1–7 (1970)

22. Camp, J.D.: Contrast myelography. Past and present. Radiology **54**, 477–505 (1950)

23. Campbell, R.L., Campbell, J.A., Heimburger, R.F., Kalsbeck, J.F., Mealey, J.: Ventriculography and myelography with absorbable radiopaque medium. Radiology **82**, 286–289 (1964)

24. Capesius, P.: Exploration radiologique d'une sciatique en 1975. J. méd Strasbourg **7**, 289–290 (1976)

25. Capesius, P., Babin, E., Maitrot, D., Dupuis, M., Haller, M., Mancs, P.: Intérêt de la radiculosaccographie dans l'exploration radiologique d'une sciatique. Bull. Soc. Sci. méd. Luxemb. **113**, 169–177 (1976)

26. Caron-Poitreau, C., Bregeon, Ch., Boasson, M., Bernat, M., Caron, J., Renier, J.-C.: Radiculographie au dimère de l'iothalamate de méthylglucamine (Dimer X). Rev. Rhum. **38**, 539–544 (1971)

27. Caron-Poitreau, C., Bregeon, Ch., Girod, F., Renier, J.C., Caron, J.: La radiculographie lombo-sacrée au Dimer X. Technique et indications actuelles. J Radiol. Électrol. **52**, 394–396 (1971)

28. Cécile, J.P., Regnier, G., Guaquiere, A., Doffiny, L., Cuvelier, A.: Postural protection against complications in radiculography with Dimer X. Neuradiology **7**, 167–172 (1974)

29. Chiapuzzo, A., Merli, E.: Saccoradicologra-

fia con iocarmato di metilglucamina. Minerva ortop. (Torino) **25**, 1–6 (1974)

30. Ciambellotti, E., Gandini, G., Imassi, G.F., Sosso, A., Bramante, L., Gromo, G.: Presupposti e indicazioni della mielografia con mezzo di contrasto idrosolubile con particolare riguardo alle lombo-sciatalgie. Minerva med. (Torino) **65**, 4063–4082 (1974)

31. Colas, J., Collet, M., Lebastard-Sartre, R., Dano, H., Tendron, J.: La radiculographie lombaire dans le diagnostic des lombo-sciatiques. Réflexions à propos de 423 examens au méthiodal. J. méd. Nantes **3**, 199–209 (1963)

32. Cuvelier, A.: Action préventive de la position couchée sur les effets secondaires de la radiculographie au Dimer X. Thèse Méd Nancy, No. 181 (1974)

33. Danziger, J., Bloch, S.: A clinical evaluation of Dimer X in lumbar radiculography. Clin. Radiol. **24**, 231 (1973)

34. Ecoiffier, J.: Premiers résultats acquis en discographie et myélographie selon les méthodes suédoises. J. Radiol. Électrol. **33**, 568 (1952)

35. Ecoiffier, J.: La radiculographie lombaire dans la sciatique. Paris: Masson & Cie. 1960

36. Ferrand, J., D'Eshougues, J.R., Barsotti, J.: La radiculographie lombo-sacrée par substance iodée hydrosoluble et résorbable. Paris: Expansion, 1961

37. Fischer, F.K.: Neue Methode zur Darstellung von Bandscheibenveränderungen bei Lumbago and Ischias. Schweiz. med. Wschr. **79**, 213–217 (1949)

38. Fischer, H.W., Revier, S.R., Moscow, N.P.: Further toxicity studies with methyl-glucamine contrast agents. Invest. Radiol. **3**, 324–329 (1968)

39. Geller, G.: Komplikationen bei der lumbalen Myelographie mit Conray 282 (Contrix 28). Fortschr. Röntgenstr. **114**, 568–569 (1971)

40. Gonsette, R.: An experimental and clinical assessment of water-soluble contrast medium in neuroradiology. A new medium – Dimer X. Clin. Radiol. **22**, 44–56 (1971)

41. Gonsette, R.E.: Metrizamide as contrast medium for myelography and ventriculography. Preliminary clinical experiences. Acta radiol. (Diagn.), Suppl. **355**, 346–358 (1973)

42. Gonsette, R., André-Balisaux, G.: Nouvelle technique de radiculographie lombo-sacrée par produit hydrosoluble résorbable, sans rachianesthésie. Ann. Radiol. **11**, 141–145 (1968)

43. Gonsette, R., André-Balisaux, G.: Utilisation des produit de contraste hydrosolubles en neuroradiologie. 8e Symposium Neuroradiologicum, Paris 1967. Acta radiol. (Diagn.) **9**, 49–53 (1969)

44. Gonsette, R., André-Balisaux, G.: Etude expérimentale et clinique de quelques produits de contraste hydrosolubles en vue de leur utilisation pour la radiculographie, la myélographie et le ventriculographie. J. Radiol. Électrol. **51**, 19–28 (1970)

45. Gottesleben, A., Selle, G.: Die lumbosacrale Radiculographie mit Dimer X. Nervenarzt **43**, 646–648 (1972)

46. Grainger, R.G., Gumpert, J., Sharpe, D.M., Carson, J.: Water-soluble lumbar radiculography. A clinical trial of Dimer X. A new contrast medium. Clin. Radiol. **22**, 57–62 (1971)

47. Guerbet, M.: Radiculographie lombosacrée au Dimer X. Une table ronde dans le service de neuroradiologie de la Pitié, 16 novembre 1970. Presse méd. **79**, 414 (1971)

48. Guerbet, M.: La radiculographie lombosacrée au Dimer X. Une mise en garde du Laboratoire Guerbet? Nouv. Presse méd. **5**, 1110 (1976)

49. Haase, J., Jepsen, B.V., Bech, H., Langeback, E.: Spinal fracture following radiculography using meglumine iothalamate (Conray). Neuroradiology **6**, 65–70 (1973)

50. Hammer, B.: Die lumbosakrale Radikulographie. Klinische Erfahrungen an 1000 Untersuchungen. Klinisch-experimentelle Untersuchungen. Wien. med. Wschr., Suppl. **17**, 1–15 (1974)

51. Hayes, C.W., Foster, J.M., Sewel, R., Killen, D.A.: Experimental evaluation of concentrated solutions of iotalamic acid derivatives as angiographic media. Amer. J. Roentgenol. **97**, 755–761 (1966)

52. Heimburger, R.F., Campbell, R.L., Kalsbeck, J.E., Mealy, J., Goodell, C.L.: Positive contrast cerebral ventriculography using water soluble media. I. Animal studies. Confin. neurol. (Basel) **28**, 97–116 (1966)

53. Heimburger, R.F., Kalsbeck, J.E., Campbell, R.L., Mealy, J.: Positive contrast cerebral ventriculography using water soluble

media. Clinical evaluation of 102 procedures using methyl-glucamine iothalamate 60%. J. Neurol. Neurosurg. Psychiat. **29**, 281–290 (1966)

54. Hilal, S.K.: Hemodynamic changes associated with the intraarterial injection of contrast media: new toxicity tests and new experimental contrast medium. Radiology **86**, 615–633 (1966)

55. Hindmarsh, T.: Methiodal sodium and metrizamide in lumbar myelography. Acta radiol. (Diagn.), Suppl. **335**, 359–366 (1973)

56. Hindmarsh, T.: Lumbar myelography with meglumine iocarmate and metrizamide. Acta radiol. (Diagn.) **16**, 209–222 (1975)

57. Hindmarsh, T.: Myelography with the non-ionic water-soluble contrast medium metrizamide. Acta radiol. (Diagn.) **16**, 417–435 (1975)

58. Hindmarsh, T., Grepe, A., Widén, L.: Metrizamide-phenothiazine interaction. Report of a case with seizures following myelography. Acta radiol. (Diagn.) **16**, 129–134 (1975)

59. Irstam, L.: Side effects of water-soluble contrast media in lumbar myelography. Acta radiol. (Diagn.) **14**, 647–656 (1973)

60. Knutsson, F.: Lumbar myelography with water soluble contrast in cases of disc prolapse. Acta orthop. scand. **20**, 294–302 (1951)

61. Kodama, J.K., Butler, W.M., Tusing, T.W., Hallet, F.P.: Iothalamate 5 acetamido N methyl 2, 4, 6, triiodo-isophtalmate, a new intravascular radiopaque medium with pharmacotoxic inertness. Exp. molec. Path. Suppl. **2**, 65–80 (1963)

62. Kosary, I.Z., Tadmor, R., Ouaknine, G., Braham, J.: Lumbosacral myelography with Dimer-X. Report of 100 cases. J. Neurosurg. **39**, 359–361 (1973)

63. Legré, J., Salamon, G., Dufour, M., Guidicelli, G.: La radiographie lombo-sacrée au Dimer X. Premiers résultats après 80 examens. Marseille méd. **2**, 135–136 (1970)

64. Lindblöm, K.: Lumbar myelography by abrodil. Acta radiol. (Stockh.) **27**, 1–7 (1946)

65. Lindblöm, K.: Complications of myelography by abrodil. Acta radiol. (Stockh.) **28**, 69–73 (1947)

66. Lorencic, M., Kumar, H., Vidakovic, Z., Popov, N.: Dimer X – a new contrast medium for subarachnoidal myelography of lumbo-sacral area. Preliminary report. Radiol. iugosl. **5**, 139–140 (1971)

67. Maitrot, D.: Hernies discales lombo-sacrées. Analyse clinique, radiologique et chirurgicale à propos de 700 cas. Thèse méd. Strasbourg, No. 5, 1973

68. Metrizamide – a non-ionic water-soluble contrast medium. Experimental and preliminary clinical investigations. Acta radiol. (Stockh.) Suppl. **335**, (1973)

69. Monroe, D.: Lumbar and sacral compression radiculitis (herniated lumbar disc syndrome). New Engl. J. Med. **254**, 243–251 (1956)

70. Perrigot, M., Pierrot-Deseilligny, E., Bussel, B., Held, J.P.: Paralysies survenues dans les suites d'une radiculographie au Dimer X. Nouv. Presse méd. **5**, 1120–1122 (1976)

71. Piguet, B., Verspyck, R., Coste, F.: Les accidents neurologiques à type radiculaire de syndrome de la queue de cheval après sacco-radiculographie au méthiodal. J. Radiol. Électrol. **5**, 165–176 (1964)

72. Reinhardt, K., Panter, K.: Les procédés myélographiques, résultats et risques. J. Radiol. Électrol. **36**, 159–170 (1955)

73. Rittmeyer, K., Freyschmidt, J.: Neue Aspekte zur Untersuchungstechnik bei der lumbosakralen Myelographie mit dem wasserlöslichen Kontrastmittel Dimer X. Röntgen-Bl. **26**, 3–11 (1973)

74. Serrano, V.R.: La radiculografia lombosacra. El dimero del iotalamato de metiglucamina (Dimer X). Radiologia (Roma) **14**, 159–166 (1972)

75. Séze, S., de, Djian, A.: Comment radiographier un cas de lombo-sciatique et comment interpréter le résultat. Rev. méd. franç **36**, 539–556 (1955)

76. Séze, S., de, Levernieux, J., Cayla, G., Jurmand, S.: Les indications de la sacco-radiculographie au Methiodal. Presse méd. **73**, 1341–1344 (1965)

77. Sicard, A., Lavarde, Gh.: La radiculographie dans le diagnostic des lombo-sciatiques (1330 cas). Acta orthop. belg. **35**, 631–635 (1969)

78. Skalpe, I.O., Amundsen, P.: Lumbar radiculography with metrizamide. A nonionic water-soluble contrast medium. Radiology **115**, 91–95 (1975)

79. Skalpe, I.O., Torbergsen, T., Amundsen, P.,

Presthus, J.: Lumbar myelography with metrizamide. Acta radiol. (Diagn.) Suppl. 335, 367–379 (1973)

80. Slätis, P., Autio, E., Suolanen, J., Norrbäck, S.: Hyperosmolarity of the cerebrospinal fluid as a cause of adhesive arachnoiditis in lumbar myelography. Acta radiol. (Diagn.) 15, 619–629 (1974)

81. Söderberg, L., Sjöberg, S., Langeland, P.: Neurological complications following myelography with water-soluble contrast medium. Acta orthop. scand. 28, 220–223 (1959)

82. Svare, A., Talle, K.: Lumbar myelography with metrizamide: an evaluation of 15 cases. Acta radiol. (Diagn.) Suppl. 335, 387–390 (1973)

83. Thun, F.: Die lumbale Dimer-X-Myelographie (Ergebnisse bei 660 Untersuchungen). Röntgen-Bl. 27, 549–560 (1974)

84. Vogelsang, H., Busse, O., Schmidt, R.: Die zervikale Myelographie mit wasserlöslichem Kontrastmittel (Metrizamide). Fortschr. Röntgenstr. 125, 225–228 (1976)

85. Walker, N., Egli, M., Wellauer, J.: Nebenreaktionen nach lumbaler Myelographie mit Dimer-X. Z. Orthop. 114, 793–804 (1976)

86. Wellauer, J.: Die Myelographie mit positiven Kontrastmitteln. Stuttgart: Georg Thieme 1961

87. Woringer, E., Baumgartner, J., Braun, J.P.: Le diagnostic de la hernie discale lombosacrée par la myélographie au mono-iodo-méthane sulfonate de sodium (à propos de 500 cas). Presse méd. 63, 1584–1586 (1955)

88. Woringer, E., Langs, A.: Dépistage systématique des hernies discales par une nouvelle substance de contraste résorbable. Rev. neurol. 80, 518 (1948)

89. Woringer, E., Langs, A.: La myélographie au Kontrast U Léo, moyen de diagnostic de la sciatique discale. J. Radiol. Électrol. 31, 450–452 (1950)

90. Zarski, E., Adynowski, J., Leo, W., Styczynski, T., Kozina, W.: Przydatnosc radykulografü w rozpoznawaniu dyskopatü ledzwiowego odcinka kregoslupa. Reumatologia (Warsz.) 11, 205–227 (1973)

Chapter 2

1. Agnoli, A.: Myelotomography in the diagnosis of lumbo-sacral disc prolapse. Acta neurochir. 32, 113–123 (1975)

2. Ahlgren, P.: Lumbale Myelographie mit Conray Meglumin 282. Fortschr. Röntgenstr. 111, 270–276 (1969)

3. Ahlgren, P.: Long term side effects after myelography with watersoluble contrast media: Conturex, Conray Meglumin 282 and Dimer-X. Neuroradiology 6, 206–211 (1973)

4. Ahlgren, P.: Amipaque myelography. The side effects compared with Dimer-X. Neuroradiology 9, 197–202 (1975)

5. Ahlgren, P., Praestholm, J.: Komplikationer ved myelografi med methiodalum. Nord. Med. 82, 1600–1604 (1969)

6. Almen, T., Wiedeman, M.P.: Application of monomers and polymers to the external surface of the vasculature. Effects on microcirculation in the bat-wing. Invest. Radiol. 3, 408 (1968)

7. Autio, E., Suolanen, J., Norrback, S., Slatis, P.: Adhesive arachnoiditis after lumbar myelography with meglumine iothalamate (Conray). Acta radiol. (Diagn.) 12, 17–24 (1972)

8. Babin, E., Maitrot, D., Dirheimer, Y., Haller, M., Mugel, J.-L., Buchheit, F.: L'intérêt de la zonographie frontale en saccoradiculographie. Sem Hôp. Paris 50, 2081–2087 (1974)

9. Babin, E., Maitrot, D., Haller, M., Dirheimer, Y., Buchheit, F.: The value of frontal zonographic sections in saccoradiculography. Neuroradiology 7, 161–166 (1974)

10. Baumgartner, J., Bonte, G., Braun, J.-P., Caron, J., Cécile, J.-P., Fischgold, H., Gonsette, R., Hirsch, J.-F., Legré, J., Metzger, J., Serre, H., Simon, J.: La radiculographie lombo-sacrée à l'iothalamate de méthyl-glucamine (Contrix 28). Bilan de 847 examens. Rev. Rhum. 36, 549–554 (1969)

11. Baumgartner, J., Bonte, G., Braun, J.-P., Caron, J., Cécile, J.-P., Fischgold, H., Gonsette, R., Hirsch, J.-F., Legré, J., Metzger, J., Serre, H., Simon, L.: Confrontation critique de 847 examens radiculographiques lombo-sacrés à l'iothalamate de méthylglucamine. Neuro-chirurgie 15, 503–507 (1969)

12. Bidstrub, P.: A case of chronic adhesive arachnoiditis after lumbar myelography with methiodal sodium. Neuroradiology 3, 157–158 (1972)

13. Capesius, P., Babin, E.: Tomographic exploration in radiculosaccography.

Proceedings of the Symposium Actualitatis Tomographiae, Genova, 11, 12, 13 September 1975. Amsterdam: Excerpta Medica 1976

14. Caron-Poitreau, C., Bregeon, Ch., Boasson, M., Bernat, M., Caron, J., Renier, J.-C.: Radiculographie au dimère de l'iothalamate de méthyl-glucamine (Dimer X). Rev. Rhum. **38**, 539–544 (1971)

15. Cécile, J.-P., Regnier, G., Guaquiere, A., Doffiny, L., Cuvelier, A.: Postural protection against complications in radiculography with Dimer X. Neuroradiology **7**, 167–172 (1974)

16. Christensen, A.B!: Fractura colli femoris som komplikation til Conray-Myelografi. Ugeskt. Laeg. **136**, 1579–1580 (1974)

17. Clement, J.-C., Neagu, S., Deshayes, P.: Notre expérience de la saccoradiculographie avec l'iothalamate de méthylglucamine. Rev. Rhum. **36**, 391–398 (1969)

18. Cuvelier, A.: Action préventive de la position couchée sur les effets secondaires de la radiculographie au Dimer X. Thèse méd. Nancy, No. 181 (1974)

19. Davis, F.M., Llewellyn, R.-C., Kirgis, H.D.: Water-soluble contrast myelography using meglumine iothalamate (Conray) with methylprednisolone acetate (Depo-Medrol). Radiology **90**, 705–710 (1968)

20. De Graaf, A.S.: Epileptiske anfall som komplikasjon til Conray-myelografi. Nord. Med. **85**, 673 (1971)

21. De Graaf, A.S., Kayed, K.S.: Epileptic seizures and EEG changes after radiculography with meglumine iothalamate (Conray) and meglumine iocarmate (Dimer X). Psychiat. neurol. Neurochir. **76**, 77 (1973)

22. Deisenhammer, E., Hammer, B.: Clinical and experimental studies on headache after myelography. Neuroradiology **9**, 99–102 (1975)

23. Dullerud, R., Morland, T.J.: Adhesive arachnoiditis after lumbar radiculography with Dimer-X and Depo-Medrol. Radiology **119**, 153–155 (1976)

24. Ferrand, J., D'Eshougues, R., Barsotti, J.: La radiculographie lombo-sacrée par substance iodée hydrosoluble et résorbable. Paris: L'expansion 1961

25. Gass, H., Goldstein, A.S., Ruskin, R., Leopold, N.A.: Chronic postmyelogram headache. Isotopic demonstration of dural leak and surgical cure. Arch. Neurol. **25**, 168–170 (1971)

26. Gonsette, R.: An experimental and clinic assessment of water-soluble contrast medium in neuroradiology. A new medium-Dimer X. Clin. Radiol. **22**, 44–56 (1971)

27. Gonsette, R.: Metrizamide as contrast medium for myelography and ventriculography. Preliminary clinical experiences. Acta radiol. (Stockh.) Suppl. **335**, 346–358 (1973)

28. Guerbet, M.: Radiculographie lombo-sacrée au Dimer X. Une table ronde dans le service de neuroradiologie de la Pitié, 16 novembre 1970. Presse méd. **79**, 414 (1971)

29. Guerbet, M.: La radiculographie lombo-sacrée au Dimer-X. Une mise en garde du Laboratoire Guerbet? Nouv. Presse méd. **5**, 1110 (1976)

30. Haase, J., Jepsen, B.V., Bech, H., Langebaek: Spinal fracture following radiculography using meglumine iothalamate (Conray). Neuroradiology **6**, 65–70 (1973)

31. Halaburt, H., Lester, J.: Leptomeningeal changes following lumbar myelography with water-soluble contrast media (meglumine iothalamate and methiodal sodium). Neuroradiology **5**, 70–76 (1973)

32. Hammer, B.: Delayed resorption of contrast media and radioelements in cases of lumbosacral malformations. Neuroradiology **3**, 97–101 (1971)

33. Hammer, B.: Die lumbosakrale Radikulographie. Klinische Erfahrungen an 1000 Untersuchungen. Klinisch-experimentelle Untersuchungen. Wien med. Wschr., Suppl. **17**, 1–15 (1974)

34. Hammer, B., Scherrer, H.: Choice of contrast medium in lumbosacral myelography. Neuroradiology **4**, 114–117 (1972)

35. Hilal, S.K.: Hemodynamic changes associated with the intraarterial injection of contrast media. New toxicity tests and a new experimental contrast medium. Radiology **86**, 615–633 (1966)

36. Hindmarsh, T.: Methiodal sodium and metrizamide in lumbar myelography. Acta radiol. (Stockh.), Suppl. **335**, 359–366 (1973)

37. Hindmarsh, T.: Myelography with a non-ionic water-soluble contrast medium (Metrizamide). Thesis, Stockholm 1974

38. Hindmarsh, T.: Lumbar myelography with

meglumine iocarmate and metrizamide. Acta radiol. (Diagn.) 16, 209–222 (1975)

39. Hindmarsh, T.: Myelography with the non-ionic water-soluble contrast medium metrizamide. Acta radiol. (Diagn.) 16, 417–435 (1975)

40. Hindmarsh, T., Grepe, A., Widen, L.: Metrizamide-phenothiazine interaction. Report of a case with seizures following myelography. Acta radiol. (Diagn.) 16, 129–134 (1975)

41. Irstam, L.: Side effects of water-soluble media in lumbar myelography. Acta radiol. (Diagn.) 14, 647–656 (1973)

42. Irstam, L.: Adverse effects of water-soluble contrast media in lumbar myelography. Thesis, Gothenburg, 1974

43. Irstam, L., Rosencrantz, M.: Water-soluble contrast media and adhesive arachnoiditis. I. Reinvestigation of nonoperated cases. Acta radiol. (Diagn.) 14, 497–506 (1973)

44. Irstam, L., Rosencrantz, M.: Water-soluble contrast media and adhesive arachnoiditis. II. Reinvestigation of operated cases. Acta radiol. (Diagn.) 15, 1–15 (1974)

45. Irstam, L., Selldén, U.: Side effects after lumbar myelography with dimeglumine iocarmate (Dimer X). Further experiences. Acta radiol. (Diagn.) 16, 449–462 (1975)

46. Irstam, L., Sundström, R., Sigstedt, B.: Lumbar myelography and adhesive arachnoiditis. Acta radiol. (Diagn.) 15, 356–368 (1974)

47. Jorgensen, J., Hansen, P.H., Steenskov, V., Ovesen, N.: A clinical and radiological study of chronic lower spinal arachnoiditis. Neuradiology 9, 139–144 (1975)

48. Kaada, B.: Transient EEG abnormalities following lumbar myelography with metrizamide. Acta radiol. (Stockh.), Suppl. 335, 380–386 (1973)

49. Kitov, D.: La radiculosaccographie au Dimer X dans le diagnostic et le traitement opératoire des hernies discales lombaires. Travail d'habilitation, Plovdiv, Dec. 1973

50. Knutsson, F.: Volum- und Formvariationen des Wirbelkanals bei Lordosierung bzw. Kyphosierung und ihre Bedeutung für die myelographische Diagnostik. Acta radiol. (Stockh.) 23, 431–443 (1942)

51. Legré, J., Dufour, M., Giudicelli, G.: Radiculographie par contraste hydrosoluble. In: Traité de Radiodiagnostic. Neuroradiologie. Canal Rachidien, Moelle et Racines, Vol. XV/3, Chap. V, pp. 73–84. Paris: Masson Cie, 1971

52. Lethinen, E., Seppänen, S.: Side effects of Conray Meglumin 282 and Dimer X in lumbar myelography. Acta radiol. (Diagn.) 12, 12–16 (1972)

53. Levine, M.C., White, D.W.: Chronic post-myelographic headache. A result of persistent epidural cerebrospinal fluid fistula. J. Amer. med. Ass. 229, 684–686 (1974)

54. Liliequist, B., Lundstrom, B.: Lumbar myelography and arachnoiditis. Neuroradiology 7, 91–94 (1974)

55. McLennan, J.E., Rosenbaum, A.E., Tyler, H.R.: Prevention of postmyelographic and postpneumoencephalographic headache by single dose intrathecal methyl prednisolone acetate. Headache 13, 39–48 (1973)

56. Metrizamide. A non-ionic water-soluble contrast medium. Experimental and preliminary clinical investigations. Acta radiol. (Stockh.), Suppl. 335 (1973)

57. Movin, A.: Myelographic appearances of disk protrusions in different positions. Acta radiol. (Diagn.) 6, 524–528 (1967)

58. Nielsen, H.: Epileptic seizures following cervical myelography. Neuroradiology 10, 59–60 (1975)

59. Nyegaard & Co. A/S, Oslo: Personal communication. Reported by: P. Ahlgren, Amipaque Myelography. Neuroradiology 9, 197–202 (1975)

60. Oftedal, S.-I., Kayed, K.: Epileptogenic effect of water-soluble contrast media. An experimental investigation in rabbits. Acta radiol. (Stockh.), Suppl. 335, 45–56 (1973)

61. Oftedal, S.-I.: Meningeal reactions to water-soluble contrast media in cats. Acta radiol. (Stockh.), Suppl. 335, 153–160 (1973)

62. Perrigot, M., Pierrot-Deseilligny, E., Bussel, B., Held, J.-P.: Paralysies survenues dans les suites d'une radiculographie au Dimer-X. Nouv. Presse méd. 5, 1120–1122 (1976)

63. Praestholm, J., Lester, J.: Water-soluble contrast lumbar myelography with meglumine iothalamate (Conray). Brit. J. Radiol. 43, 303–308 (1970)

64. Radberg, C., Wennberg, F.: Late sequelae following lumbar myelography with water-soluble contrast media. Acta radiol. (Diagn.) 14, 507–512 (1973)

65. Rittmeyer, K., Freyschmidt, J., Argyrakis,

146

A., Eckel, H.: Radikulotomographie bei der lumbosakralen Myelographie. Fortschr. Röntgenstr. **123**, 436–441 (1975)

66. Salamon, G., Louis, R., Guerinel, G.: Le fourreau dural lombo-sacré. Etude radio-anatomique. Acta radiol. (Diagn.) **5**, 1107–1123 (1966)

67. Skalpe, I.O.: Animal experimental and clinical investigations of a non-ionic water-soluble contrast media (Metrizamide). Thesis, Oslo 1973

68. Skalpe, I.O.: Myelography with metrizamide, meglumine iothalamate and meglumine iocarmate. An experimental investigation in cats. Acta radiol. (Stockh.), Suppl. **335**, 57–66 (1973)

69. Skalpe, I.O., Amundsen, P.: Lumbar radiculography with metrizamide. A non-ionic water-soluble contrast medium. Radiology **115**, 91–95 (1975)

70. Skalpe, I.O., Torbergsen, T., Amundsen, P., Presthus, J.: Lumbar myelography with metrizamide. Acta radiol. (Stockh.) Suppl. **335**, 367–379 (1973)

71. Skalpe, I.O., Torvik, A.: Toxicity of metrizamide and meglumine iocarmate in the spinal subarachnoid space. An experimental study in rats with special reference to long-term effects. Invest. Radiol. **10**, 154–159 (1975)

72. Slätis, P., Autio, E., Suolanen, J., Norrbäck, S.: Hyperosmolality of the cerebrospinal fluid as a cause of adhesive arachnoiditis in lumbar myelography. Acta radiol. (Diagn.) **15**, 619–629 (1974)

73. Suolanen, J.: Adhesive arachnoiditis following myelography with various water-soluble contrast media. Neuroradiology **9**, 73–78 (1975)

74. Svare, A., Talle, K.: Lumbar myelography with metrizamide: an evaluation of 15 cases. Acta radiol. (Stockh.), Suppl. **335**, 387–390 (1973)

75. Vik-Mo, H., Maurer, H.J.: Meningeal reactions following myelography. Effects of detergent washing agent. Acta radiol. (Diagn.) **16**, 39–42 (1975)

76. Vogelsang, H., Busse, O., Schmidt, R.: Die zervikale Myelographie mit wasserlöslichem Kontrastmittel (Metrizamide). Fortschr. Röntgenstr. **125**, 225–228 (1976)

77. Von Essen, C., Thulin, C.A.: The potential risk of myelography with positive contrast medium in cases with traumatic injuries of the lower spinal canal (a case report). Neurochirurgia (Stuttg.) **12**, 208–212 (1969)

78. Walker, N., Egli, M., Wellauer, J.: Nebenreaktionen nach lumbaler Myelographie mit Dimer-X. Z. Orthop. **114**, 793–804 (1976)

79. Wiggli, U., Oberson, R.: Die Häufigkeit extra-arachnoidalen Liquorausflusses nach Lumbalpunktion. Schweiz. med. Wschr. **105**, 235–239 (1975)

Chapter 3

1. Blau, J.N., Logue, V.: Intermittent claudication of the cauda equina. An unusual syndrome resulting from central protrusion of a lumbar intervertebral disc. Lancet **1961 I**, 1081–1086

2. Bloch-Michel, H., Cauchoix, J., Benoist, M.: A propos de 60 observations de sciatique paralysante. Sem. Hôp. Paris **43**, 2640–2646 (1967)

3. Buchheit, F., Maitrot, D., Philippides, D., Babin, E.: Les formes topographiques de hernies discales. Apports de la saccoradiculographie avec zonographie. Neuro-chirurgie **21**, 43–54 (1975)

4. Cauchoix, J., Bloch-Michel, H., Benoist, M., Deburge, A., Chassaing, V., Savary, L.: Sciatiques "arthrosiques" par compression radiculaire d'origine ostéophytique dans le récessus latéral. A propos de 18 observations. Rev. Rhum. **43**, 475–480 (1976)

5. Charbonnel, A.: La sciatique par hernie discale. Rev. Prat. (Paris) **22**, 3139–3149 (1972)

6. Charcot, J.M.: Sur la claudication intermittente. C. R. Soc Biol. (Paris) **5**, 225–238 (1853)

7. Collard, M.: Sciatique paralysante (41 observations). Thèse méd. Strasbourg, No. 14, 1967

8. Creissard, P.: Anatomie des racines du sciatique dans le canal lombaire. La hernie discale en tant qu'agent de compression radiculaire. Rev. Prat. (Paris) **22**, 3095–3105 (1972)

9. Danforth, M.S., Wilson, P.D.: The anatomy of the lumbo-sacral region in relation to sciatic pain. J. Bone Jt Surg. **7**, 109–160 (1925)

10. Dejerine, J.: La claudication intermittente de la moelle épinière. Presse méd. **19**, 981–984 (1911)

11. DePalma, A.F., Rothman, R.H.: Lumbar disc lesions: Anatomic and pathologic features and the clinic syndrome. In: The Intervertebral Disc, Chap. 3, pp. 58–84. Philadelphia: W.B. Saunders Co. 1970

12. DePalma, A.F., Rothman, R.H.: Salient clinical features of lumbar disc lesions. In: The Intervertebral Disc, Chap. 11, pp. 181–202. Philadelphia: W.B. Saunders Co. 1970

13. DePalma, A.F., Rothman, R.H.: Clinical manifestations of lumbar disc syndrome. In: The Intervertebral Disc, Chap. 12, pp. 203–248. Philadelphia: W.B. Saunders Co. 1970

14. D'Eshougues, J.R., Laine, E., Bonte, G., Galibert, P., Lemaitre, G., Lebeurre, R.: Confrontation des données cliniques, radiculographiques et opératoires dans 171 observations de pathologie douloureuse lombo-sacrée. Lille méd. 9, 333–349 (1964)

15. Epstein, B.: The spine: a radiological text and atlas. Philadelphia: Lea & Febiger, 1969

16. Epstein, B.S., Epstein, J.A., Lavine, L.: The effect of anatomic variations in the lumbar vertebrae and spinal canal on cauda equina and nerve root syndromes. Amer. J. Roentgenol. 91, 1055–1063 (1964)

17. Epstein, J.A., Epstein, B.S., Rosenthal, A.D., Carras, R., Lavine, L.S.: Sciatica caused by nerve root entrapment in the lateral recess: the superior facet syndrome. J. Neurosurg. 36, 584–589 (1972)

18. Evans, J.G.: Neurogenic intermittent claudication. Brit. med. J. 2, 985–987 (1964)

19. Ferrand, J., D'Eshougues, J.R.: Les enseignements de la sacco-radiculographie lombo-sacrée dans les névralgies crurales (sur 15 observations personelles). Sem. Hôp. Paris 57, 2825–2836 (1963)

20. Finneson, B.E.: Low back pain. In: Lumbar Disc Disease, pp. 141–216. Philadelphia: Lippincott Co. 1973

21. French, J.D., Paine, J.T.: Cauda equina compression syndrome with herniated nucleus pulposus. A report of eight cases. Ann. Surg. 120, 73–87 (1944)

22. Godlewski, S.: Examen clinique d'un malade atteint de sciatique ou de lombosciatique. Rev. Prat. (Paris) 22, 3107–3117 (1972)

23. Hakelius, A., Hindmarsh, J.: The comparative reliability of preoperative diagnostic methods in lumbar disc surgery. Acta orthop. scand. 43, 234–238 (1972)

24. Hudgins, W.B.: The predictive value of myelography in the diagnosis of ruptured lumbar discs. J. Neurosurg. 32, 152–162 (1970)

25. Jacobson, R.E., Gargano, F.P., Rosomoff, H.L.: Transverse axial tomography of the spine. Part 1. Axial anatomy of the normal lumbar spine. J. Neurosurg. 42, 406–411 (1975)

26. Jeanmart, L., Retif, J.: Confrontation des résultats de l'examen myélographique avec les données cliniques et les constatations opératoires à propos de 150 cas de hernies discales lombaires. J. belge Radiol. 50, 415–423 (1967)

27. Kavanaugh, G.J., Svien, H.J., Holman, C.B., Johnson, R.M.: "Pseudoclaudication" syndrome produced by compression of the cauda equina. J. Amer. med. Ass. 206, 2477–2481 (1968)

28. Kissel, P., Tridon, P.: Les syndromes de la queue de cheval d'origine discale. Gaz. méd. Fr. 67, 1789–1795 (1960)

29. Kirkaldy-Willis, W.H., McIvor, G.W.D.: Lumbar spinal stenosis. Editorial comment. Clin. Orthop. 115, 2–3 (1976)

30. Kirkaldy-Willis, W.H., Paine, K.W.E., Cauchoix, J., McIvor, G.W.D.: Lumbar spinal stenosis. Clin. Orthop. 99, 30 (1974)

31. Maitrot, D.: Hernies discales lombo-sacrées. Analyse clinique, radiologique et chirurgicale à propos de 700 cas. Thèse méd. Strasbourg, No. 5, 1973

32. Middleton, L.: Contribution à l'étude des syndromes de compression des racines de la queue de cheval d'origine osseuse: le canal lombaire étroit et le canal radiculaire étroit. Thèse méd. Strasbourg, No. 194, 1976

33. Mixter, W.J., Barr, J.S.: Rupture of the intervertebral disc with involvement of the spinal canal. New Engl. J. Med. 211, 210–215 (1934)

34. Paillas, J.E., Bille, J., Louis, R.: Le syndrome de la queue de cheval par hernie discale. Sur une série de 31 cas vérifiés. Marseille méd. 7–8, 513–517 (1964)

35. Piganiol, G., Bonnal, J., Herve, H.: Sciatiques discales pseudo-tumorales et tumeurs

de la queue de cheval à début sciatalgique. Marseille chir. **7**, 610–614 (1955)

36. Ramadier, J.O., Vermeulen, H.: Sciatiques paralysantes. Acta orthop. belg. **35**, 620–630 (1969)
37. Salamon, G., Louis, R., Guerinel, G.: Le fourreau dural lombo-sacré. Etude radio-anatomique. Acta radiol. (diagn.) **5**, 1107–1123 (1966)
38. Salibi, B.S.: Neurogenic intermittent claudication and stenosis of the lumbar spinal canal. Surg. Neurol. **5**, 269–272 (1976)
39. Schlesinger, P.T., Falls, G.: Incarceration of the first sacral nerve in a lateral bony recess of the spinal canal as a cause of sciatica. J. Bone Jt Surg. **37A**, 115–124 (1955)
40. Serre, H., Simon, L., Baumelou, H., Bouvier, J.P.: Le syndrome de la queue de cheval d'origine discale en pratique rhumatologique. Sem. Hôp. Paris **46**, 3302–3310 (1970)
41. Sèze, S. de: La sciatique dite banale essentielle ou rhumatismale et le disque lombosacré. Rev. Rhum. **10**, 986–1037 (1939)
42. Sèze, S. de, Guillaume, J., Desproges-Gotteron, R., Jurmand, S., Maitre, M.: Sciatique paralysante (étude clinique, pathogénique, thérapeutique) d'après 100 observations. Sem. Hôp. Paris **33**, 1773–1795 (1957)
43. Sèze, S. de, Ryckewaert, A.: Sciatique vertébrale commune. In: Maladies des Os et des Articulations, Vol. II, pp. 1104–1155. Paris: Editions Médicales Flammarion
44. Sicard, A., Touzard, R.: La forme pseudotumorale des hernies discales lombaires. Presse méd. **78**, 2453–2456 (1970)
45. Verbiest, H.: A radicular syndrome from developmental narrowing of the lumbar vertebral canal. J. Bone Jt Surg. **36B**, 230–237 (1954)
46. Verbiest, H.: Neurogenic intermittent claudication in cases with absolute and relative stenosis of the lumbar vertebral canal, in cases with narrow lumbar intervertebral foramina, and in cases with both entities. Clin. Neurosurg. **20**, 204–214 (1973)
47. Wilson, C.B., Ehni, G., Grollmus, J.: Neurogenic intermittent claudication. Clin. Neurosurg. **18**, 62–85 (1971)

Chapter 4

1. Agnoli, A.: Myelotomography in the diagnosis of lumbo-sacral disc prolapse. Acta neurochir. (Wien) **32**, 113–123 (1975)
2. Agnoli, A.: Anormale Wurzelabgänge im lumbosacralen Bereich und ihre klinische Bedeutung. J. Neurol. (Brux.) **211**, 217–228 (1976)
3. Arnell, S.: Myelography with water-soluble contrast, with special regard to the normal roentgen-picture. Acta radiol. (Stockh.) Suppl. **75** (1948)
4. Babin, E., Maitrot, D., Dirheimer, Y., Haller, M., Mugel, J.L., Buchheit, F.: L'intérêt de la zonographie frontale en saccoradiculographie. Sem. Hôp. Paris **50**, 2081–2087 (1974)
5. Babin, E., Maitrot, D., Haller, M., Dirheimer, Y., Buchheit, F.: The value of frontal zonographic sections in saccoradiculography. Neuroradiology **7**, 161–166 (1974)
6. Breig, A., Marions, O.: Biomechanics of the lumbosacral nerve roots. Acta radiol. (Diagn.) **1**, 1141–1160 (1963)
7. Capesius, P., Babin, E.: Tomographic exploration in radiculosaccography. Proceedings of the Symposium Actualitatis Tomographiae, Genova, 11, 12, 13 September 1975. Amsterdam: Excerpta Medica 1976
8. Diemath, H.E.: Die lumbale Funktionsmyelographie mit Conray 60. Schweiz. Arch. Neurol. Psychiat. **108**, 7–12 (1971)
9. Ecoiffier, J.: Séméiologie radiographique des images. In: La Radiculographie Lombaire dans la Sciatique, Chap. IV, pp. 53–61. Paris: Masson & Cie. 1960
10. Ethelberg, S., Riishede, J.: Malformation of lumbar spinal roots and sheaths in the causation of low backache and sciatica. J. Bone Jt Surg. **34B**, 442–446 (1952)
11. Ferrand, J., D'Eshougues, J.R., Barsotti, J.: Les images normales. In: La Radiculographie Lombo-sacrée par Substance Iodée Hydrosoluble et Résorbable, pp. 19–25. Paris: Expansion 1961
12. Heon, M.: Les malformations radiculaires lombaires dans la chirurgie discale. Laval méd. **34**, 536–539 (1963)
13. Heon, M.: Incidence des malformations radiculaires lombairs lors de la chirurgie discale lombaire. Un. méd. Can. **101**, 1146–1149 (1972)
14. Knutsson, F.: Volum- und Formvariationen des Wirbelkanals bei Lordosierung bzw. Kyposierung und ihre Bedeutung für

die myelographische Diagnostik. Acta radiol. (Stockh.) **23**, 431–443 (1942)

15. Komminoth, R., Woringer, E., Philippi, R.: Méga cul-de-sac dural. Etude clinique de 60 cas. Neuro-chirurgie **14**, 607–616 (1968)

16. Legré, J., Dufour, M., Giudicelli, G.: Radiculographie par contraste hydrosoluble. In: Traité de Radiodiagnostic, Vol. XV, pp. 73–82. Paris: Masson & Cie. 1971

17. Manelfe, C., Treil, J., Lestrade, M., Fardou, H., Roulleau, J.: Elargissement de l'espace épidural antérieur en regard de la charnière lombo-sacrée. (Son interprétation au cours des radiculosaccographies.) J. Radiol. Électrol. **54**, 864–865 (1973)

18. Movin, A.: Myelographic appearances of disk protrusions in different positions. Acta Radiol. (Diagn.) **6**, 524–528 (1967)

19. Ortner, W.D.: Über die lumbale Funktionsmyelographie. Radiologe **12**, 69–73 (1972)

20. Pecker, J., Simon, J., Bou-Salah, A., Pivault, Ch.: L'accolement en canon de fusil des racines rachidiennes. Piège diagnostique. Nouv. Presse méd. **3**, 1155–1156 (1974)

21. Salamon, G., Louis, R., Guerinel, G.: Le fourreau dural lombo-sacré. Etude radioanatomique. Acta radiol. (Diagn.) **5**, 1107–1123 (1966)

22. Sassaroli, S., Urso, S.: Normal lumbosacral radiculography. In: Lumbosacral Radiculography by Means of Hydrosoluble Contrast Media. An anatomical and functional outline, pp. 13–15. Padua: Piccin Medical Books 1974

23. Sassaroli, S., Urso, S.: Functional lumbosacral radiculography. In: Lumbosacral Radiculography by Means of Hydrosoluble Contrast Media. An Anatomical and functional outline, pp. 15–21. Padua: Piccin Medical Books 1974

24. Wellauer, J.: Das normale lumbale Myelogramm mit wasserlöslichen Kontrastmitteln. In: Die Myelographie mit positiven Kontrastmitteln, pp. 46–49. Stuttgart: Georg Thieme 1961

Chapter 5

1. Ahlgren, P.: Long term side effects after myelography with watersoluble contrast media: Conturex, Conray Meglumin 282

and Dimer X. Neuroradiology **6**, 206–211 (1973)

2. Babin, E., Maitrot, D., Dirheimer, Y., Haller, M., Mugel, J.L., Buchheit, F.: L'intérêt de la zonographie frontale en saccoradiculographie. Sem. Hôp. Paris **50**, 2081–2087 (1974)

3. Babin, E., Maitrot, D., Haller, M., Dirheimer, Y., Buchheit, F.: The value of frontal zonographic sections in saccoradiculography. Neuroradiology **7**, 161–166 (1974)

4. Capesius, P., Babin, E.: Tomographic exploration in radiculosaccography. In: Procedings of the Symposium Actualitatis Tomographiae. Genoa, September 11–13, 1975. Amsterdam: Excerpta Medica 1976

5. Capesius, P., Babin, E.: Exploration radiculosaccographique des canaux lombaires étroits. Ann. Radiol. **20**, 501–507 (1977)

6. Capesius, P., Babin, E., Soutter, J.W., Middelton, L., Maitrot, D., Wackenheim, A.: Compression of the dural sac by anomalous lumbar articular processes as demonstrated by radiculosaccography. Bull. Soc. Sci. méd. Luxemb. (in press)

7. Capesius, P., Babin, E., van Damme, W., Touitou, D., Haller, M., Ammerich, H.: Deux formes radiculosaccographiques des neurinomes de la queue de cheval. J. méd. Strasbourg **8**, 23–26 (1977)

8. Cronqvist, S.: The postoperative myelogram. Acta radiol. (Stockh.) **52**, 45–51 (1959)

9. Cronqvist, S., Fuchs, W.: Lumbar myelography in complete obstruction of the spinal canal. Acta Radiol. (Diagn.) **2**, 145–152 (1964)

10. D'Eshougues, J.R., Ferrand, J., Barsotti, J.: La radiculographie lombo-sacrée par substance iodée, hydrosoluble et résorbable. I. Données séméiologiques. Entretiens de Bichat — Médecine, 417–426 (1960)

11. Ecoiffier, J.: Séméiologie radiographique des images. In: La Radiculographie Lombaire dans la Sciatique, pp. 53–61. Paris: Masson & Cie. 1960

12. Epstein, J.A., Epstein, B.S., Lavine, L.S.: Surgical treatment of nerve root compression caused by scoliosis of the lumbar spine. J. Neurosurg. **41**, 449–454 (1974)

13. Ferrand, J., D'Eshougues, J.R., Barsotti, J.: Les images anormales. In: La Radiculographie Lombo-sacrée par Substance

Iodée Hydrosoluble et Résorbable. Paris: Expansion, 1961

14. Gulati, D.R., Rout, D.: Myelographic block caused by redundant lumbar nerve root. Case report. J. Neurosurg. **38**, 504–505 (1973)

15. Jeanmart, L., Retif, J., Brihaye, J.: Syndrome de la queue de cheval par compression d'origine tumorale et discale: apport de l'examen myélographique. J. Radiol. Électrol. **51**, 561–566 (1970)

16. Hirsch, C., Rosencrantz, M., Wickbom, I.: Lumbar myelography with water-soluble contrast media. With special reference to the appearances of root pockets. Acta radiol. (Diagn.) **8**, 54–64 (1969)

17. Komminoth, R., Woringer, E., Philippi, R.: Méga cul-de-sac dural. Etude clinique de 60 cas. Neuro-chirurgie **14**, 607–616 (1968)

18. Maitrot, D.: Hernies discales lombosacrées. Analyse clinique, radiologique et chirurgicale à propos de 700 cas. Thèse méd. Strasbourg, No. 5, 1973

19. Moiel, R., Ehni, G.: Cauda equina compression due to spondylolisthesis with intact neural arch. Report of two cases. J. Neurosurg. **28**, 262–265 (1968)

20. Retif, J., Jeanmart, L.: Etude myélographique des hernies discales lombaires et dorsales avec arrêt complet du produit de contraste. Acta neurol. psychiat. belg. **68**, 543–551 (1968)

21. Rothman, R.H., Campbell, R.E., Menkowitz, E.: Myelographic patterns in lumbar disk degeneration. Clin. Orthop. **99**, 18–29 (1974)

22. Sassaroli, S., Urso, S.: Radiculografia lombosacrale con mezzo di contrasto idrosolubile. Dati anatomici e funzionali. Lumbosacral radiculography by means of hydrosoluble contrast media. An anatomical and functional outline. Padua: Piccin Medical Books 1974

23. Schut, L., Groff, R.A.: Redundant nerve roots as a cause of complete myelographic block. Case report. J. Neurosurg. **28**, 394–395 (1968)

24. Shapiro, R.: The pathologic myelogram. In: Myelography, 3rd ed., pp. 136–151. Chicago: Year Book Medical Publishers, Inc. 1976

25. Smith, R.W., Loeser, J.D.: A myelographic variant in lumbar arachnoiditis. J. Neurosurg. **36**, 441–446 (1972)

26. Tenner, M.S.: Myelography of nonmass lesions in the spinal canal. Sem. Roentgenol. **7**, 277–296 (1972)

27. Wellauer, J.: Der röntgenologische Nachweis von Protrusion und Bandscheibenprolaps durch die Myelographie. In: Die Myelographie mit positiven Kontrastmitteln, pp. 98–114. Stuttgart: Georg Thieme 1961

Chapter 6

1. Abdullah, A.F., Ditto, E.W., Byrd, E.B., Williams, R.: Extreme lateral lumbar disc herniations. Clinical syndrome and special problems of diagnosis. J. Neurosurg. **41**, 229–234 (1974)

2. Babin, E., Maitrot, D., Dirheimer, Y., Haller, M., Mugel, J.L., Buchheit, F.: L'intérêt de la zonographie frontale en sacco-radiculographie. Sem. Hôp. Paris **50**, 2081–2087 (1974)

3. Babin, E., Maitrot, D., Haller, M., Dirheimer, Y., Buchheit, F.: The value of frontal zonographic sections in saccoradiculography. Neuroradiology **7**, 161–166 (1974)

4. Balaparameswara, Rao S., Dinakar, I., Sreenivasa, Rao K.: Extraosseous extradural tuberculous granuloma simulating a herniated lumbar disc. Case report. J. Neurosurg. **35**, 488–490 (1971)

5. Blikra, G.: Intradural herniated lumbar disc. J. Neurosurg. **31**, 676–679 (1969)

6. Brish, A., Payan, H.M.: Lumbar intraspinal extradural ganglion cyst. J. Neurol. Neurosurg. Psychiat. **35**, 771–775 (1972)

7. Buchheit, F., Maitrot, D., Philippides, D., Babin, E.: Les formes topographiques de hernies discales. Apports de la saccoradiculographie avec zonographie. Neurochirurgie **21**, 43–54 (1975)

8. Capesius, P., Babin, E.: Tomographic exploration in radiculosaccography. In: Procedings of the Symposium Actualitatis Tomographiae, Genoa, September 11–13, 1975. Amsterdam: Excerpta Medica 1976

9. Capesius, P., Babin, E., Soutter, J.W., Middelton, L., Maitrot, D., Wackenheim, A.: Compression of the dural sac by anomalous lumbar articular processes as demonstrated by radiculosaccography. Bull. Soc. Sci. méd. Luxemb. (in press)

10. Capesius, P., Babin, E., van Damme, W., Touitou, D., Haller, M., Ammerich, H.: Deux formes radiculosaccographiques des neurinomes de la queue de cheval. J. méd. Strasbourg **8**, 23–26 (1977)

11. Cohen, J.: Extradural varix simulating herniated nucleus pulposus. J. Mt Sinai Hosp. **8**, 136–138 (1949)

12. DePalma, A.F., Rothman, R.H.: Lumbar disc lesions: anatomic and pathologic features and the clinic syndrome. In: The Intervertebral Disc, Chap. 3, pp. 58–84. Philadelphia: W.B. Saunders Co, 1970

13. Devadiga, K.V., Gass, H.H.: Chronic lumbar extradural haematoma simulating disc syndrome. J. Neurol. Neurosurg. Psychiat. **36**, 255–259 (1973)

14. Epstein, B.S.: Low back pain associated with varices of the epidural veins simulating herniations of the nucleus pulposus. Amer. J. Roentgenol. **57**, 736–742 (1947)

15. Ferrand, J., D'Eshougues, J.R.: Les enseignements de la sacco-radiculographie lombosacrée dans les névralgies crurales (sur 15 observations personnelles). Sem. Hôp. Paris **57**, 2825–2836 (1963)

16. Finneson, B.E.: Lumbar disc disease. In: Low Back Pain, Chap. 6, pp. 141–216. Philadelphia: Lippincott Company 1973

17. Gümbel, U., Pia, H.W., Vogelsang, H.: Lumbosacrale Gefäßanomalien als Ursache von Ischialgien. Acta neurochir. (Wien) **20**, 131–151 (1969)

18. Gutterman, P., Shenkin, H.A.: Syndromes associated with protrusion of upper lumbar intervertebral discs. Results of surgery. J. Neurosurg. **38**, 499–503 (1973)

19. Kao, C.C., Uihlein, A., Bickel, W.H., Soule, E.H.: Lumbar intraspinal extradural ganglion cyst. J. Neurosurg. **29**, 168–172 (1968)

20. Keon-Cohen, B.T.: Epidural abscess simulating disc hernia. J. Bone Jt Surg. **50 B**, 128–130 (1968)

21. Kulowski, J.: Subdural rupture of an intervertebral lumbar disc. Case report. Missouri Med. **64**, 715–716 (1967)

22. Legré, J., Dufour, M., Giudicelli, G.: Hernies discales. In: Traité de Radiodiagnostic. Vol. 15. Neuroradiologie. Canal Rachidien, Moelle et Racines, pp. 199–211. Paris: Masson & Cie. 1971

23. Maitrot, D.: Hernies discales lombo sacrées. Analyse clinique, radiologique et chirurgicale à propos de 700 cas. Thèse méd. Strasbourg, No. 5, 1973

24. Patrick, B.S.: Extreme lateral ruptures of lumbar intervertebral discs. Surg. Neurol. **3**, 301–304 (1975)

25. Piguet, B., Ramadier, J.O., Mazabraud, A., Coste, F.: A propos des sciatiques par anomalies veineuses épidurales (sciatique paralysante et syndrome de la queue de cheval postmyélographique à recrudescences menstruelles, avec angiomatose épidurale). Rev. Rhum. **31**, 101–108 (1964)

26. Reina, A.: Tuberculous epidural granuloma simulating a herniated lumbar disc. Surg. Neurol. **4**, 336–338 (1975)

27. Rengachary, S.S., Murphy, D.: Subarachnoid hematoma following lumbar puncture causing compression of the cauda equina. Case report. J. Neurosurg. **41**, 252–254 (1974)

28. Roth, J.A., Kaufman, H.H.: Hypertrophy of the ligamentum flavum. In: Handbook of Clinical Neurology. Vinken, P.J., Bruyn, G.W. (eds.). Tumors of the spine and spinal cord. Vol. XX, pp. 809–817. Amsterdam: North-Holland Publishing Co. 1976

29. Rothman, R.H., Campbell, R.E., Menkowitz, E.: Myelographic patterns in lumbar disk degeneration. Clin. Orthop. **99**, 19–29 (1974)

30. Shapiro, R.: The herniated intervertebral disk. In: Myelography, 3rd ed., Chap. 16, pp. 348–413. Chicago: Yearbook Medical Publishers 1975

31. Sicard, A., Touzard, R.: Les sciatiques bilatérales par hernie discale. Presse méd. **79**, 1895–1897 (1971)

32. Svien, H.J., Adson, A.W., Dodge, H.W.: Lumbar extradural hematoma: report of a case simulating protruded disk syndrome. J. Neurosurg. **7**, 587–588 (1950)

33. Taptas, J.N., Andreadis, A., Kordiolis, N.I.: Les hernies discales lombaires sousdurales. Neuro-chirurgie **17**, 51–56 (1971)

34. Thomalske, G., Mohr, G.: Intradurale Sequestrierung lumbaler Diskushernien unter besonderer Berücksichtigung der Achondroplasie. Nervenarzt **45**, 376–379 (1974)

Chapter 7

1. Ahlgren, P.: Long term side effects after myelography with watersoluble contrast

media: Conturex, Conray Meglumin 282 and Dimer-X. Neuroradiology **6**, 206–211 (1973)
2. Brodsky, A.E.: Post-laminectomy and post-fusion stenosis of the lumbar spine. Clin. Orthop. **115**, 130–139 (1976)
3. Cauchoix, J., Taussig, G., Nordin, J.Y.: Sciatique et syndrome de la queue de cheval par rétrécissement du canal rachidien après arthrodèse lombo-sacrée postérieure. Sem. Hôp. Paris **45**, 2023–2025 (1969)
4. Cronqvist, S.: The postoperative myelogram. Acta radiol. (Stockh.) **52**, 45–51 (1959)
5. DePalma, A.F., Rothmann, R.H.: Complications, failures and tragedies of operative treatment of lumbar disc disease. In: The Intervertebral Disc, Chap. 16, pp. 324–353. Philadelphia: W.B. Saunders Company 1970
6. De Villiers, P.D., Booysen, E.L.: Fibrous spinal stenosis. A report on 850 myelograms with a water-soluble contrast medium. Clin. Orthop. **115**, 140–144 (1976)
7. Fahrenkrug, A., Gottschalck, B., Hojgaard: Myelography with water-soluble media in lumbo-sciatica after operation for herniated lumbar disk. Acta radiol. (Stockh.) **2**, 138–152 (1964)
8. Finneson, B.E.: Lumbar disc discase. In: Low Back Pain, Chap. 6, pp. 141–216. Philadelphia: J.B. Lippincott Company 1973
9. Grumme, Th., Bingas, B., Knupling, R.: Meningozele nach lumbalen Bandscheibenoperationen. Acta neurochir. (Wien) **27**, 177–187 (1972)
10. Irstam, L., Rosencrantz, M.: Water-soluble contrast media and adhesive arachnoiditis. II. Reinvestigation of operated cases. Acta radiol. (Diagn.) **15**, 1–15 (1974)
11. Jain, K.K.: Nerve root scarring and arachnoiditis as a complication of lumbar intervertebral disc surgery-surgical treatment. Neurochirurgia (Stuttg.) **17**, 185–192 (1974)
12. Jorgensen, J., Hansen, P.H., Steenskov, V., Ovesen, N.: A clinical and radiological study of chronic lower spinal arachnoiditis. Neuroradiology **9**, 139–144 (1975)
13. Maitrot, D.: Les réinterventions. In: Hernies Discales Lombo-sacrées. Analyse Clinique, Radiologique et Chirurgicale à Propos de 700 Cas, Chap. V, pp. 125–131. Thèse méd. Strasbourg, 1973

14. Rinaldi, I., Hodges, T.O.: Iatrogenic lumbar meningocele: report of three cases. J. Neurol. Neurosurg. Psychiat. **33**, 484–492 (1970)
15. Rinaldi, I., Peach, W.P.: Postoperative lumbar meningocele. Report of two cases. J. Neurosurg. **30**, 504–507 (1969)
16. Sassaroli, S., Urso, S.: Radiculografia lombosacrale con mezzo di contrasto idrosolubile. Dati anatomici e funzionali. Lumbosacral radiculography by means of hydrosoluble contrast media. An anatomical and functional outline. Padua: Piccin Medical Books 1974
17. Seaman, W.B., Marder, S.N., Rosenbaum, H.E.: The myelographic appearance of adhesive spinal arachnoiditis. J. Neurosurg. **10**, 145–153 (1953)
18. Sèze, S., de: Les ennuis de la chirurgie discale. Complications, opérations "blanches", échecs, récidives. Rev. Prat. (Paris) **22**, 3177–3182 (1972)
19. Smith, R.W., Loeser, J.D.: A myelographic variant in lumbar arachnoiditis. J. Neurosurg. **36**, 441–446 (1972)
20. Smolik, E.A., Nash, F.P.: Lumbar spinal arachnoiditis. A complication of the intervertebral disc operation. Ann. Surg. **133**, 490–495 (1951)
21. Tarlov, I.M.: Spinal perineurial and meningeal cysts. J. Neurol. Neurosurg. Psychiat. **33**, 833–843 (1970)
22. Tedeschi, N., Benini, A.: Leptomeningitis chronica fibroplastica der Cauda equina als Ursache ischias-ähnlicher Beschwerden. Neurochirurgia (Stuttg.) **19**, 84–90 (1976)

Chapter 8

1. Alker, G.J., Glasauer, F.E., Zoll, J.G.: Myelographic demonstration of lumbosacral nerve root avulsion. Radiology **89**, 101–104 (1967)
2. Archer, V., Cooper, G., Cimmino, C.: Occult meningocele of the sacrum: report of three cases. Radiology **51**, 691–696 (1948)
3. Baker, G., Webb, J.: Intrasacral meningocele causing backache and sacral nerve pain: Report of case. Proc. Mayo Clin. **27**, 231–234 (1952)
4. Basauri, L., Hudson, H., Bardales, A.: Diverticuli of the nerve root sheaths. J. Neurosurg. **31**, 580–582 (1969)

5. Bechar, M., Beks, J.W.F., Penning, L.: Intradural arachnoid cysts with scalloping of vertebrae in the lumbosacral region. Acta neurochir. (Wien) **26**, 275–283 (1972)
6. Benini, A.: Lumbale und sakrale Wurzeltaschendivertikel als Ursache ischias ähnlicher Beschwerden. Neurochirurgia (Stuttg.) **16**, 1–8 (1973)
7. Bowie, E.A., Glasgow, G.I.: Cauda equina lesions associated with ankylosing spondylitis: report of three cases. Brit. med. J. **2**, 24–27 (1961)
8. Braun, J.P., Babin, E.: Les formations kystiques et diverticulaires des méninges rachidiennes. Sem. Hôp. Paris **46**, 2750–2754 (1970)
9. Brish, A., Payan, H.M.: Lumbar intraspinal extradural ganglion cyst. J. Neurol. Neurosurg. Psychiat. **35**, 771–775 (1972)
10. Brown M.H., Powell, L.D.: Anterior sacral meningocele. J. Neurosurg. **2**, 535–538 (1945)
11. Bryant, Th.: Case of deficiency of the anterior part of the sacrum with a thecal sac in the pelvis, similar to the tumour of spina bifida. Lancet **1837–38 I**, 358
12. Calihan, R.J.: Anterior sacral meningocele. Radiology **58**, 104–108 (1952)
13. Campbell, J.B.: Congenital anomalies of neural axis. Surgical management based on embryologic considerations. Amer. J. Surg. **75**, 231–236 (1948)
14. Carlson, D.H., Hoffman, H.B.: Lumbosacral traumatic meningocele. Neurology (Minneap.) **21**, 174–176 (1971)
15. Chaouat, Y.: Lombosacroradiculalgies par canaux larges. (Variété de dysharmonie médullo-radiculo-méningo-rachidienne lombosacrée d'origine dure-mérienne). In: L'Actualité Rhumatologique Présentée au Praticien. Sèze, S., de, Ryckewaert, A. (eds.), pp. 95–106. Paris: Expansion Scientifique Edit. 1974
16. Chaouat, Y., Kanovitch, B., Faures, B., Ginet, Cl., Piatecki, A., Vignaud, J.: Lomboradiculalgies par canaux larges. Une variété de dysharmonie médullo-radiculo-méningo-rachidienne d'origine dure-mérienne. Rev. Rhum. **41**, 491–499 (1974)
17. Crellin, R.Q., Jones, E.R.: Sacral extradural cysts. A rare cause of low backache and sciatica. J. Bone Jt Surg. **55B**, 20–31 (1973)
18. Derreumaux, L.L., Delcambre, B., Chris-tiaens, J.L., Zylberberg, G., Cornille, Ch.: Les dilatations du cul-de-sac dural et les anomalies des gaines radiculaires. Lille méd. **14**, 410–418 (1969)
19. Eder, D.: Anterior sacral meningocele; survey of literature and report of cases. Bull. Los Angeles neurol. Soc. **14**, 104–112 (1949)
20. Enderle, C.: Meningocele intrasacre occulto (rivelato con la myelographie). Riv. Neurol. **5**, 418–423 (1932)
21. Ferrand, J., D'Eshougues, R., Barsotti, J.: La "columnisation" longitudinale et médiane du "gros cul-de-sac dural" (opération de Hanraets). Presse méd. **68**, 1401 (1960)
22. Ferrand, J., D'Eshougues, R., Barsotti, J.: La radiculographie lombo-sacrée par substance iodée hydrosoluble et résorbable. Paris: Expansion éd. 1961
23. Finkemeyer, H., Grubel, G.: Eine seltene Komplikation nach Bandscheibenoperationen. Beitr. Neurochir. **15**, 71–76 (1968)
24. Finney, L.A., Wulfman, W.A.: Traumatic intradural lumbar nerve root avulsion with associated fraction injury to the common peroneal nerve. Amer. J. Roentgenol. **84**, 952–957 (1960)
25. Florez, G., Ucar, S.: The occult intrasacral meningocele. Neurochirurgia (Stuttg.) **19**, 46–53 (1976)
26. Gardner, V.J.: Embryology origin of spinal malformations. Acta radiol. (Stockh.) **5**, 1013–1023 (1960)
27. Goodell, C.: Neurological deficits associated with pelvic fractures. J. Neurosurg. **24**, 837–842 (1966)
28. Gordon, A.L., Yudell, A.: Cauda equina lesion associated with rheumatoid spondylitis. Ann. intern. Med. **78**, 555–557 (1973)
29. Grumme, Th., Bingas, B., Knüpling, R.: Meningozele nach lumbalen Bandscheibenoperationen. Acta neurochir. (Wien) **22**, 177–187 (1972)
30. Gurdjian, E.A., Webster, J.E., Ostrowski, A.Z., Hardy, W.G., Lindner, D.W., Thomas, L.M.: Herniated lumbar intervertebral discs. An analysis of 1176 operated cases. J. Trauma **1**, 158–176 (1961)
31. Hammer, B.: Delayed resorption of contrast media and radio-elements in cases of lumbosacral malformations. Neuroradiology **3**, 97–101 (1971)
32. Hanraets, P.R.: Degenerative back and its

154

differential diagnosis. Amsterdam: Elsevier 1959

33. Hauge, T.: Chronic rheumatoid polyarthritis and spondylarthritis associated with neurological symptoms and signs and occasionally simulating an intraspinal expansive process. Acta chir. scand. **120**, 395–401 (1961)

34. Howieson, J., Norrell, H., Wilson, C.: Expansion of the subarachnoid space in the lumbosacral region. Radiology **90**, 488–492 (1968)

35. Joseph, R.A., McKenzie, T.: Occult intrasacral meningocele. J. Neurol. Neurosurg. Psychiat. **33**, 493–496 (1970)

36. Kak, V.K., Chugh, K.S., Sodhi, J.S.: Occult intrasacral meningocele. Neurochirurgia (Stuttg.) **4**, 148–152 (1972)

37. Kao, C.C., Uihlein, A., Bickel, W.H., Soule, E.H.: Lumbar intraspinal extradural ganglion cyst. J. Neurosurg. **29**, 168–172 (1968)

38. Keen, J.: Genesis of spina bifida and allied congenital defect. Clin. Proc. **7**, 162–172 (1948)

39. Kennedy, R.L.J.: An unusual rectal polyp: anterior sacral meningocele. Surg. Gynec. Obstet. **43**, 803 (1926)

40. Komminoth, R., Woringer, E., Philippi, R.: Méga cul-de-sac dural. Etude clinique de 60 cas. Neuro-chirurgie **14**, 607–616 (1968)

41. Lazorthes, G., Espano, J., Arbus, L., Lacapere, J.P., Lazorthes, Y.: Les malformations du cul-de-sac spinal. Essai de classification. Neuro-chirurgie **12**, 503–509 (1966)

42. Lee, M.L.H., Watters, D.J.: Neurological complications of ankylosing spondylitis. Brit. med. J. **1**, 798 (1962)

43. Leigh, J.F., Rogers, J.V.: Anterior sacral meningocele. Amer. J. Roentgenol. **71**, 808–812 (1954)

44. Lombardi, G., Passerini, A.: Spinal cord diseases. A radiologic and myelographic analysis, pp. 161–170. Baltimore: Williams and Wilkins 1964

45. Martin, P., Hasaerts, R., Thumerelle, G.: La méningocèle sacrée antérieure. Acta chir. belg. **48**, 437–443 (1956)

46. Matthews, W.B.: The neurological complications of ankylosing spondylitis. J. neurol. Sci. **6**, 561–573 (1968)

47. McGill, I.G.: An unusual neurological syndrome associated with ankylosing spondylitis. Guy's Hosp. Rep. **115**, 33–36 (1966)

48. McLennan, J.E., McLaughlin, W.T., Skillicorn, S.A.: Traumatic lumbar nerve root meningocele. Case report. J. Neurosurg. **39**, 528–532 (1973)

49. Paleirac, R., Temple, J.P., Janicot, J.Y., Givaudand, A.: Etude des variations morphologiques du cul-de-sac dural au moyen de la radiculographie au méthiodal. J. Radiol. Électrol. **41**, 837–840 (1960)

50. Payne, R.F., Thomson, J.L.G.: Myelography in lumbo-sacral plexus injury. Brit. J. Radiol. **42**, 840–845 (1969)

51. Perret, G., Green, D., Keller, J.: Diagnosis and treatment of intradural arachnoid cysts of the thoracic spine. Radiology **79**, 425–429 (1962)

52. Pia, H.W.: Megacauda. Eine angeborene Erweiterung des Caudasackes im Lumbosakralbereich. Langenbecks Arch. klin. Chir. **290**, 429–439 (1959)

53. Pool, J.: Spinal cord and local signs secondary to occult sacral meningoceles in adults. Bull. N.Y. Acad. Med. **28**, 655–663 (1952)

54. Rhoton, A.L., Jr., Kao, C.C., Uihlein, A.: Extradural ganglion cyst. In: Handbook of Clinical Neurology, Part II: Tumours of the Spine and Spinal Cord. Vinken, P.J., Bruyn, G.W. (eds.), Vol. XX, pp. 605–609. Amsterdam: North-Holland Publishing Co. 1976

55. Rinaldi, I., Hodges, T.O.: Iatrogenic lumbar meningocele: report of three cases. J. Neurol. Neurosurg. Psychiat. **33**, 484–492 (1970)

56. Rinaldi, I., Peach, W.F.: Postoperative lumbar meningocele. Report of two cases. J. Neurosurg. **30**, 504–507 (1969)

57. Rosenkranz, W.: Ankylosing spondylitis: cauda equina syndrome with multiple spinal arachnoid cysts. Case report. J. Neurosurg. **34**, 241–243 (1971)

58. Rowlands, B.C.: Anterior sacral meningocele. Report of two cases. Brit. J. Surg. **43**, 301–304 (1955)

59. Schober, R.: Klinische und diagnostische Bedeutung cystischer Wurzeltaschenerweiterungen. Acta radiol. (Diagn.) **1**, 754–761 (1963).

60. Schreiber, F., Haddad, B.: Lumbar and sacral cysts causing pain. J. Neurosurg. **8**, 504–509 (1951)

61. Schurr, P.H.: Sacral extradural cyst: an uncommon cause of low back pain. J. Bone Jt Surg. **37 B**, 601–605 (1955)

62. Sherman, R.M., Caylor, H.D., Long, L.: Anterior sacral meningocele. Amer. J. Surg. **79**, 743–747 (1950)

63. Sole-Llenas, J.: Les kystes des racines sacrées et leur valeur pathologique. Acta radiol. (Diagn.) **1**, 782–796 (1963)

64. Sutton, D.: Sacral cysts. Acta radiol. (Diagn.) **1**, 787–795 (1963)

65. Swanson, H.S., Fincher, E.F.: Extradural arachnoidal cysts of traumatic origin. J. Neurosurg. **4**, 530–538 (1947)

66. Sypert, G.W., Leech, R.W., Harris, A.B.: Posttraumatic lumbar epidural true synovial cyst. Case report. J. Neurosurg. **39**, 246–248 (1973)

67. Tarlov, I.M.: Perineurial cysts of the spinal nerve roots. Arch. Neurol. Psychiat. (Chic.) **40**, 1067–1074 (1938)

68. Tarlov, I.M.: Cysts (perineurial) of the sacral roots. J. Amer. med. Ass. **138**, 740–744 (1948)

69. Tarlov, I.M.: Sacral nerve-root cysts: another cause of the sciatic and cauda equina syndrome. Springfield: Charles C. Thomas, 1953

70. Tarlov, I.M.: Spinal perineurial and meningeal cysts. J. Neurol. Neurosurg. Psychiat. **33**, 833–843 (1970)

71. Thierry, A., Archimbaud, J.P., Fischer, G., Freidel, M., Mansuy, L.: La méningocèle sacrée antérieure. Revue de la littérature et présentation d'un cas. Neuro-chirurgie **15**, 389–412 (1969)

72. Wilkins, R.H., Odom, G.L.: Spinal intradural cysts. In: Handbook of Clinical Neurology. Vinken, P.J., Bruyn, G.W. (eds.), Vol. XX, pp. 55–102. Tumours of the Spine and Spinal Cord. Amsterdam: North-Holland Publishing Company 1976

73. Young, I., Bruwer, A.: The occult intrasacral meningocele. Amer. J. Roentgenol. **105**, 390–399 (1969)

74. Zumpano, B.J., Saunders, R.L.: Lumbar intradural arachnoid diverticulum with cauda equina compression. Surg. Neurol. **5**, 349–353 (1976)

Chapter 9

1. Abbott, W.D.: Compression of the cauda equina by the ligamentum flavum. J. Amer. med. Ass. **106**, 2129–2130 (1936)

2. Alexander, E.: Significance of the small lumbar spinal canal: cauda equina compression syndromes due to spondylosis. Part 5: Achondroplasia. J. Neurosurg. **31**, 513–519 (1969)

3. Arnoldi, C.C., Brodsky, A.E., Cauchoix, J., Crock, H.V., Dommisse, G.F., Edgar, M.A., Gargano, F.P., Jacobson, R.E., Kirkaldy-Willis, W.H., Kurihara, A., Langenskiold, A., Macnab, I., McIvor, W.D., Newman, P.H., Paine, K.W.E., Russin, L.A., Sheldon, J., Tile, M., Urist, M.R., Wilson, W.E., Wiltse, L.L.: Lumbar spinal stenosis and nerve root entrapment syndromes. Definition and classification. Clin. Orthop. **115**, 4–5 (1976)

4. Auquier, L., Hirsch, J.F., Paolaggi, J.B., Rouques, Cl., Ghozian, R.: Sténose du canal rachidien lombaire et claudication sciatique. A propos de 29 cas dont 12 opérés. Rev. Rhum. **39**, 429–437 (1972)

5. Babin, E., Capesius, P., Maitrot, D.: Signes radiologiques osseux des variétés morphologiques de canaux lombaires étroits. Ann. Radiol. **20**, 491–499 (1977)

6. Boussens, J.: Syndromes "contenant-contenu". A propos d'un rétrécissement aigu osseux du canal rachidien lombaire, complication de discoidectomies avec greffes osseuses. Orientations de recherches expérimentales. Bordeaux méd. **3**, 2301–2322 (1970)

7. Brodsky, A.: Post-laminectomy and postfusion stenosis of the lumbar spine. Clin. Orthop. **115**, 130–139 (1976)

8. Brown, H.A.: Enlargement of the ligamentum flavum: cause of low back pain with sciatic radiation. J. Bone Jt Surg. **20**, 325–338 (1938)

9. Cantore, G.P., Gambacorta, D.: Tabetic lumbar osteoarthropathy with cauda equina syndrome. Acta neurochir. (Wien) **33**, 107–112 (1976)

10. Capesius, P., Babin, E.: Tomographic exploration in radiculosaccography. Proceedings of the Symposium Actualitatis. Tomographiae, Genoa, September 11–13. Amsterdam: Excerpta Medica 1976

11. Capesius, P., Babin, E.: Exploration radiculosaccographique des canaux lombaires étroits. Ann. Radiol. **20**, 501–507 (1977)

12. Capesius, P., Babin, E., Soutter, J.W., Middelton, L., Maitrot, D., Wackenheim, A.:

Compression of the dural sac by anomalous lumbar articular processes as demonstrated by radiculosaccography. Bull. Soc. Sci. méd. Luxemb. (in press)

13. Cartlidge, N.E., McCollum, P.K., Ayyar, R.D.A.: Spinal cord compression in Paget's disease. J. Neurol. Neurosurg. Psychiat. **35**, 825–828 (1972)

14. Cauchoix, J., Benoist, M., Chassaing, V.: Degenerative spondylolisthesis. Clin. Orthop. **115**, 122–129 (1976)

15. Cauchoix, J., Benoist, M., Taussig, G., Nordin, J.Y.: Sciatique et syndrome de la queue de cheval par pseudospondylolisthésis. Sem. Hôp. Paris **45**, 2017–2022 (1969)

16. Cauchoix, J., Bloch-Michel, H., Benoist, M., Chassaing, V.: Spondylolisthésis dégénératif. Manifestations cliniques et traitement à propos de 26 cas opérés. Nouv. Presse méd. **5**, 561–564 (1976)

17. Cauchoix, J., Bloch-Michel, H., Benoist, M., Deburge, A., Chassaing, V., Savary, L.: Sciatiques "arthrosiques" par compression radiculaire d'origine ostéophytique dans le récessus latéral. A propos de 18 observations. Rev. Rhum. **43**, 475–480 (1976)

18. Cauchoix, J., Taussig, G., Nordin, J.Y.: Sciatique et syndrome de la queue de cheval par rétrécissement du canal rachidien après arthrodèse lombo-sacrée postérieure. Sem. Hôp. Paris **45**, 2023–2025 (1969)

19. Chaouat, Y.: Les canaux rachidiens étroits. Dysharmonies médullo-radiculo-rachidiennes par sténose canalaire. Concours méd. **95**, 2318–2330 (1973)

20. Clark, K.: Significance of the small lumbar canal: cauda equina compression syndromes due spondylosis. Part 2. Clinical and surgical significance. J. Neurosurg. **31**, 495–498 (1969)

21. Cressman, M.R., Pawl, R.P.: Serpentine myelographic defect caused by a redundant nerve root. Case report. J. Neurosurg. **28**, 391–393 (1968)

22. Davatchi, F., Benoist, M., Massare, Cl., Helenon, Ch., Bloch-Michel, H.: Contribution à l'étude des canaux étroits à l'étage lombaire. Technique radiologique et valeur normale. Sem. Hôp. Paris **29**, 2008–2012 (1969)

23. Davatchi, F., Benoist, M., Massare, Cl., Helenon, Ch., Bloch-Michel, H.: Etude du canal lombaire dans la sciatique vertébrale

commune. Sem. Hôp. Paris **45**, 2013–2016 (1969)

24. David-Chaussé, J.: Le rétrécissement du canal rachidien lombaire. Rev. méd. Toulouse **5**, 583–594 (1969)

25. David-Chaussé, J., Vallat, J.M., Dehais, J.: Deux cas de compression de la queue de cheval d'origine pagétique. Rôle du rétrécissement du canal lombaire osseux. In: La Maladie de Paget. Symposium International organisé par D.J. Hioco, Le Mas d'Artigny – St. Paul de Vence, 20–23 juin 1973, pp. 59–69. Paris: Laboratoires Armour Montagu 1974

26. Duvoisin, R.C., Yahr, M.D.: Compressive spinal cord and root syndrome in achondroplastic dwarfs. Neurology (Minneap.) **109**, 202–207 (1962)

27. Ehni, G.: Spondylotic cauda equina radiculopathy. Tex. St. J. Med. **61**, 746–752 (1965)

28. Ehni, G.: Significance of the small lumbar spinal canal: cauda equina compression syndromes due to spondylosis. Part 1. Introduction. J. Neurosurg. **31**, 490–494 (1969)

29. Ehni, G., Moiel, R.H., Bragg, T.G.: The "redundant" or "knotted" nerve root: a clue to spondylotic cauda equina radiculopathy. Case report. J. Neurosurg. **32**, 252–254 (1970)

30. Eisenstein, S.: Measurements of the lumbar spinal canal in 2 racial groups. Clin. Orthop. **115**, 42–46 (1976)

31. Epstein, B.S.: The spine: a radiologic text and atlas, 3rd ed. Philadelphia: Lea & Febiger 1969.

32. Epstein, B.S., Epstein, J.A., Lavine, L.: The effect of anatomic variations in the lumbar vertebrae and spinal canal on cauda equina and nerve root syndromes. Amer. J. Roentgenol. **91**, 1055–1063 (1964)

33. Epstein, J.A.: Diagnosis and treatment of painful neurological disorders caused by spondylosis of lumbar spine. J. Neurosurg. **17**, 991–1001 (1960)

34. Epstein, J.A., Epstein, B.S.: Neurological and radiologic manifestations associated with spondylosis of cervical and lumbar spine. Bull. N.Y. Acad. Med. **35**, 370–386 (1959)

35. Epstein, J.A., Epstein, B.S., Lavine, L.: Nerve root compression associated with narrowing of the lumbar spinal canal. J.

Neurol. Neurosurg. Psychiat. **25**, 165–176 (1962)

36. Epstein, J.A., Epstein, B.S., Lavine, L.S.: Surgical treatment of nerve root compression caused by scoliosis of the lumbar spine. J. Neurosurg. **41**, 449–454 (1974)
37. Epstein, J.A., Epstein, B.S., Lavine, L.S., Carras, R., Rosenthal, A.D.: Degenerative lumbar spondylolisthesis with an intact neural arch (pseudospondylolisthesis). J. Neurosurg. **44**, 139–147 (1976)
38. Epstein, J.A., Epstein, B.S., Lavine, L.S., Carras, R., Rosenthal, A.D., Sumner, P.: Lumbar nerve root compression at the intervertebral foramina caused by arthritis of the posterior facets. J. Neurosurg. **39**, 362–369 (1973)
39. Epstein, J.A., Epstein, B.S., Rosenthal, A.D., Carras, R., Lavine, L.S.: Sciatica caused by nerve root entrapment in the lateral recess: the superior facet syndrome. J. Neurosurg. **36**, 584–589 (1972)
40. Epstein, J.A., Malis, L.I.: Compression of spinal cord and cauda equina in achondroplastic dwarfs. Neurology (Minneap.) **5**, 875–881 (1955)
41. Evans, J.G.: Neurogenic intermittent claudication. Brit. med. J. **2**, 985–987 (1964)
42. Fox, J.L.: Redundant nerve roots in the cauda equina. Case report. J. Neurosurg. **30**, 74–75 (1969)
43. Friedman, E.: Narrowing of spinal canal due to thickened lamina. A cause of lowback pain and sciatica. Clin. Orthop. **21**, 190–197 (1961)
44. Gargano, F.P., Jacobson, R.E., Rosomoff, H.L.: Transverse axial tomography of the spine. Neuroradiology **6**, 254–258 (1974)
45. Gelman, M.I.: Cauda equina compression in acromegaly. Radiology **112**, 357–360 (1974)
46. Gispert, Cruz, I. de: Complicaciones neurologicas de la achondroplasia. Rev. clin. esp. **53**, 127–131 (1954)
47. Godlewski, S., Harispe, L., Fabiani, J.M.: Claudication intermittente de la queue de cheval. Sténose serrée du canal rachidien par hypertrophie pagétique de la première vertèbre lombaire. Intervention décompressive. Guérison. Nouv. Presse méd. **4**, 109 (1975)
48. Grossman, Z.D., Wistow, B.W., Wallinga, H.A., Heitzman, E.R.: Recognition of vertebral abnormalities in computed tomography of the chest and abdomen. Radiology **121**, 369–373 (1976)
49. Gulati, D.R., Rout, D.: Myelographic block caused by redundant lumbar nerve root. Case report. J. Neurosurg. **38**, 504–505 (1973)
50. Hadley, L.A.: Constriction of the intervertebral foramen. A cause of nerve root pressure. J. Amer. med. Ass. **140**, 473–475 (1949)
51. Hammerschlag, S.B., Wolpert, S.M., Carter, B.L.: Computed tomography of the spinal canal. Radiology **121**, 361–367 (1976)
52. Hartman, J.T., Dohn, D.F.: Paget's disease of the spine with cord or nerve-root compression. Report of six cases. J. Bone Jt Surg. **48A**, 1079–1084 (1966)
53. Highman, J.H.: Complete myelographic block in lumbar degenerative disease. Clin. Radiol. **16**, 106–111 (1965)
54. Hinck, V.C., Hopkins, C.E., Clark, W.M.: Sagittal diameter of the lumbar spinal canal in children and adults. Radiology **85**, 929–937 (1965)
55. Hubault, A.: Complications neurologiques de la maladie de Paget. In: Aux Confins de la Rhumatologie, pp. 303–320. Paris: Expansion 1961
56. Hubault, A.: Des complications neurologiques de la maladie de Paget. In: La Maladie de Paget. Symposion International organisé par D.J. Hioco, Le Mas d'Artigny — St. Paul de Vence, 20–23 juin 1973, pp. 43–58. Paris: Laboratoires Armour Montagu 1974
57. Jacobson, R.E., Gargano, F.P., Rosomoff, H.L.: Transverse axial tomography of the spine. Part 1. Axial anatomy of the normal lumbar spine. J. Neurosurg. **42**, 406–411 (1975)
58. Jacobson, R.E., Gargano, F.P., Rosomoff, H.L.: Transverse axial tomography of the spine. Part 2. The stenotic spinal canal. J. Neurosurg. **42**, 412–419 (1975)
59. Jones, R.A.C., Thomson, J.L.C.: The narrow lumbar canal. A clinical and radiological review. J. Bone Jt Surg. **50B**, 595–605 (1968)
60. Kaufman, H.H., Ommoya, A.K., Dopman, J.L., Roth, J.A.: Hypertrophy of the ligamentum flavum. Secondary cord syndrome

in an acromegalic. Arch. Neurol. **25**, 256–259 (1971)

61. Kirkaldy-Willis, W.K., McIvor, G.W.D.: Lumbar spinal stenosis. Editorial comment. Clin. Orthop. **115**, 2–3 (1976)
62. Kirkaldy-Willis, W.H., Paine, K.W.E., Cauchoix, J., McIvor, G.W.D.: Lumbar spinal stenosis. Clin. Orthop. **99**, 30–50 (1974)
63. Klenerman, L.: Cauda equina and spinal cord compression in Paget's disease. J. Bone Jt Surg. **48B**, 365–370 (1966)
64. Lange, S.A. de: Eine Anomalie der Cauda equina bei einer achondroplastischen Frau. Acta neurochir. (Wien) **16**, 114–121 (1967)
65. Mathé, J.F., Feve, J.R., Resche, F., Delobel, R., Carbonell, R.: Rétrécissement du canal lombaire par sténose fibreuse. Ann. Méd. Phys. **18**, 587–591 (1975)
66. McIvor, G.W.D., Kirkaldy-Willis, W.H.: Pathological and myelographic changes in the major types of lumbar spinal stenosis. Clin. Orthop. **115**, 72–76 (1976)
67. Middelton, L.: Contribution à l'étude des syndromes de compression des racines de la queue de cheval d'origine osseuse. Le canal lombaire étroit et le canal radiculaire étroit. Thèse méd. Strasbourg, No. 194, 1976
68. Moiel, R., Ehni, G.: Cauda equina compression due to spondylolisthesis with intact neural arch. Report of two cases. J. Neurosurg. **28**, 262–265 (1968)
69. Moiel, R.H., Ehni, G., Anderson, M.S.: Nodule of the ligamentum flavum as a cause of nerve root compression. Case report. J. Neurosurg. **27**, 456–458 (1967)
70. Morris, L.: Water-soluble contrast myelography in spinal canal stenosis and nerve entrapment. Clin. Orthop. **115**, 49–52 (1976)
71. Nelson, M.A.: Lumbar spinal stenosis. J. Bone Jt Surg. **55B**, 506–512 (1973)
72. Newman, P.H.: Stenosis of the lumbar spine in spondylolisthesis. Clin. Orthop. **115**, 116–121 (1976)
73. Nicola, G.C., Nizzoli, V.: Claudication intermittente des membres inférieurs par sténose totale du canal lombaire. Neurochirurgia (Stuttg.) **17**, 48–57 (1974)
74. Paillas, J.E., Recordier, A.M., Pellet, W., Serratrice, G., Peragut, J.C.: Le syndrome du canal lombaire étroit (à propos de 21 observations). Rev. méd. Toulouse **7**, 109–128 (1971)

75. Pau, A., Turtas, S.: Redundant nerve roots of the cauda equina. A case report. Acta neurochir. (Wien) **33**, 311–317 (1976)
76. Ploussard, Ch.: Atteintes radiculo-médullaires au cours de l'achondroplasie. Thèse méd. Paris., No. 35, 1967
77. Ramani, P.S., Perry, R.H., Tomlinson, B.E.: Role of ligamentum flavum in the symptomatology of prolapsed intervertebral discs. J. Neurol. Neurosurg. Psychiat. **38**, 550–557 (1975)
78. Raulin, M.: Les épaississements des lames vertébrales. Relation avec les myélopathies et divers syndrômes radiculaires. Etude clinique et anatomo-pathologique. Thèse méd. Paris, No. 1106, 1962
79. Roberson, G.H., Llewellyn, H.J., Taveras, J.M.: The narrow lumbar spinal canal syndrome. Radiology **107**, 89–97 (1973)
80. Sadar, E.S., Walton, R.J., Gossman, H.H.: Neurological dysfunction in Paget's disease of the vertebral column. J. Neurosurg. **37**, 661–665 (1972)
81. Salibi, B.S.: Neurogenic intermittent claudication and stenosis of the lumbar spinal canal. Surg. Neurol. **5**, 269–272 (1976)
82. Sarpyener, M.A.: Congenital stricture of the spinal canal. J. Bone Jt Surg. **27**, 70–79 (1945)
83. Scapinelli, R.: Sindromi da stenosi del canale vertebrale lombare (presentazione di 29 casi, di cui 17 operati). Clin. ortop. **24**, 79–103 (1973)
84. Schatzker, J., Pennal, G.F.: Spinal stenosis, a cause of cauda equina compression. J. Bone Jt Surg. **50B**, 606–618 (1968)
85. Schlesinger, P.T.: Incarceration of the first sacral nerve in a lateral bony recess of the spinal canal as a cause of sciatica. J. Bone Jt Surg. **37A**, 115–124 (1955)
86. Schreiber, F., Rosenthal, H.: Paraplegia from ruptured lumbar discs in achondroplastic dwarfs. J. Neurosurg. **9**, 642–651 (1952)
87. Schut, L., Groff, R.A.: Redundant nerve roots as a cause of complete myelographic block. Case report. J. Neurosurg. **28**, 394–395 (1968)
88. Serre, H., Gros, C., Simon, L., Baumelou, H., Lamboley, C.: Compressions radiculaires par arthropathies tabétiques du rachis. Rev. Rhum. **37**, 525–533 (1970)
89. Sèze, S. de, Hubault, A., Hamonet, Cl., Du-

dognon, P., Prost, A.: Arthropathies tabétiques avec compressions radiculaires de la queue de cheval. A propos de 4 nouvelles observations. Nouv. Presse méd. **1**, 2747–2752 (1972)

90. Shapiro, R.: Spondylosis and the narrow spinal canal. In: Myelography, 3rd ed., Chap. 17, pp. 414–438. Chicago: Year Book Medical Publishers, Inc. 1975
91. Sheldon, J.J., Russin, L.A., Gargano, F.P.: Lumbar spinal stenosis. Radiographic diagnosis with special reference to transverse axial tomography. Clin. Orthop. **115**, 53–67 (1976)
92. Shenkin, H.A., Hash, C.J.: A new approach to the surgical treatment of lumbar spondylosis. J. Neurosurg. **44**, 148–155 (1976)
93. Sicard, A., Lavarde, G.: Les lésions radiculaires au cours des arthropathies tabétiques du rachis lombaire. Presse méd. **75**, 2209–2212 (1967)
94. Sorensen, B.F., Wirthlin, A.J.: Redundant nerve roots of the cauda equina. Surg. Neurol. **3**, 177–181 (1975)
95. Spillane, J.D.: Three cases of achondroplasia with neurological complications. J. Neurol. Neurosurg. Psychiat. **15**, 246–252 (1952)
96. Stroobandt, G., Laterre, E.C., Vincent, A., Cornelis, G.: Compression radiculo-médullaire d'origine rachidienne chez un achondroplase. Neuro-chirurgie **16**, 295–306 (1970)
97. Teng, P., Papatheodorou, C.: Lumbar spondylosis with compression of the cauda equina. Arch. Neurol. **8**, 221–229 (1963)
98. Thomalske, G., Mohr, G.: Intradurale Sequestrierung lumbaler Diskushernien unter besonderer Berücksichtigung der Achondroplasie. Nervenarzt **45**, 376–378 (1974)
99. Thurel, R., Nehlil, J., Lazar, L.: Complications radiculaires et médullaires des ostéoarthropathies vertébrales tabétiques. Rev. neurol. **114**, 62–65 (1966)
100. Towne, E.B., Reichert, F.L.: Compression of the lumbosacral roots of the spinal cord by thickened ligamenta flava. Ann. Surg. **94**, 327–336 (1931)
101. Varughese, G.: Extradural extrusion of roots of the cauda equina. Surg. Neurol. **5**, 161–163 (1976)
102. Verbiest, H.: A radicular syndrome from developmental narrowing of the lumbar vertebral canal. J. Bone Jt Surg. **36B**, 230–237 (1954)

103. Verbiest, H.: Further experiences on pathological influence of developmental narrowness of bony lumbar vertebral canal. J. Bone Jt Surg. **37B**, 576–583 (1955)
104. Verbiest, H.: Neurogenic intermittent claudication in cases with absolute and relative stenosis of the lumbar vertebral canal, in cases with narrow lumbar intervertebral foramina, and in cases with both entities. Clin. Neurosurg. **20**, 204–214 (1973)
105. Verbiest, H.: Neurogenic intermittent claudication — lesions of the spinal cord and cauda equina, stenosis of the vertebral canal, narrowing of intervertebral foramina and entrapment of peripheral nerves. In: Handbook of Clinical Neurology. Vinken, P.J., Bruyn, G.W. (eds.), Vol. XX, pp. 611–807. Amsterdam: North Holland Publishing Company 1976
106. Vignon, C., Lespine, A., Calvel, V., Meunier, P., Vignon, E.: La mesure du canal lombaire. Lyon méd. **233**, 603–607 (1975)
107. Vignon, G., Lespine, A., Calvel, V., Meunier, P., Vignon, E.: Le syndrome de la sténose du canal lombaire de Verbiest. Lyon méd. **233**, 609–619 (1975)
108. Villers, P.D. de, Booysen, E.L.: Fibrous spinal stenosis. A report on 850 myelograms with a water-soluble contrast medium. Clin. Orthop. **115**, 140–144 (1976)
109. Wilson, C.B.: Significance of the small lumbar spinal canal: cauda equina compression syndromes due to spondylosis. Part 3. Intermittent claudication. J. Neurosurg. **31**, 499–506 (1969)
110. Wilson, C.B., Ehni, G., Grollmus, J.: Neurogenic intermittent claudication. Clin. Neurosurg. **18**, 62–85 (1971)
111. Yamada, H., Ohya, M., Okada, T., Shiozawa, Z.: Intermittent cauda equina compression due to narrow spinal canal. J. Neurosurg. **37**, 83–88 (1972)

Chapter 10

1. Adkins, B.W.D.: Spondylolisthesis. J. Bone Jt Surg. **37B**, 48–62 (1955)
2. Babin, E., Maitrot, D., Haller, M., Dirheimer, Y., Buchheit, F.: The value of frontal zonographic sections in saccoradiculography. Neuroradiology **7**, 161–166 (1974)

3. Bagley, C., Arnold, J.G.: Unusual symptomatology of cauda equina tumors. Report of a case of dermoid, with a review of the literature of dermoid and teratomatous tumours of the vertebral canal. Trans. Amer. neurol. Ass. **66**, 171–173 (1940)

4. Balaparameswara, Rao S., Dinakar, I., Sreenivasa, Rao K.: Extraosseous extradural tuberculous granuloma simulating a herniated lumbar disc. Case report. J. Neurosurg. **35**, 488–490 (1971)

5. Berris, H.: Tuberculous spondylitis simulating herniated intervertebral disk. Neurology (Minneap.) **4**, 710–712 (1954)

6. Bobroff, L.M., Leeds, N.E.: Minimal terminal irregularities of the distal subarachnoid space as a sign of epidural seeding. Amer. J. Radiol. **118**, 601–604 (1973)

7. Boudin, G., Pepin, B., Hubault, A., Labet, R.: Sur quelques aspects particuliers du rachis chez le tabétique. Bull. Soc. méd. Hôp. Paris **113**, 439–443 (1962)

8. Capesius, P., Babin, E., van Damme, W., Touitou, D., Haller, M., Ammerich, H.: Deux formes radiculosaccographiques des neurinomes de la queue de cheval. J. méd. Strasbourg **8**, 23–26 (1977)

9. Cauchoix, J., Benoist, M., Chassaing, V.: Degenerative spondylolisthesis. Clin. Orthop. **115**, 122–129 (1976)

10. Cauchoix, J., Benoist, M., Taussig, G., Nordin, J.Y.: Sciatique et syndrome de la queue de cheval par pseudospondylolisthésis. Sem. Hôp. Paris **45**, 2017–2022 (1969)

11. Cauchoix, J., Bloch-Michel, H., Benoist, M., Chassaing, V.: Spondylolisthésis dégén - ératif. Manifestations cliniques et traitement à propos de 26 cas opérés. Nouv. Presse méd. **5**, 561–564 (1976)

12. Chadduck, W.M.: Intraspinal tuberculous abscess simulating lumbar disc disease. Virginia med. Mth. **99**, 968–971 (1972)

13. Charpentier, J., Messimy, R., Dalage, C., Gozlan, R.: Contribution à l'étude du filum terminale intradural et de ses tumeurs. Presse méd. **78**, 175–178 (1970)

14. Cophignon, J., Julian, H., Houdart, R.: Les épidurites tuberculeuses dites primitives ou associées à une tuberculose de l'arc postérieur. A propos de 13 observations personnelles. Neuro-chirurgie **14**, 783–797 (1968)

15. Cronqvist, S., Fuchs, W.: Lumbar myelography in complete obstruction of the spinal canal. Acta radiol. (Diagn.) **2**, 145–152 (1964)

16. Decker, R.E., Gross, S.W.: Intraspinal dermoid tumor presenting as chemical meningitis. Report of a case without dermal sinus. J. Neurosurg. **27**, 60–62 (1967)

17. Decker, H.G., Shapiro, S.W., Porter, H.R.: Epidural tuberculous abscess simulating herniated lumbar intervertebral disc: a case report. Ann. Surg. **149**, 294–296 (1959)

18. Dubowitz, V., Lober, J., Zachary, R.B.: Lipoma of the cauda equina. Arch. Dis. Childh. **40**, 207–213 (1965)

19. Epstein, B.S.: Myelographic diagnosis of epidural metastases in lumbosacral spinal canal. Amer. J. Roentgenol. **68**, 730–735 (1952)

20. Epstein, J.A., Epstein, B.S., Lavine, L.S., Carras, R., Rosenthal, A.D.: Degenerative lumbar spondylolisthesis with an intact neural arch (pseudospondylolisthesis). J. Neurosurg. **44**, 139–147 (1976)

21. Finneson, B.E.: Spondylolysis and spondylolisthesis. In: Low Back Pain, Chap. XI, pp. 276–288. Philadelphia: Lippincott Co. 1973

22. Fourrier, X.: Contribution à l'étude du traitement chirurgical du spondylolisthésis. Thèse méd. Paris, No. 773, 1969

23. Freeman, R.E., Onofrio, B.M., Layton, D.D.: An unusual compressive syndrome of the cauda equina. Mayo Clin. Proc. **50**, 139–140 (1975)

24. Frenay, J., Lambooy, N.: Syndrome de la queue de cheval secondaire à un spondylolisthésis par atteinte lombaire basse d'une polyarthrite chronique évolutive. Neuro-chirurgie **20**, 431–440 (1974)

25. Gill, G.G., Manning, J.G., White, H.L.: Surgical treatment of spondylolisthesis without spine fusion. Excision of the loose lamina with decompression of the nerve roots. J. Bone Jt Surg. **37 A**, 493–520 (1955)

26. Giuffre, R.: Intradural spinal lipomas: review of the litterature (99 cases) and report of an additional case. Acta neurochir. (Wien) **14**, 69–95 (1966)

27. Griffiths, R.W., Rose, M.J.: Acute vertebral collapse and cauda equina compression in tertiary syphilis. J. Neurol. Neurosurg. Psychiat. **38**, 558–560 (1975)

28. Gros, C., Vlahovitch, B., Mohasseb, G.: Les tumeurs géantes intrarachidiennes de la

région de la queue de cheval. Montpellier méd. **56**, 72–73 (1959)

29. Gros, C., Vlahovitch, B., Mohasseb, G.: Importance des signes radiographiques dans les tumeurs géantes du canal lombo-sacré. Montpellier méd. **102**, 268–273 (1960)

30. Gros, C., Vlahovitch, B., Mossaheb, G., Roilgen, A.: Kystes épidermoides intra-rachidiens par greffe épithéliale après ponctions lombaires. Neurochirurgie **7**, 163–165 (1961)

31. Guyot, J.F.: Compressions de la queue de cheval. Rev. Prat. (Paris) **20**, 1843–1853 (1970)

32. Hewlett, R.H., Ganz, J.C.: Histiocytosis X of the cauda equina. Neurology (Minneap.) **26**, 472–476 (1976)

33. Jeanmart, L., Retif, J., Brihaye, J.: Syndrome de la queue de cheval par compression d'origine tumorale et discale: apport de l'examen myélographique. J. Radiol. Électrol. **51**, 561–566 (1970)

34. Junghanns, H.: Spondylolisthesen ohne Spalt im Zwischengelenkstück. Arch. orthop. Unfall-Chir. **29**, 118–127 (1930)

35. Kaplan, E.S.: Post-discectomy tuberculous abscess. Case report. J. Neurosurg. **38**, 358–361 (1973)

36. Keon-Cohen, B.T.: Epidural abscess simulating disc hernia. J. Bone Jt Surg. **50B**, 128–130 (1968)

37. Langue, J.P.: Contribution à l'étude des syndromes de la queue de cheval par ostéo-arthropathie vertébrale tabétique (à propos d'une observation personnelle et de huit observations de la littérature). Thèse méd. Lyon, No. 280, 1971

38. Liebeskind, A., Jacobson, R., Anderson, R., Schechter, M.M.: Unusual neurologic and roentgenographic manifestations of eosinophilic granuloma. Arch. Neurol. **28**, 131–133 (1973)

39. Loeser, J.D., Lewin, R.J.: Lumbosacral lipoma in the adult. Case report. J. Neurosurg. **29**, 405–409 (1968)

40. Lusskin, R.: Pain patterns in spondylolisthesis. Clin. Orthop. **40**, 123–136 (1965)

41. Massare, C., Bernegeau, J.: Le spondylolisthésis lombo-sacré. Examen radiologique. Rev. Chir. orthop. **57** (Suppl. I), 110–114 (1971)

42. McNab, I.: Spondylolisthesis with an intact neural arch—the so-called pseudospondylolisthesis. J. Bone Jt Surg. **32B**, 325–333 (1950)

43. McNeel, D.P., Ehni, G.: Charcot joint of the lumbar spine. J. Neurosurg. **30**, 55–61 (1969)

44. Moiel, R., Ehni, G.: Cauda equina compression due to spondylolisthesis with intact neural arch. Report of two cases. J. Neurosurg. **28**, 262–265 (1968)

45. Monpetit, G.: Radiculalgies et tumeurs intra-rachidiennes. Thèse méd. Paris, No. 976, 1956

46. Montrieul, B., Georget, A.M., Tournilhac, M., Chabannes, J.: L'intradurographie comme élément du diagnostic des métastases dans la queue de cheval de néoplasmes viscéraux. Neuro-chirurgie **20**, 458–461 (1974)

47. Natarajan, M., Rajagopal, T., Srinivasan, K.: A giant schwannoma of cauda equina. Surg. Neurol. **4**, 367–368 (1975)

48. Newman, P.H.: The etiology of spondylolisthesis. J. Bone Jt Surg. **45B**, 39–59 (1963)

49. Newman, P.H.: Stenosis of lumbar spine in spondylolisthesis. Clin. Orthop. **115**, 116–121 (1976)

50. Pecker, J., Simon, J., Guy, G., Carsin, M., Jan, M.: Radiological features of the meningo-radicular metastases of tumors of the central nervous system. J. Neurosurg. **38**, 627–630 (1973)

51. Pettersson, G., Werkmäster, K.: Intraspinal dermoid cysts in children; survey of literature and own cases. Acta paediat. (Uppsala) **52**, 187–189 (1963)

52. Picault, Ch.: Le spondylolisthésis lombo-sacré. Introduction. Rev. Chir. orthop. **57** (Suppl. I), 88–89 (1971)

53. Piera, J.B., Durand, J., Pannier, S., Guiot, G., Grossiord, A.: Dix cas de neurinomes géants lombo-sacrés. Ann. Méd. interne (Paris) **5**, 315–330 (1975)

54. Piganiol, G., Bille, J., Berard, M., Paillas, J.E.: Tumeurs géantes de la queue de cheval. Neuro-chirurgie **10**, 221–229 (1964)

55. Prentice, W.B., Kieffer, S.A., Gold, L.H., Bjornson, R.G.: Myelographic characteristics of metastasis to the spinal cord and cauda equina. Amer. J. Roentgenol. **118**, 682–689 (1973)

56. Ramani, P.S., Sengupta, R.P.: Cauda equina compression due to tabetic arthro-

pathy of the spine. J. Neurol. Neurosurg. Psychiat. **36**, 260–264 (1973)

57. Reina, A.: Tuberculous epidural granuloma simulating a herniated lumbar disc. Surg. Neurol. **4**, 336–338 (1975)

58. Riddel, D.M.: Spondylolisthesis in a Charcot spine. Proc. roy. Soc. Med. **54**, 823–824 (1961)

59. Roger, H., Poursines, Y., Recordier, M.: L'ostéoarthropathie vertébrale tabétique. Etude de 16 cas personnels. Marseille méd. **70**, 65–136 (1933)

60. Rogers, H.M., Long, D.M., Chou, S.N., French, L.A.: Lipomas of the spinal cord and cauda equina. J. Neurosurg. **34**, 349–354 (1971)

61. Rosenberg, N.J.: Degenerative spondylolisthesis. Predisposing factors. J. Bone Jt Surg. **57 A**, 467–474 (1975)

62. Rouques, L., Israel, J., Passelecq, A., Lacroix-coutry, M., Plainfossé, M.C.: A propos des ostéo-arthropathies vertébrales tabétiques. Presse méd. **70**, 693–696 (1962)

63. Ruprecht, E.: Zur Pathogenese der Wurzelläsion bei der Spondylolisthesis. Z. Orthop. **94**, 196–206 (1961)

64. Sans-Jofre, M.: Contribution à l'étude du spondylolisthésis avec manifestations radiculaires. (Résultats de 26 interventions par voie postérieure). Thèse méd. Rouen No. 342, 1974

65. Sassaroli, S., Urso, S.: Radiculografia lombosacrale con mezzo di contrasto idrosolubile (dati anatomici e funzionali). — Lumbosacral radiculography by means of hydrosoluble contrast media (an anatomical and functional outline). Padua: Piccin Medical Books 1974

66. Serre, H., Gros, C., Simon, L., Baumelou, H., Lamboley, C.: Compressions radiculaires par arthropathies tabétiques du rachis. Rev. Rhum. **37**, 525–533 (1970)

67. Sèze, S., de: Sciatique par neurinome de la queue de cheval. La forme sciatalgique pure des tumeurs de la queue de cheval, avec 4 observations. Bull. Soc. méd. Hôp. Paris **59**, 249–252 (1943)

68. Sèze, S. de, Hubault, A., Hamonet, Cl., Dudognon, P., Prost, A.: Arthropathies tabétiques avec compressions radiculaires de la queue de cheval. A propos de 4 nouvelles observations. Nouv. Presse méd. **1**, 2747–2752 (1972)

69. Sèze, S. de, Hubault, A., Lasserre, P.P., Monpetit, G.: Les compression par tumeurs intra-rachidiennes. A propos de 106 cas observés dans un service de rhumatologie. Rev. Rhum. **41**, 83–91 (1974)

70. Sèze, S. de, Petit-Dutaillis, B.: Trois neurinomes de la queue de cheval à symptomatologie purement douloureuse. Rev. neurol. **75**, 75–145 (1943)

71. Sèze, S., de, Ryckewaert, A.: Sciatique et neurinome radiculaire. In: Maladies des Os et des Articulations, Vol. II, pp. 1170–1172. Paris: Flammarion 1954

72. Shapiro, R.: Tumors. In: Myelography, 3rd ed., Chap. XV, pp. 279–347. Chicago: Year Book Medical Publishers, Inc. 1975

73. Sicard, A., Lavarde, G.: Les lésions radiculaires au cours des arthropathies tabétiques du rachis lombaire. Presse méd. **75**, 2209–2212 (1967)

74. Simonin, J.L.: Le spondylolisthésis lombaire. (Etude de 727 cas). Thèse méd. Paris, No. 711, 1966

75. Taillard, W.: Les spondylolisthésis. Paris: Masson et Cie. 1957

76. Thurel, R.: Tumeurs intra-rachidiennes. Les précis du Praticien. Paris: Baillières 1964

77. Thurel, R., Nehlil, J., Lazar, L.: Complications radiculaires et médullaires des ostéoarthropathies vertébrales tabétiques. Rev. neurol. **114**, 62–65 (1966)

78. Vigouroux, R.P., Choux, M., Baurand, C., Chamant, J.H.: A propos des lombo-sciatiques tumorales (24 cas observés dans une statistique de 1000 lombo-sciatiques opérées). Neuro-chirurgie **13**, 761–770 (1967)

Subject Index

Advances in Neurosurgery

Volume 1

Brain Edema – Cerebello Pontine Angle Tumors

Pathophysiology and Therapy – Diagnosis and Surgery
Editors: K. Schürmann, M. Brock, H.-J. Reulen, D. Voth
187 figures. XVII, 385 pages. 1973
ISBN 3-540-06486-9

Volume 2

Meningiomas. Multiple Sclerosis. Forensic Problems in Neurosurgery

Proceedings of the 25th Annual Meeting of the
"Deutsche Gesellschaft für Neurochirurgie"
Bochum, September 22–25, 1974
Editors: W. Klug, M. Brock, M. Klinger, O. Spoerri
200 figures, 86 tables. XXI, 444 pages. 1975
ISBN 3-540-07237-3

Volume 3

Brain Hypoxia. Pain

Proceedings of the 26th Annual Meeting of the
"Deutsche Gesellschaft für Neurochirurgie"
Heidelberg, May 1–3, 1975
Editors: H. Penzholz, M. Brock, J. Hamer, M. Klinger, O. Spoerri
160 figures, 110 tables. XIX, 460 pages. 1975
ISBN 3-540-07466-X

Volume 4

Lumbar Disc Adult Hydrocephalus

Proceedings of the 27th Annual Meeting of the
"Deutsche Gesellschaft für Neurochirurgie"
Berlin, September 12–15, 1976
Editors: R. Wüllenweber, M. Brock, J. Hamer, M. Klinger, O. Spoerri
154 figures, 67 tables. XXIII, 338 pages
(18 pages in German). 1977
ISBN 3-540-08100-3

V. Chan-Palay

Cerebellar Dentate Nucleus

Organization, Cytology, and Transmitters
293 figures including 79 plates, some in color.
XXI, 548 pages. 1977
ISBN 3-540-07958-0

Cranial Computerized Tomography

Proceedings of the Symposium Munich,
June 10–12, 1976
Editors: W. Lanksch, E. Kazner,
Editorial Board: T. Grumme, F. Marguth,
H. R. Müller, H. Steinhoff, S. Wende
620 figures. XIV, 478 pages. 1976
ISBN 3-540-07938-6
Distribution rights for Japan:
Nankodo Co. Ltd., Tokyo

H. V. Crock, H. Yoshizawa

The Blood Supply of the Vertebral Column and Spinal Cord in Man

120 figures, 44 color plates. XIII, 130 pages.
1977
ISBN 3-211-81402-7
Distribution rights for Japan:
Nankodo Co. Ltd., Tokyo

H. M. Duvernoy

Human Brainstem Vessels

Preface by R. Warwick
Illustrations by J. L. Vannson
108 figures, 2 folding plates. Approx. 195 pages.
1977
ISBN 3-540-08336-7

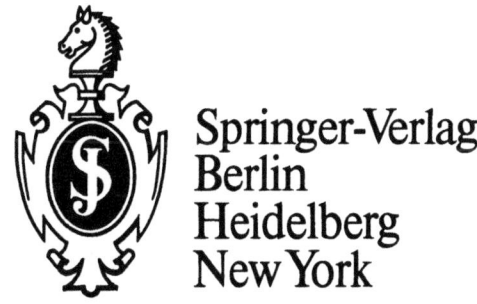

Springer-Verlag
Berlin
Heidelberg
New York

H. M. Duvernoy

The Superficial Veins of the Human Brain

Veins of the Brain Stem and of the Base of the Brain
71 figures (138 separate illustrations).
VI, 110 pages. 1975
ISBN 3-540-06876-7
Distribution rights for Japan:
Nankodo Co. Ltd., Tokyo

Dynamics of Brain Edema

Proceedings of the 3rd International Workshop on Dynamic Aspects of Cerebral Edema, Montreal, Canada, June 25–29, 1976
Editors: H. M. Pappius, W. Feindel
83 figures, 81 tables. III, 404 pages. 1976
ISBN 3-540-08009-0

Handbuch der medizinischen Radiologie
6. Band

Röntgendiagnostik der Wirbel-säule – Roentgen Diagnosis of the Vertebral Column

3 Bandteile. Redigiert von L. Diethelm
1. Teil
864 Abbildungen (in 1269 Einzeldarstellungen)
XVI, 867 Seiten. 1974
ISBN 3-540-06463-X
2. Teil
486 Abbildungen in 677 Einzeldarstellungen.
XIV, 800 Seiten. 1974
ISBN 3-540-06993-3
3. Teil: K. Reinhardt:
Krankhafte Haltungsänderungen – Skoliosen und Kyphosen
444 Abbildungen in 730 Einzeldarstellungen.
83 Tabellen. XIX, 880 Seiten. 1976
ISBN 3-540-07523-2

H. W. Kölmel

Atlas of Cerebrospinal Fluid Cells

2nd, enlarged edition
251 figures, 139 in color. VIII, 142 pages. 1977
ISBN 3-540-08186-0

G. Salamon, Y. P. Huang

Radiologic Anatomy of the Brain

In cooperation with numerous experts
282 figures in 463 separate illustrations.
XIII, 404 pages. 1976
ISBN 3-540-07528-3
Distribution rights for Japan:
Nankodo Co. Ltd., Tokyo

B. Schlesinger

The Upper Brainstem in the Human

Its Nuclear Configuration and Vascular Supply
With a Foreword by H. Ferner
326 figures some in color, 10 tables.
XVI, 266 pages. 1976
ISBN 3-540-07497-X

A. Wackenheim

Roentgen Diagnosis of the Craniovertebral Region

500 figures. XXII, 601 pages. 1974
ISBN 3-540-06615-2
Distribution rights for Japan:
Igaku Shoin Ltd., Tokyo

A. Wackenheim, J. P. Braun

The Veins of the Posterior Fossa

Normal and Pathologic Findings
171 figures. Approx. 170 pages. 1977
ISBN 3-540-08337-5

S. Wende, E. Zieler, N. Nakayama

Cerebral Magnification Angiography

Physical Basis and Clinical Results
With the collaboration of K. Schindler
141 figures. VII, 150 pages. 1974
ISBN 3-540-06651-9
Distribution rights for Japan:
Igaku Shoin Ltd., Tokyo

GPSR Compliance

The European Union's (EU) General Product Safety Regulation (GPSR)
is a set of rules that requires consumer products to be safe and our
obligations to ensure this.

If you have any concerns about our products, you can contact us on
ProductSafety@springernature.com

In case Publisher is established outside the EU, the EU authorized
representative is:

Springer Nature Customer Service Center GmbH
Europaplatz 3
69115 Heidelberg, Germany

Batch number: 09635766

Printed by Printforce, the Netherlands